# ACCESS TO SURGERY: 500 SINGLE BEST ANSWER QUESTIONS IN GENERAL AND SYSTEMIC PATHOLOGY

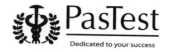

PasTest
Dedicated to your success

# DEDICATION

To my mother for her struggle in life and for leading her children into intellectual pursuits.

To my father for never compromising on principles and for providing his children with the best of everything possible within his limited resources.

# ACCESS TO SURGERY: 500 SINGLE BEST ANSWER QUESTIONS IN GENERAL AND SYSTEMIC PATHOLOGY

**Shahzad G. Raja**

BSc, MBBS, MRCS

Specialist Registrar Cardiothoracic Surgery

Department of Cardiothoracic Surgery

Western Infirmary

Glasgow

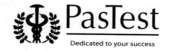

PasTest

Dedicated to your success

© 2007 PASTEST LTD

Egerton Court
Parkgate Estate
Knutsford
Cheshire
WA16 8DX

Telephone: 01565 752000

First published 2007

ISBN: 1905635362

ISBN: 9781905635368

A catalogue record for this book is available from the British Library.

The information contained within this book was obtained by the author from reliable sources. However, while every effort has been made to ensure its accuracy, no responsibility for loss, damage or injury occasioned to any person acting or refraining from action as a result of information contained herein can be accepted by the publishers or author.

Text prepared by Carnegie Book Production, Lancaster, UK

Printed and bound in the UK by Athenaeum Press, Gateshead

# CONTENTS

# Answers

# PREFACE

Recent reforms in medical education in the United Kingdom have prompted the replacement of multiple choice questions (MCQs) with single best answer questions (SBAs). *Access to Surgery: 500 Single Best Answer Questions in General and Systemic Pathology* is the first book of its kind and provides 500 practice SBAs in general and systemic pathology for candidates taking the surgical examinations. As the title indicates, it is primarily written for surgical trainees, with an emphasis mainly on the surgical aspects of human pathology. However, it can be used as a practice tool by undergraduate medical students and by trainees in other medical disciplines (for whom pathology can often be a major examination hurdle).

Each question has been carefully formulated to cover a given topic in pathology. All the major aspects of pathology are dealt with, and are organised in sequence in the following sections: Cell Injury and Wound Healing, Inflammation and Immunology, Neoplasia, Microbiology, Disorders of Fluids and Electrolytes, Bleeding and Haemostasis, Cardiovascular Pathology, Pulmonary Pathology, Renal Pathology, Gastrointestinal and Hepatobiliary Pathology, Haematopathology, Endocrine Pathology, Breast and Female Reproductive Pathology, Male Reproductive Pathology, Bone and Joint Pathology and Central Nervous System Pathology; a section on Pharmacology has also been included. The questions also cover the complete MRCS applied pathology syllabus and are also expected to be useful for specialty FRCS candidates.

This book contains a substantial number of patient-based questions or clinical scenarios that will enable prospective candidates to test their ability to integrate key basic pathological concepts with relevant clinical problems. In addition, factual recall questions have also been included that probe for basic recall of facts. Detailed and comprehensive explanations, rather than just brief answers, have been provided so that candidates do not have to consult textbooks for clarification, as is the case with most MCQ books.

The questions in this book can be used in a number of ways: (i) as a diagnostic tool (ie a pre-test), (ii) as a guide and focus for further study, and (iii) for self-assessment. The least effective use of these questions is to 'study' them by reading them one at a time, and then looking at the correct answer. These 500 practice questions are intended to be an integral part of a well-planned review as well as an isolated resource. If used appropriately, these questions can provide self-assessment information beyond a numerical score. Furthermore, the questions have been planned in such a way that this book can be used as companion to any textbook of pathology.

I am hopeful that this book will prove a useful revision and self-assessment tool for all those involved in learning pathology.

Shahzad G. Raja

2007

# ABBREVIATIONS

| | |
|---|---|
| ACE | angiotensin-converting enzyme |
| ACTH | adrenocorticotrophic hormone |
| ADH | antidiuretic hormone |
| ADP | adenosine diphosphate |
| AFP | alpha-fetoprotein |
| AIDS | acquired immune deficiency syndrome |
| AJCC | American Joint Committee on Cancer |
| ALT | alanine aminotransferase |
| AST | aspartate aminotransferase |
| ATP | adenosine triphosphate |
| BCG | bacillus Calmette–Guérin |
| CEA | carcinoembryonic antigen |
| CIN | cervical intraepithelial neoplasia |
| CIS | carcinoma in situ |
| CLL | chronic lymphocytic leukaemia |
| CML | chronic myelogenous leukaemia |
| CNS | central nervous system |
| CPP | cerebral perfusion pressure |
| CREST | calcinosis, Raynaud's phenomenon, (o)esophageal dysmotility, sclerodactyly and telangiectasia |
| CSF | cerebrospinal fluid |
| CT | computed tomography |
| DIC | disseminated intravascular coagulation |
| $D_{LCO}$ | diffusing capacity of the lung for carbon monoxide |
| DNA | deoxyribonucleic acid |
| EBV | Epstein–Barr virus |
| ECG | electrocardiography |
| EEG | electroencephalogram |
| EF-2 | elongation factor 2 |
| ELISA | enzyme-linked immunosorbent assay |

| EMG | electromyography |
| ESR | erythrocyte sedimentation rate |
| FFP | fresh frozen plasma |
| FSH | follicle-stimulating hormone |
| GABA | gamma-aminobutyric acid |
| GFAP | glial fibrillary acidic protein |
| GFR | glomerular filtration rate |
| GGT | gamma-glutamyl transpeptidase |
| GM-CSF | granulocyte–macrophage colony-stimulating factor |
| GP | general practitioner |
| GTP | guanosine-5-triphosphate |
| GVHD | graft-versus-host disease |
| H&E | haematoxylin and eosin (stain) |
| hCG | human chorionic gonadotrophin |
| HDL | high-density lipoprotein |
| HIV | human immunodeficiency virus |
| HLA | human leukocyte antigen |
| HPETE | hydroperoxyeicosatetraenoic acid |
| HPV | human papillomavirus |
| HSV | herpes simplex virus |
| ICP | intracranial pressure |
| Ig | immunoglobulin |
| IL | interleukin |
| INR | international normalised ratio |
| LAP | leukocyte alkaline phosphatase |
| LDH | lactate dehydrogenase |
| LDL | low-density lipoprotein |
| LMWH | low-molecular-weight heparin |
| MAP | mean arterial pressure |
| MCH | mean corpuscular haemoglobin |
| MCHC | mean corpuscular haemoglobin concentration |
| MCV | mean corpuscular volume (or red blood cells) |
| MEN | multiple endocrine neoplasia |

| | |
|---|---|
| MRI | magnetic resonance imaging |
| NADPH | nicotinamide-adenine dinucleotide phosphate |
| NK | natural killer |
| NSAID | non-steroidal anti-inflammatory drug |
| PCR | polymerase chain reaction |
| PEEP | peak end-expiratory pressure |
| PPD | purified protein derivative |
| PSA | prostate-specific antigen |
| PT | prothrombin time |
| PTH | parathyroid hormone |
| PTT | partial thromboplastin time |
| Rh | rhesus |
| RNA | ribonucleic acid |
| RTA | renal tubular acidosis |
| SHO | senior house officer |
| SIADH | syndrome of inappropriate ADH secretion |
| SLE | systemic lupus erythematosus |
| SSRI | selective serotonin-reuptake inhibitor |
| TB | tuberculosis |
| TF | tissue factor |
| TNF | tumour necrosis factor |
| TNM | tumour-node-metastasis |
| TSH | thyroid-stimulating hormone |
| TTP | thrombotic thrombocytopenic purpura |
| UICC | Union Internationale Contre le Cancer |
| VDRL | Venereal Disease Research Laboratories (test, for syphilis) |
| VLDL | very-low-density lipoprotein |
| VSD | ventricular septal defect |
| vWD | von Willebrand's disease |
| vWF | von Willebrand factor |
| WBC | white blood cell |

# QUESTIONS

# SECTION 1:
# CELL INJURY AND WOUND HEALING — QUESTIONS

For each question given below choose the ONE BEST option.

**1.1**  **A 65-year-old man suffered a massive myocardial infarction that was complicated by shock and prolonged hypotension. On arrival in the emergency department he was found to have focal neurological signs in addition to features consistent with low-output cardiac failure. Despite the best efforts of the medical team he died the next day. At autopsy, the most likely change you would expect to see in a brain biopsy would be:**

- ○ A  Acute haemorrhagic change
- ○ B  Coagulative necrosis
- ○ C  Granulomatous change
- ○ D  Lacunar infarct
- ○ E  Liquefactive necrosis

**1.2**  **A 45-year-old woman with a chronic infective lesion on her leg underwent a full-thickness biopsy of the lesion. During histological examination of this lesion a rim of multinuclear giant cells is seen. The central region is most likely to show:**

- ○ A  Caseous necrosis
- ○ B  Eosinophilic necrosis
- ○ C  Fibrinous necrosis
- ○ D  Foam cells
- ○ E  Pyogenic necrosis

**1.3** **A skin biopsy from an anorexic 16-year-old girl showed cellular atrophy. During atrophy:**

O A The cell disappears

O B Cellular organelles swell

O C Cell size decreases

O D Cell size increases

O E Protein synthesis increases

**1.4** **A 35-year-old man is a habitual smoker. If a biopsy is taken from the respiratory tract in this man, the epithelium of respiratory tract is most likely to show:**

O A Mucous hyperplasia

O B Smooth-muscle hyperplasia

O C Squamous cell anaplasia

O D Squamous cell hypertrophy

O E Stratified squamous metaplasia

**1.5** **Hypertrophy can be physiological or pathological and is caused by increased functional demand or by specific hormonal stimulation. Hypertrophy can be best described as:**

O A Abnormal deposition in a cell

O B Change in cell morphology

O C Decrease in cell size

O D Increase in cell number

O E Increase in cell size and in its organelles

**1.6**  **Apoptotic cells usually exhibit distinctive morphological features. Which one of the following morphological features is usually seen in pure apoptosis?**

○  A  Cellular swelling
○  B  Chromatin condensation
○  C  Early disruption of the plasma membrane
○  D  Nuclear stabilisation
○  E  Phagocytosis of apoptotic bodies by neutrophils

**1.7**  **A histopathologist reports fat necrosis after examining a slide. Fat necrosis might be found in which one of the following situations?**

○  A  Brain injury
○  B  Muscle injury
○  C  Trauma to the abdomen
○  D  Trauma to the breast
○  E  Trauma to the bowel

**1.8**  **A healthy 26-year-old man fractured his right tibia in a road traffic accident. His right leg was immobilised in a plaster cast. The cast was removed from his leg after 8 weeks of immobilisation. Which of the following changes is most likely to have taken place in his gastrocnemius muscle after this time?**

○  A  Decrease in the number of muscle fibres
○  B  Decrease in the number of nerve fibres
○  C  Increase in the number of fast fibres
○  D  Increase in the mitochondrial content
○  E  Increase in the number of satellite cells

cell injury

**1.9** **A 21-year-old man sustained a severe soft-tissue injury following a road traffic accident. Which of the following metabolic effects is most likely to follow this injury?**

O   A   Decreased aldosterone secretion

O   B   Inhibition of gluconeogenesis

O   C   Mobilisation of fat stores

O   D   Protein anabolism

O   E   Respiratory alkalosis

**1.10** **A 32-year-old man, working in a power plant, was exposed to radioactive material. He is most likely to suffer radiation injury due to:**

O   A   Decreased intracellular $Na^+$

O   B   Decreased intracellular $Ca^{2+}$

O   C   Free radical formation

O   D   Increased adenosine triphosphate (ATP) production

O   E   Inhibition of protein synthesis

**1.11** **A 15-year-old girl with haemophilia A has had episodes of pain in her knees for the past 6 years. Over time, there has been an increase in size of her knee joints, with deformity. Laboratory studies show decreased levels of coagulation factor VIII activity. Which of the following is most likely to be seen within the joint space following episodes of pain?**

O   A   Anthracotic pigment

O   B   Cholesterol crystals

O   C   Lipofuscin

O   D   Neutrophils

O   E   Russell bodies

**1.12**  A 42-year-old woman has complained of mild, burning, substernal or epigastric pain following meals for the past 3 years. Upper gastrointestinal endoscopy is performed and biopsies are taken of an erythematous area of the lower oesophageal mucosa 3 cm above the gastro-oesophageal junction. There is no mass lesion, no ulceration, and no haemorrhage is noted. The biopsies demonstrate the presence of columnar epithelium with goblet cells. Which of the following mucosal alterations is most likely to be represented by these findings?

    ○  A  Carcinoma
    ○  B  Dysplasia
    ○  C  Hyperplasia
    ○  D  Ischaemia
    ○  E  Metaplasia

**1.13**  A 62-year-old diabetic and hypertensive man suffered a stroke which affected his speech and movement in the right arm and leg. A cerebral angiogram revealed an occlusion of his left middle cerebral artery. Months later, a computed tomographic (CT) scan shows a large, 5-cm cystic area in his left parietal lobe cortex. This CT finding most likely demonstrates a lesion that is the consequence of resolution of which of the following events?

    ○  A  Apoptosis
    ○  B  Atrophy
    ○  C  Caseous necrosis
    ○  D  Coagulative necrosis
    ○  E  Liquefactive necrosis

**1.14**  **A 25-year-old woman breastfed her first baby for almost 1 year with no difficulties and no complications. Which of the following cellular processes that occurred in the breast during pregnancy allowed her to nurse the infant for this period of time?**

○  A  Ductal epithelial metaplasia

○  B  Epithelial dysplasia

○  C  Lobular hyperplasia

○  D  Stromal hypertrophy

○  E  Steatocyte atrophy

**1.15**  **An 80-year-old woman was found dead in her room in a nursing home one morning. An autopsy was carried out and her death was reported as being secondary to old age. At autopsy, her heart was small (250 g) and dark-brown in colour on section. Microscopically, there was light-brown perinuclear pigment seen after haematoxylin and eosin (H&E) staining of the cardiac muscle fibres. Which of the following substances is most likely to be increased in the myocardial fibres to produce this cardiac appearance?**

○  A  Calcium, following necrosis

○  B  Cholesterol, as a consequence of atherosclerosis

○  C  Glycogen, resulting from a storage disease

○  D  Haemosiderin, resulting from iron overload

○  E  Lipochrome, from 'wear and tear'

**1.16** A histopathologist examining a slide used a series of immunohistochemical stains to identify different cellular components. One particular stain identified the presence of intermediate filaments within cells. This cytokeratin stain is most likely to be useful for which of the following diagnostic purposes?

   A  Confirmation of a history of chronic alcoholism

   B  Confirmation that a neoplasm is a carcinoma

   C  Determination of the contractile properties of cells

   D  Visualisation of cytoskeletal alterations with impending cell death

   E  Assessment of the degree of metaplasia or dysplasia

**1.17** A 73-year-old woman with long-standing hypertension and aortic stenosis died suddenly one morning. An autopsy was performed on her body. At autopsy, her heart weighed 540 g. The size of her heart is most likely to be the result of which of the following processes involving the myocardial fibres?

   A  Fatty degeneration

   B  Fatty infiltration

   C  Hyperplasia

   D  Hypertrophy

   E  Oedema

cell injury

cell injury

**1.18** **A 28-year-old woman developed a darker skin complexion after returning from a holiday trip to Goa. Her skin did not show warmth, erythema or tenderness. Her skin tone faded to its original appearance within 1 month. Which of the following substances contributes most to the biochemical process leading to these skin changes?**

- A Glycogen
- B Haem
- C Homogentisic acid
- D Lipofuscin
- E Tyrosine

**1.19** **Metaplasia is a reversible change in which one adult cell type (epithelial or mesenchymal) is replaced by another adult cell type. In which of the following situations is the process of epithelial metaplasia most likely to have occurred?**

- A Acute myocardial infarction
- B Lactation following pregnancy
- C Tanning of the skin following sunlight exposure
- D Urinary obstruction due to an enlarged prostate
- E Vitamin A deficiency

**1.20** A histopathologist reviewing a slide noticed a disease process which has led to scattered loss of individual cells, with the microscopic appearance of karyorrhexis and cell fragmentation. The overall tissue structure, however, has remained intact. This process is most typical of which of the following diseases?

○ A  Barbiturate overdose
○ B  Brown atrophy of the heart
○ C  Chronic alcoholic liver disease
○ D  Renal transplant rejection
○ E  Viral hepatitis

**1.21** A 55-year-old woman with chronic atrial fibrillation suddenly developed an acute abdomen and was rushed to the emergency department. At emergency laparoscopy most of the small-bowel loops were dusky to purple-red in colour. Her mesenteric veins were patent. The most probable underlying pathological process is:

○ A  Coagulative necrosis
○ B  Dry gangrene
○ C  Gas gangrene
○ D  Liquefactive gangrene
○ E  Wet gangrene

cell injury

**1.22** **A 13-year-old girl complained of redness and pain in her cheeks after spending a sunny day on the beach. Her GP told her that she was suffering from sunburn on the cheeks. What is the most probable underlying cause of her complaint?**

○ A Antigen–antibody reaction
○ B Damage to DNA
○ C Free radical injury
○ D Ischaemic injury
○ E Vasoconstriction

**1.23** **A 25-year-old male worker involved in an accident in a dry-cleaning facility was brought to the emergency department following exposure to massive amounts of carbon tetrachloride, both on the skin and by inhalation. Severe damage to which of the following organs is most likely to occur in this man?**

○ A Heart
○ B Intestine
○ C Kidney
○ D Liver
○ E Stomach

**1.24** **Adenosine triphosphate (ATP) depletion and decreased ATP synthesis are frequently associated with both hypoxic and chemical (toxic) injury. Which of the following is most likely to result from depletion of ATP?**

○ A Decreased rate of anaerobic glycolysis
○ B Decreased influx of calcium
○ C Increased activity of ouabain-sensitive $Na^+$, $K^+$-ATPase
○ D Increased glycogen synthesis
○ E Increased unfolded protein response

**1.25** **Accumulation of which of the following substances indicates ageing at a cellular level in a biopsy taken from an elderly person?**

○ A Beta carotene
○ B Bilirubin
○ C Haemosiderin
○ D Lipofuscin
○ E Melanin

**1.26** **A 36-year-old man sustained a 5-cm-long incised wound on his forearm during a bar fight. Which of the following is NOT likely to be seen as a complication of healing in this patient?**

○ A Cicatrisation and disfigurement
○ B Keloid
○ C Malignancy
○ D Proud flesh
○ E Wound dehiscence

**1.27** **A 26-year-old woman suffered serious burns to her hands and chest. Which of the following factors is NOT likely to influence wound healing in this woman?**

○ A Blood supply
○ B Infection
○ C Steroids
○ D Vitamin A deficiency
○ E Zinc

cell injury

**1.28** **A rugby player sustained a laceration to his right forearm as a result of a rough tackle. This wound was closed with sutures. Wound healing proceeded over the next week. Which of the following factors will be most likely to aid wound healing in this patient?**

○ A Corticosteroid therapy
○ B Hypoalbuminaemia
○ C Presence of sutures
○ D Poor tissue perfusion
○ E Secondary wound infection

**1.29** **In a clinical study, patients undergoing laparoscopic procedures are followed to document the postsurgical wound-healing process. The port site incisions are closed with sutures. Over the 4 weeks following surgery, the wounds are observed to regain tensile strength and there is re-epithelialisation. Which of the following substances is most likely to be identified as functioning intracellularly in cells involved in this wound-healing process?**

○ A Collagen
○ B Fibronectin
○ C Hyaluronic acid
○ D Laminin
○ E Tyrosine kinase

**1.30** An SHO accidentally stabbed himself with a surgical blade while assisting in an exploratory laparotomy. He sustained a small, 0.5-cm-long laceration to his right index finger. Which of the following substances, on contact with injured vascular basement membrane, will activate both the coagulation sequence and the kinin system as an initial response to this injury?

- O A Hageman factor
- O B Histamine
- O C Plasmin
- O D Platelet activating factor
- O E Thromboxane

**1.31** A histopathology report describes 'hyaline degeneration'. Which of the following microscopic descriptions is most characteristic of hyaline degeneration?

- O A Accumulation of lipids in cells
- O B Homogeneous, ground-glass, pink-staining appearance of cells
- O C Presence of calcium salts with destruction of cellular detail
- O D Pyknotic, densely stained nucleus
- O E Totally amorphous appearance with no cell membrane discernable

**1.32 Which of the following findings will be most striking in a microscopic slide showing atrophy of an organ?**

○ A  A greater number of autophagic vacuoles

○ B  A greater number of myofilaments

○ C  A greater number of mitochondria

○ D  A greater number of rough endoplasmic reticulum

○ E  A greater number of smooth endoplasmic reticulum

**1.33 Which of the following cells is an example of a permanent cell, on the basis of a classification according to regenerative ability?**

○ A  Acinar cell of the pancreas

○ B  Colonic mucosal cell

○ C  Erythrocyte

○ D  Hepatocyte

○ E  Osteocyte

**1.34 Which of the following provides an example of concomitant hyperplasia and hypertrophy?**

○ A  Breast enlargement at puberty

○ B  Cystic hyperplasia of the endometrium

○ C  Enlargement of skeletal muscle in athletes

○ D  Left ventricular cardiac hypertrophy

○ E  Uterine growth during pregnancy

**1.35** You are looking at a histopathology slide that shows changes associated with cell injury. Which of the following cell changes associated with injury is most likely to be accompanied by disruption of the cell membrane?

○ A Apoptosis
○ B Cloudy swelling
○ C Coagulative necrosis
○ D Hydropic change
○ E Pyknosis

**1.36** The histopathologist reported the presence of 'epithelioid cells' in a biopsied cervical lymph node from a patient with tuberculosis. Epithelioid cells are transformed from:

○ A Epithelial cells
○ B Eosinophils
○ C Lymphocytes
○ D Macrophages
○ E Neutrophils

**1.37** A lump was excised and sent for histopathological examination. The histopathologist reported seeing what appeared to be an abnormal amount and arrangement of normal tissue than is appropriate or normal for the area in which the tissue arises. This is best described as:

○ A Carcinosarcoma
○ B Embryonal tumour
○ C Hamartoma
○ D Mixed tumour
○ E Teratoma

**1.38** **A histopathology report states that the periphery of a haematoma is infiltrated by new capillaries, fibroblasts, and collagen. What is this process called?**

O   A   Embolisation

O   B   Lysis of the clot

O   C   Organisation of the haematoma

O   D   Recanalisation

O   E   Thrombosis

**1.39** **Which of the following terms best describes the passage of leukocytes through the blood vessel wall?**

O   A   Diapedesis

O   B   Euperiporesis

O   C   Migration

O   D   Phagocytosis

O   E   Pavement

**1.40** **A 62-year-old man suffered a small myocardial infarction involving the inferior wall of the heart. The length of time required for a scar of a small myocardial infarct to reach full strength is approximately:**

O   A   3 days

O   B   1 week

O   C   2 weeks

O   D   6 weeks

O   E   Several months

# SECTION 2:
# INFLAMMATION AND
# IMMUNOLOGY — QUESTIONS

For each question given below choose the ONE BEST option.

**2.1**  **A 45-year-old woman with carcinoma of right breast and enlarged axillary lymph nodes on the same side underwent mastectomy with axillary clearance. Histological examination of the axillary lymph nodes showed no evidence of metastasis. This enlargement of lymph nodes is most probably due to:**

○  A  Lymphoma

○  B  Paracortical lymphoid hyperplasia

○  C  Secondary deposits

○  D  Sinus histiocytosis

○  E  Tuberculosis

**2.2**  **A 6-year-old boy has a history of repeated pyogenic infections. He had normal antibody responses following childhood immunisations and showed normal recovery from chickenpox and measles. Decreased numbers or functional defects in which of the following cells best explains the cause of his repeated pyogenic infections?**

○  A  B lymphocytes

○  B  Eosinophils

○  C  Macrophages

○  D  Neutrophils

○  E  T lymphocytes

**2.3** **A 26-year-old woman developed haemolytic anaemia after taking an over-the-counter analgesic. The foremost step in the mechanism of cell injury in this condition is:**

○  A   Activation of T lymphocytes
○  B   Formation of IgG/IgM antibodies
○  C   Formation of B lymphocytes
○  D   Formation of IgE antibodies
○  E   Release of cytokines

**2.4** **A woman is stung by a bee. Within 5 minutes, she develops a raised, red, swollen lesion at the site of injury, 2 cm in size. Which of the following findings is most likely to be seen in this lesion?**

○  A   Foreign body reaction
○  B   Haemorrhage
○  C   Lymphocytic infiltration
○  D   Neutrophilic migration
○  E   Vasodilation

**2.5** **What is the function of ICAM-1 and VCAM-1 in inflammation?**

○  A   Chemotaxis
○  B   Leukocyte adhesion
○  C   Leukocyte margination
○  D   Leukocyte transmigration
○  E   Phagocytosis

**2.6**   A 25-year-old woman develops nasal discharge and itching of the eyes each year in the Spring. She was referred by her GP for allergy testing. Fifteen minutes after skin testing with a mixture of grass pollens, she developed erythema and a 15-mm wheal at the site. The skin test response is most likely to be a result of which of the following mechanisms?

○   A   Antigen–antibody complexes being formed in blood vessels in the skin

○   B   Influx of phagocytic cells in response to injection of foreign proteins

○   C   Release of histamine from mast cells

○   D   Release of lymphokines by sensitised lymphocytes reacting with antigens

○   E   Release of lymphokines from mast cells

**2.7**   Platelet-derived growth factor binds to its receptor, activating cell growth. The receptor–growth factor complex uses which of the following mechanisms to signal to the cell to divide?

○   A   Activation of tyrosine kinase

○   B   Binding of GTP to a G protein

○   C   Binding to DNA

○   D   Increase in intracellular calcium concentration

○   E   Opening of an ion channel

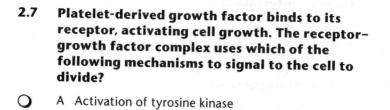

inflammation

**2.8** **A 35-year-old woman with a renal transplant received antilymphocyte globulins. A week later she experienced fever and hypotension. Which of the following mechanisms is responsible for these manifestations?**

- ○ A Granuloma formation
- ○ B Type I hypersensitivity
- ○ C Type II hypersensitivity
- ○ D Type III hypersensitivity
- ○ E Type IV hypersensitivity

**2.9** **A 42-year-old woman is anaesthetised for elective cholecystectomy. She was given an antibiotic injection, following which she developed a rash and her airway pressures became very high. Which of the following mechanisms is responsible for these manifestations?**

- ○ A Arthus reaction
- ○ B Type I hypersensitivity
- ○ C Type II hypersensitivity
- ○ D Type III hypersensitivity
- ○ E Type IV hypersensitivity

**2.10** **A newborn baby developed features of rhesus incompatibility. Rhesus incompatibility is an indication of:**

- ○ A Arthus reaction
- ○ B Type I hypersensitivity
- ○ C Type II hypersensitivity
- ○ D Type III hypersensitivity
- ○ E Type IV hypersensitivity

**2.11** **Which of the following cytokines is produced by T lymphocytes that express class II MHC antigen?**

○ A Alpha interferon

○ B Beta interferon

○ C Gamma interferon

○ D Interleukin-1

○ E Tumour necrosis factor

**2.12** **A 12-year-old boy was brought to the emergency department by his parents because he had developed marked right lower quadrant abdominal pain over the past 24 hours. On physical examination there was rebound tenderness on palpation over the right lower quadrant. Laparoscopic surgery was performed, and the appendix was swollen, erythematous, and partly covered by a yellowish exudate. It was removed, and a microscopic section showed infiltration with numerous neutrophils. The pain experienced by this patient was predominantly the result of the formation of which of the following pairs of chemical mediators?**

○ A Complement C3b and IgG

○ B Histamine and serotonin

○ C Interleukin-1 and tumour necrosis factor

○ D Leukotriene and HPETE

○ E Prostaglandin and bradykinin

inflammation

inflammation

**2.13** A 35-year-old man was seen in a surgical outpatient clinic complaining of a tender lump which had appeared on his right forearm about 3 weeks previously. On enquiry, he revealed that he had been involved in a road traffic accident about 6 months before, when several pieces of windscreen entered his forearm which were removed at the time of initial presentation in the emergency department. At elective surgery a further fragment of glass was recovered from his right forearm. Which of the following cell types is would be most characteristic of the inflammatory response in this situation?

- A Eosinophil
- B Giant cell
- C Mast cell
- D Neutrophil
- E Plasma cell

**2.14** Cultured sputum from a 55-year-old man with a 4-day history of cough and fever grew *Streptococcus pneumoniae*. Clearance of these organisms from the lung parenchyma would be most effectively accomplished through generation of which of the following substances by the major inflammatory cell type responding to this infection?

- A Hydrogen peroxide
- B Kallikrein
- C Leukotriene
- D Platelet-activating factor
- E Prostaglandins

**2.15** A 64-year-old man with a history of inhaling silica dust for many years in his job has become increasingly dyspnoeic over the last 3 years. A chest X-ray now shows increased intersitital markings and nodules ranging in size from 1 cm to 3 cm in the parenchyma. His pulmonary problems are most likely to be caused by which of the following inflammatory processes?

    ○  A  Foreign-body giant-cell formation
    ○  B  Histamine release by mast cells
    ○  C  Neutrophilic infiltration with release of leukotrienes
    ○  D  Production of immunoglobulin by plasma cells
    ○  E  Release of growth factors by macrophages

**2.16** A 16-year-old boy with a 1-day history of sore throat was seen by his GP. On physical examination, the most prominent finding was a pharyngeal purulent exudate. Which of the following types of inflammation does this boy have?

    ○  A  Acute inflammation
    ○  B  Abscess formation
    ○  C  Chronic inflammation
    ○  D  Granulomatous inflammation
    ○  E  Resolution of inflammation

inflammation

**2.17** A 15-year-old girl presented to the emergency department complaining of chronic cough with fever and weight loss for the past month. A chest X-ray revealed multiple nodules, ranging from 1 cm to 4 cm in size, some of which demonstrated cavitation (in the upper lobes). A sputum sample revealed the presence of acid-fast bacilli. Which of the following cells is the most important cell in the development her lung lesions?

A Fibroblast

B Neutrophil

C Macrophage

D Mast cell

E Platelet

**2.18** A sexually active 21-year-old man has experienced pain when passing urine for 3 days. Urethritis is suspected, and *Neisseria gonorrhoeae* is cultured. Numerous neutrophils are present in a smear of the exudate from the penile urethra. These neutrophils are most likely to have undergone diapedesis to reach the organisms as a consequence of release of which of the following chemical mediators?

A Bradykinin

B Complement C5a

C Hageman factor

D Histamine

E Prostaglandin

**2.19** A 58-year-old man with osteoarthritis of 4 years' duration feels better after taking acetylsalicylic acid (aspirin) as his pain is markedly reduced. This pain reduction is most likely to be the result of a reduction in which of the following inflammatory responses?

○ A  Anticoagulation by Hageman factor inhibition
○ B  Fever resulting from interleukin-1
○ C  Neutrophil chemotaxis by leukotriene B4
○ D  Pain resulting from bradykinin generation
○ E  Prostaglandin-mediated vasodilation

**2.20** In an experiment, *Streptococcus pneumoniae* organisms are added to a solution containing leukocytes. Engulfment and phagocytosis of the microbes is observed to occur. A substance is then added that enhances engulfment. Which of the following substances is most likely to produce this effect?

○ A  Complement C3b
○ B  Glutathione peroxidase
○ C  Immunoglobulin M
○ D  P-selectin
○ E  NADPH oxidase

**2.21** **A healthy 25-year-old man with no major medical problems says that he breaks out with blotchy areas of erythema that are pruritic over the skin of his arms, legs and trunk within an hour every time he eats strawberries, this is followed by diarrhoea. These problems abate within a few hours, and physical examination reveals no abnormal findings. Which of the following immunological abnormalities is he most likely to have?**

- A   Cell-mediated hypersensitivity
- B   Hypergammaglobulinaemia
- C   Immune complex deposition
- D   Localised anaphylaxis
- E   Release of complement C3b

**2.22** **A 28-year-old lawyer has experienced episodes of myalgia, pleural effusions, pericarditis, and arthralgia without joint deformity over the course of the past 12 months. He has continued working at his job. A full blood count reveals a mild normocytic anaemia. Which of the following laboratory screening tests is most appropriate to begin the investigation of his condition?**

- A   Antinuclear antibody test
- B   Blood culture
- C   CD4 lymphocyte count
- D   Creatine phosphokinase
- E   Sedimentation rate

**2.23** A 15-month-old boy with failure to thrive has recently been falling ill with one bacterial pneumonia after another, with both *Haemophilus influenzae* and *Streptococcus pneumoniae* cultured from his sputum. He was born at term with no congenital anomalies. Which of the following diseases is he most likely to have?

- ○ A  Acute leukaemia
- ○ B  DiGeorge syndrome
- ○ C  Epstein–Barr virus (EBV) infection
- ○ D  Selective IgA deficiency
- ○ E  X-linked agammaglobulinaemia

**2.24** While presenting an audit of outcomes involving patients who received renal allografts in a renal transplant unit, the SHO highlighted the fact that patients who received renal allografts with matching to the donor by tissue typing for HLA-DR (class II) antigens had a low rate of complications. Which of the following immunological abnormalities is most likely to be diminished by tissue typing?

- ○ A  Amyloidosis
- ○ B  Cell lysis by CD8 lymphocytes
- ○ C  CD4 lymphocyte activation
- ○ D  Graft-versus-host disease
- ○ E  Serum sickness

inflammation

**2.25** **Which of the following is most likely to be found in a 10-year-old girl showing type I hypersensitivity response of the immune system accompanied by eosinophilia?**

○ A   Amyloidosis
○ B   Dust inhalation
○ C   Liver flukes
○ D   Neoplasm
○ E   Spirochaetes

**2.26** **A 28-year-old nurse has had a chronic cough with fever for 2 months. On physical examination, her temperature is 37.9 ˚C. A chest X-ray reveals a diffuse bilateral reticulonodular pattern. A transbronchial biopsy is performed. On microscopic examination of the biopsy, focal areas of inflammation containing epithelioid macrophages, Langhans giant cells and lymphocytes are found. These findings are most typical for which of the following immunological responses?**

○ A   Graft-versus-host disease
○ B   Polyclonal B-cell activation
○ C   Type I hypersensitivity
○ D   Type II hypersensitivity
○ E   Type IV hypersensitivity

**2.27** **Tumour necrosis factor (TNF) is a cytokine involved in systemic inflammation. Which of the following statements about TNF is true?**

○ A   It inhibits apoptotic cell death
○ B   It inhibits the acute phase reaction
○ C   It is a soluble intracytoplasmic peptide
○ D   It is an appetite suppressant
○ E   It is mainly produced by basophils

**2.28** **Interleukin-1 (IL-1) is one of the first cytokines ever described. Its initial discovery was as a factor that could induce fever. Which of the following statements about interleukin-1 is correct?**

○ A   It increases the expression of adhesion factors on endothelial cells
○ B   It is a lipopolysaccharide
○ C   It is an anti-inflammatory cytokine
○ D   It is produced by endothelial cells
○ E   It suppresses bone marrow cells

**2.29** **Ciclosporin is an immunosuppressant drug that is widely used after allogeneic organ transplantation to reduce the activity of the patient's immune system and so the risk of organ rejection. Which of the following statements about ciclosporin is correct?**

○ A   It binds to a cytosolic protein (cyclophilin) of immunocompetent lymphocytes
○ B   It is a glycoprotein produced from horse serum
○ C   It is associated with enhanced lymphokine production
○ D   It is associated with cytokine release syndrome
○ E   It is responsible for enhanced function of effector T cells

inflammation

**2.30** **A 36-year-old man developed hyperacute rejection following kidney transplantation. Hyperacute rejection:**

○ A  Is a T-cell-mediated response in recipients with pre-existing antibodies to the donor

○ B  Is best treated by a large dose of methylprednisolone

○ C  Is complement-mediated

○ D  Is characterised by profuse bleeding

○ E  Occurs within the first day or so after transplantation

**2.31** **The histopathology report for a granulomatous lesion suggests chronic inflammation. Which cell types are most commonly seen in tissue undergoing chronic inflammation?**

○ A  Eosinophils

○ B  Lymphocytes

○ C  Mast cells

○ D  Neutrophils

○ E  Platelets

**2.32** **A histopathology report describes the presence of granulation tissue in a lesion. Which of the following features is characteristic of granulation tissue?**

○ A  Giant cells and fibroblasts

○ B  Giant cells and lymphocytes

○ C  Giant cells, plasma cells and lymphocytes

○ D  Neutrophils and necrotic tissue

○ E  Proliferation of new capillaries, with fibroblasts and new collagen formation

**2.33** **Which of the following terms best describes the unidirectional migration of leukocytes towards a target?**

○ A  Chemotaxis
○ B  Diapedesis
○ C  Endocytosis
○ D  Margination
○ E  Meiosis

**2.34** **What is the origin of the cells of the mononuclear phagocyte system?**

○ A  Bone marrow
○ B  Liver
○ C  Lymph nodes
○ D  Thymus
○ E  Spleen

**2.35** **Which of the following types of inflammation is most likely to be characterised by Langhans giant cells?**

○ A  Fibrinous inflammation
○ B  Granulomatous inflammation
○ C  Purulent inflammation
○ D  Serous inflammation
○ E  Suppurative inflammation

inflammation

**2.36** A 42-year-old woman with end-stage renal disease is prepared to receive a kidney from her husband. Assays for HLA antigens indicate that the donor and recipient are not 100% compatible. The patient is given an immunosuppressive drug regimen. Three months after transplantation, laboratory tests indicate that the patient's kidney function is declining. There is a rapid decrease in urine output and the urine contains blood cells and a high level of protein. The transplanted kidney is enlarged and tender. After treatment with antilymphocyte globulin, the patient's critical condition is reversed. What type of graft did this patient receive?

○ A Allograft
○ B Autograft
○ C Isograft
○ D Syngraft
○ E Xenograft

**2.37** A 45-year-old man with end-stage renal disease is prepared to receive a kidney from his best friend. Assays for HLA antigens indicate that the donor and recipient are not 100% compatible. The patient is given an immunosuppressive drug regimen. Thirteen weeks after transplantation, laboratory tests indicate that the patient's kidney function is declining. There is a rapid decrease in urine output and the urine contains blood cells and a high level of protein. The transplanted kidney is enlarged and tender. After treatment with antilymphocyte globulin, the patient's critical condition is reversed. During the crisis period, the patient was most likely experiencing:

○ A Acute rejection
○ B Chronic rejection

○   C  Graft-versus-host disease

○   D  Hyperacute rejection

○   E  Toxicity to the drugs

**2.38**  **Following a major traffic accident, a wife (blood group B) and husband (blood group A) are rushed to the emergency department. Donor blood for the wife is erroneously transfused into the husband. Within minutes, he develops a fever, chills, dyspnoea and a dramatic decrease in blood pressure. This reaction is most likely to have been caused by:**

○   A  A cell-mediated response against the A antigen of the recipient

○   B  Anti-A isohaemagglutinin of the immunoglobulin M (IgM) class present in the recipient

○   C  Anti-B isohaemagglutinin of the IgM class preformed in the recipient

○   D  Immunoglobulin G (IgG) production by the recipient in response to the infused red blood cells

○   E  IgM production by the recipient in response to the B antigen

**2.39**  **A 26-year-old woman with blood group type A, Rh-negative, is pregnant with her second child. Her first child is Rh-positive, and the father is also Rh-positive. The second child is most likely to be at risk of developing:**

○   A  An autoimmune disease

○   B  ABO incompatibility

○   C  Drug-induced haemolytic anaemia

○   D  Neutropenia

○   E  Haemolytic disease of the newborn

inflammation

**2.40** **A Rh-negative woman with a Rh-positive husband and a Rh-positive firstborn child is pregnant for the second time. The midwife tells the woman that the second baby is at risk of developing haemolytic disease of the newborn. Which of the following agents would be most likely to protect the baby from developing the disease?**

- A  Albumin from Rh-positive donors
- B  Anti-Rh antibody (Rh immunoglobulin)
- C  A transfusion of platelets
- D  Plasma from randomly selected donors
- E  Rh-positive erythrocytes

**2.41** **A 25-year-old man with persistent low-grade fever and cough had a blood smear which showed a marked increase in the number of cells with a large bi-lobed nucleus. Which of the following cell types was seen in the smear?**

- A  Basophils
- B  Eosinophils
- C  Lymphocytes
- D  Monocytes
- E  Neutrophils

**2.42** **Which of the following white blood cells will be the predominant cell type seen under the microscope if a blood smear is made from a normal healthy individual?**

- A  Basophils
- B  Eosinophils
- C  Lymphocytes
- D  Monocytes
- E  Neutrophils

**2.43** **A 58-year-old farmer with a hydatid cyst in the liver was admitted for elective surgery to remove the cyst. Which of the following white blood cell types will be raised in this patient's preoperative full blood count?**

○ A Basophils
○ B Eosinophils
○ C Lymphocytes
○ D Monocytes
○ E Neutrophils

**2.44** **Which of the following pro-inflammatory cytokines secreted by macrophages is also secreted by muscle?**

○ A Interleukin-3
○ B Interleukin-4
○ C Interleukin-5
○ D Interleukin-6
○ E Interleukin-9

**2.45** **Which of the following cytokines has anti-inflammatory properties?**

○ A Granulocyte macrophage colony-stimulating factor
○ B Interleukin-2
○ C Interleukin-3
○ D Interleukin-10
○ E Tumour necrosis factor (TNF)

inflammation

**2.46 Which of the following cytokines is a major regulator of eosinophil accumulation in tissues?**

- A Granulocyte macrophage colony-stimulating factor
- B Interleukin-1
- C Interleukin-5
- D Interleukin-10
- E Tumour necrosis factor (TNF)

**2.47 Arachidonic acid is one of the essential fatty acids required by most mammals. It is essential for the synthesis of which of the following mediators of inflammation?**

- A Bradykinin
- B Interferon-gamma
- C Interleukin-1
- D Prostaglandins
- E Tumour necrosis factor

**2.48 Leukotrienes are involved in asthmatic and allergic reactions and act to sustain inflammatory reactions. Blockage of which one of the following enzymes will inhibit the synthesis of leukotrienes?**

- A 5-alpha-reductase
- B 5-lipoxygenase
- C Cyclooxygenase-1
- D Cyclooxygenase-2
- E Peroxidase

inflammation

**2.49** **Which one of the following is a primary function of the Kupffer cells in the liver?**

○ A Protein synthesis
○ B Recycling of old red blood cells
○ C Secretion of mucus
○ D Storage of fat-soluble vitamins
○ E Synthesis of intrinsic factor

**2.50** **Which of the following immune cells has perforin in its granules?**

○ A B lymphocyte
○ B Eosinophil
○ C Kupffer cell
○ D Mast cell
○ E Natural killer cell

inflammation

# SECTION 3: NEOPLASIA — QUESTIONS

For each question given below choose the ONE BEST option.

**3.1** A 42-year-old woman noted a lump in her right breast while taking a shower. Her GP confirmed the presence of a 3-cm, firm, irregular, non-movable mass located in the upper outer quadrant of her right breast on physical examination. A fine-needle aspiration of this mass was performed. Cells obtained from the mass were examined cytologically and were consistent with infiltrating ductal carcinoma. The mass was excised in a lumpectomy procedure, and an axillary lymph node dissection was performed. Which of the following findings will best predict a better prognosis for this patient?

○ A Flow cytometric analysis demonstrates aneuploidy and a high S-phase

○ B No metastases are found in the sampled lymph nodes

○ C She has one relative who had a similar type of breast cancer

○ D The tumour cells are strongly oestrogen receptor-positive

○ E The tumour has a high grade

**3.2** A change in bowel habits prompted a 58-year-old man to see his GP. On physical examination, there were no lesions noted on digital rectal examination, but his stool was positive for occult blood. A colonoscopy was performed and revealed a 6-cm friable mass located in the caecum. A biopsy of this mass was performed and microscopic examination showed a moderately differentiated adenocarcinoma. Which of the following findings is most likely to be present in this patient?

○ A  A high titre of DNA topoisomerase I autoantibody

○ B  A K-*ras* mutation in the neoplastic cells

○ C  An immunoperoxidase stain positive for vimentin in the neoplastic cells

○ D  A plasma HIV-1 RNA level of 40,000 copies/ml

○ E  A stool culture positive for *Shigella flexneri*

**3.3** A healthy 45-year-old woman has a routine health check. She has no chest pain, cough, or fever. A chest X-ray is taken, however, which shows a peripheral 'coin lesion', 2.5 cm in diameter, in the right mid-lung field. Which of the following biological characteristics would best distinguish this lesion as a neoplasm, rather than a granuloma?

○ A  Necrosis

○ B  Rapid increase in size

○ C  Recurrence following excision

○ D  Sensitivity to radiation or chemotherapy

○ E  Uncontrolled (autonomous) growth

**3.4** A histopathologist reported on a biopsy specimen obtained from a patient with a malignant neoplasm. The histopathology report stated that the specimen showed a neoplasm composed predominantly of cells with a spindle shape and a high nuclear/cytoplasmic ratio, with marked pleomorphism. These cells were found to be vimentin-positive, cytokeratin-negative and CD45-negative on immunohistochemical staining. This type of neoplasm is most likely to have been diagnosed in which of the following patients?

○ A A 25-year-old man with an enlarged left testis

○ B A 35-year-old woman with a left breast mass and enlarged axillary lymph nodes

○ C A 55-year-old woman with massive ascites and multiple peritoneal metastases

○ D A 15-year-old boy with a mass in the left femur and lung metastases

○ E A 55-year-old man with a right renal mass

**3.5** A 45-year-old woman was found to have a 4-cm-diameter, non-tender mass in her right breast. The mass appeared to be fixed to the chest wall. Another 2-cm, non-tender mass was palpable in the left axilla. A chest X-ray reveals multiple nodules in both lungs, ranging in size from 0.5 cm to 2 cm. Which of the following classifications best describes the stage of her disease?

○ A T1 N1 M0

○ B T1 N0 M1

○ C T2 N1 M0

○ D T3 N0 M0

○ E T4 N1 M1

neoplasia

**3.6** **A study was performed to analyse characteristics of malignant neoplasms in biopsy specimens. The biopsies were performed on patients who had palpable mass lesions in the breast. Of the following microscopic findings, which is most likely to indicate that the neoplasm is malignant?**

○ A   Atypia
○ B   Increased nuclear/cytoplasmic ratio
○ C   Invasion
○ D   Necrosis
○ E   Pleomorphism

**3.7** **Review of a series of surgical pathology reports indicates that a certain type of neoplasm is graded as grade I on a scale of I to IV. Clinically, some of the patients with this neoplasm are found to be stage I. Which of the following is the best interpretation of a neoplasm with this stage I designation?**

○ A   It has an in-situ component
○ B   It has probably arisen from epithelium
○ C   It is unlikely to be malignant
○ D   It is well differentiated and localised
○ E   It could spread via lymphatics

neoplasia

**3.8** **A 48-year-old woman has had a painless mass in the right parotid gland for the past 8 months. A 2-cm-diameter, discrete, solid mass is enucleated from the parotid gland. Histological examination shows a neoplastic lesion with uniform epithelial and myoepithelial cells forming acini, tubules and ducts and supported by a myxoid and chondroid stroma. Which of the following is the most likely complication of this type of parotid lesion?**

○ A  Contralateral immune-mediated parotitis
○ B  Haematogenous metastases to lungs and bone
○ C  Ipsilateral submaxillary salivary gland neoplasm
○ D  Local recurrence
○ E  Regional lymph node metastases

**3.9** **A 76-year-old man with back pain was diagnosed with metastatic prostatic carcinoma involving his lumbar spine. High serum levels of which of the following tumour markers will aid the diagnosis of prostatic carcinoma?**

○ A  Acid phosphatase
○ B  Alkaline phosphatase
○ C  Alpha-fetoprotein
○ D  CEA
○ E  PSA

neoplasia

**3.10** **During an oncology department multidisciplinary meeting the consultant oncologist mentions that a patient has a very radiosensitive tumour. Which of the following tumours is this consultant most likely to be referring to?**

○ A Chondrosarcoma
○ B Endometrial carcinoma
○ C Gastric carcinoma
○ D Ovarian malignancy
○ E Seminoma

**3.11** **During an oncology department multidisciplinary meeting the consultant oncologist mentions that a patient has a hormone-producing tumour. Which of the following tumours is this consultant most likely to be referring to?**

○ A Arrhenoblastoma
○ B Lipoma
○ C Nephroblastoma
○ D Seminoma
○ E Teratoma

**3.12** **A farmer is diagnosed with hepatic angiosarcoma. Exposure to which of the following agents is responsible for the occurrence of this neoplasm?**

○ A Aflatoxin
○ B Arsenic
○ C Dust particles
○ D Mouldy hay
○ E Pollen

**3.13** A 35-year-old woman is very anxious about her tendency to develop breast cancer as both her mother and grandmother died of it. She has no lump palpable on examination. The best way to assess her risk of developing breast cancer is to perform:

○ A  Mammography

○ B  Magnetic resonance imaging

○ C  *TP53* gene analysis

○ D  *BRCA1* and *BRCA2* gene analysis

○ E  Fine-needle aspiration cytology

**3.14** Hypercalcaemia is probably the most common paraneoplastic syndrome. The most likely mechanism by which cancer causes this abnormality is:

○ A  Bone metastasis

○ B  Increased level of vitamin D

○ C  Increased level of parathyroid hormone (PTH)

○ D  Increased level of PTH-related protein

○ E  Renal failure

**3.15** You are reading a histopathology report which describes the excised tumour as benign. Which one of the following is a benign tumour?

○ A  Adenocarcinoma

○ B  Fibrosarcoma

○ C  Haematoma

○ D  Osteogenic sarcoma

○ E  Warthin's tumour

neoplasia

**3.16** **Which of the following features is taken into account when staging a cancer?**

○ A  Basophilia
○ B  Local invasion
○ C  Nuclear/cytoplasmic ratio
○ D  Number of mitotic figures
○ E  Pleomorphism

**3.17** **A 50-year-old woman has got a 7-cm-diameter mass in her right breast, with one enlarged right axillary lymph node. The most likely stage of disease is:**

○ A  IA
○ B  IB
○ C  IIB
○ D  IIIA
○ E  IIIB

**3.18** **You are reading a histopathology report which describes an excised lesion as a premalignant condition. Which of the following is a premalignant condition?**

○ A  Acne
○ B  Familial polyposis
○ C  Keloid
○ D  Solar keratosis
○ E  Villous adenoma of colon

neoplasia

**3.19** **During an oncology department's multidisciplinary meeting the consultant oncologist mentions that a patient has a radioresistant tumour. Which of the following tumours is this consultant most likely to be referring to?**

○ A  Adenocarcinoma of breast
○ B  Liposarcoma
○ C  Lymphoma
○ D  Medulloblastoma
○ E  Osteogenic sarcoma

**3.20** **A 52-year-old woman with carcinoma of left breast and left axillary lymph node involvement underwent successful mastectomy with axillary clearance. The histopathology report described the tumour to be 3.5 cm in its maximum diameter, with three axillary lymph nodes showing microscopic evidence of tumour. The most likely stage of disease in this patient is:**

○ A  I
○ B  IIA
○ C  IIB
○ D  IIIA
○ E  IIIB

**3.21** **A 60-year-old woman with suspected carcinoma of cervix is seen by the gynaecologist. The most reliable and easy method to confirm the diagnosis is:**

○ A  Blood culture
○ B  Colposcopy
○ C  Laparotomy
○ D  Pap smear
○ E  Ultrasound

neoplasia

**3.22** **A 5-year-old child has been diagnosed with a tumour. Which of the following tumours is most likely to be found in this child?**

○ A Lymphangiosarcoma

○ B Melanoma

○ C Meningioma

○ D Nephroblastoma

○ E Pleomorphic adenoma

**3.23** ***BRCA1* and *BRCA2* genes are used as tumour markers for the diagnosis of a tumour of which of the following organs?**

○ A Bladder

○ B Breast

○ C Kidney

○ D Lung

○ E Rectum

**3.24** **A 56-year-old man presents in the surgical outpatient clinic complaining of increasing pain in the mid-epigastrium, with occasional radiation to the back. He also mentions that he has lost nearly 5 kg in weight over the past 3 months. The consultant suspects pancreatic carcinoma. Which of the following tumour markers would aid in confirming this diagnosis?**

○ A Alpha-fetoprotein (AFP)

○ B Carcinoembryonic antigen (CEA)

○ C CA-125

○ D Human chorionic gonadotrophin (hCG)

○ E Prostate-specific antigen (PSA)

neoplasia

**3.25** **A 38-year-old woman presented with an enlarging pelvic mass that extended to the umbilicus. On clinical examination, no pathological abnormalities of the gastrointestinal tract were revealed. Which tumour marker is likely to be raised?**

○ A CA-125
○ B CEA
○ C hCG
○ D HER2
○ E p53s

**3.26** **Industrial exposure to which of the following substances has been correlated with the occurrence of malignant mesothelioma?**

○ A Asbestos
○ B Beryllium
○ C Coal dust
○ D Nitrogen dioxide
○ E Silica

**3.27** **Which one of the following tumours is associated with Paget's disease of bone?**

○ A Ewing's sarcoma
○ B Giant-cell tumour
○ C Metastatic duct carcinoma of the breast
○ D Osteosarcoma
○ E Multiple enchondromas

neoplasia

**3.28  Which of the following is the most common primary malignant tumour of the thyroid?**

○  A  Anaplastic carcinoma
○  B  Follicular carcinoma
○  C  Large-cell carcinoma
○  D  Medullary carcinoma
○  E  Papillary carcinoma

**3.29  A patient presents in the surgical outpatient clinic with carcinoma of the oral cavity. Carcinoma of the oral cavity:**

○  A  Is more common in women
○  B  Is predisposed to by erythroplasia
○  C  Is predisposed to by hairy leukoplakia
○  D  Is predominantly adenocarcinoma in type
○  E  Occurs most frequently on the hard palate

**3.30  Which of the following is the most common benign bone tumour affecting individuals under the age of 21 years?**

○  A  Chondromyxoid fibroma
○  B  Osteochondroma
○  C  Giant-cell tumour
○  D  Aneurysmal bone cyst
○  E  Osteogenic sarcoma

neoplasia

**3.31** **A 6-year-old child has been diagnosed with medulloblastoma. In children, medulloblastomas usually originate in the region of the:**

○ A Cerebellar vermis
○ B Cerebral hemispheres
○ C Fourth ventricle
○ D Filum terminale
○ E Pons

**3.32** **Which of the following is the most common benign germ-cell tumour of the ovaries in premenopausal woman?**

○ A Brenner tumour
○ B Dysgerminoma
○ C Dermoid cyst
○ D Hilus-cell tumour
○ E Mucinous cystadenoma

**3.33** **A 12-year-old boy complains of leg pain and swelling, and an X-ray of the affected limb shows the classic sign of Codman's triangle. Which of the following is the most likely diagnosis?**

○ A Aneurysmal bone cyst
○ B Chondrosarcoma
○ C Multiple myeloma
○ D Osteomyelitis
○ E Osteosarcoma

neoplasia

**3.34 Which of the following cancer–oncogene pairings is correct?**

- A Breast cancer – *ras* oncogene
- B Burkitt's lymphoma – *c-myc* oncogene
- C Chronic myelogenous leukaemia – N-*myc* oncogene
- C Colon cancer – *erb*-B3 oncogene
- E Neuroblastoma – c-*abl* oncogene

**3.35 Which of the following cancer–paraneoplastic syndrome associations is correct?**

- A Breast carcinoma – acanthosis nigricans
- B Gastric carcinoma – dermatomyositis
- C Pancreatic carcinoma – hypertrophic osteoarthropathy
- D Small-cell carcinoma of the lung – hypercalcaemia
- E Thymoma – pure red blood cell aplasia

**3.36 Which of the following tumour-chromosome associations is correct?**

- A Neuroblastoma – chromosome 1
- B Neurofibromas – chromosome 13
- C Osteogenic sarcoma – chromosome 8
- D Retinoblastoma – chromosome 11
- E Wilms' tumour – chromosome 7

**3.37 In which of the following sites is a tumour more likely to occur in adults than in children?**

- A Bone
- B Central nervous system
- C Kidney
- D Lung
- E Soft tissue

neoplasia

**3.38** **Which of the following types of cancers is most common in organ transplant recipients?**

○   A   Breast cancer

○   B   Lung cancer

○   C   Pancreatic cancer

○   D   Prostate cancer

○   E   Skin cancer

**3.39** **For which of the following tumours is the malignant potential most often associated with tumour size?**

○   A   Breast adenocarcinoma

○   B   Colon adenocarcinoma

○   C   Prostate adenocarcinoma

○   D   Renal adenocarcinoma

○   E   Squamous cell carcinoma of the lung

**3.40** **Which of the following sites in newborns most commonly gives rise to tumours derived from all three germ-cell layers?**

○   A   Central nervous system

○   B   Mediastinum

○   C   Ovaries

○   D   Sacrococcygeal area

○   E   Testis

neoplasia

**3.41** **A 52-year-old heavy smoker with complaints of cough, dyspnoea, wheezing and haemoptysis was found to have a 4-cm tumour involving the chest wall. Biopsy of the tumour revealed it to be a non-small-cell lung cancer. What is the stage of this primary lung cancer?**

○ A TX
○ B T1
○ C T2
○ D T3
○ E T4

**3.42** **A 53-year-old-old patient with non-small-cell lung cancer involving the left upper lobe had a staging computed tomographic scan which revealed enlarged ipsilateral mediastinal lymph nodes. What is the nodal staging according to TNM staging system for this patient?**

○ A N0
○ B N1
○ C N2
○ D N3
○ E N4

**3.43** **Which of the following is the most common predisposing factor for adenocarcinoma of the oesophagus?**

○ A Exposure to nitrosamines
○ B Gastro-oesophageal reflux disease
○ C Human papilloma virus infection
○ D Smoking
○ E Tylosis palmaris

**3.44** **A 52-year-old man had a stage III colon cancer resected successfully, followed by adjuvant chemotherapy. What is the most likely 5-year survival rate for this patient?**

○ A 90%

○ B 70%–85%

○ C 30%–60%

○ D 5%

○ E <1%

**3.45** **Which of the following types of lung cancer is most likely to present as disseminated disease at the time of initial presentation?**

○ A Adenocarcinoma

○ B Bronchoalveolar carcinoma

○ C Large-cell carcinoma

○ D Small-cell carcinoma

○ E Squamous cell carcinoma

**3.46** **Lambert–Eaton myasthenic syndrome is a recognised paraneoplastic syndrome that is most commonly associated with which of the following malignancies?**

○ A Breast cancer

○ B Lung cancer

○ C Malignant melanoma

○ D Oesophageal cancer

○ E Phaeochromocytoma

neoplasia

**3.47 A 68-year-old man with haematuria was diagnosed with bladder cancer. The primary tumour involved the perivesical fat. What is the primary tumour (T) stage of this patient's cancer?**

   A  Ta

   B  T1

   C  T2

   D  T3

   E  T4

**3.48 Which of the following is the most commonly associated risk factor for bladder cancer?**

   A  Alcohol

   B  Coffee

   C  Human papilloma virus infection

   D  Radon

   E  Smoking

**3.49 A 52-year-old man was diagnosed with renal cell carcinoma. The tumour was seen to be extending into the inferior vena cava on computed tomography. What is the clinical stage of this tumour?**

   A  Stage 0

   B  Stage I

   C  Stage II

   D  Stage III

   E  Stage IV

neoplasia

**3.50** **A 53-year-old woman was diagnosed with a squamous cell carcinoma on the forehead measuring more than 2 cm but less than 4 cm in its greatest dimension. What is the tumour stage of this primary tumour according to the TNM staging system for head and neck cancers?**

- ○ A  T1
- ○ B  T2
- ○ C  T3
- ○ D  T4
- ○ E  TX

neoplasia

# SECTION 4: MICROBIOLOGY — QUESTIONS

For each question given below choose the ONE BEST option.

**4.1** **A 4-year-old child was brought to the emergency department with fever, hypotension, erythema and neck stiffness. Which of the following toxins is most likely to be responsible for this child's condition?**

- ○ A Botulinum toxin
- ○ B Endotoxin
- ○ C Erythrotoxin
- ○ D Exotoxin
- ○ E Neurotoxin

**4.2**  A 55-year-old man was brought to the emergency department 2 hours after the onset of delirium. On arrival, he was confused and uncooperative. His vital signs were: temperature 39.4 °C, blood pressure 95/50 mmHg, pulse 140/minute and regular, respiratory rate 24/minute. Clinical examination was unremarkable. Laboratory investigations showed: serum glucose 3.9 mmol/l, serum creatinine 1.4 mg/dl; urinary glucose 0, urinary protein 2+, urinary white blood cell count >200 cells/high-power field, and no urinary casts. Which of the following organisms is most likely to be grown from blood cultures in this patient?

○  A  *Bacteroides fragilis*
○  B  *Candida albicans*
○  C  *Escherichia coli*
○  D  *Pseudomonas aeruginosa*
○  E  *Staphylococcus aureus*

microbiology

**4.3** A sexually active 19-year-old male university student has had fatigue and malaise for the past 10 days. Early in the course he had a mild pharyngitis. On physical examination, he has enlarged and tender posterior cervical, axillary and inguinal lymph nodes. His liver edge is slightly tender and the spleen tip is palpable. He has mild scleral icterus. A full blood count shows: haemoglobin 13.5 g/dl, haematocrit 40%, mean corpuscular volume (MCV) 93 fl, platelet count 263 × 10⁹/l, and white blood cell count (WBC) 13 × 10⁹/l, with a WBC differential count of 45 neutrophils, 3 bands, 25 lymphocytes, 15 atypical lymphocytes, 10 monocytes, and 2 eosinophils. Which of the following infectious agents is most likely responsible for these findings?

- A  Epstein–Barr virus
- B  Hepatitis A virus
- C  Human immunodeficiency virus
- D  Rubella virus
- E  Rubeola virus

**4.4** The vaginal culture of a 28-year-old woman with excessive vaginal discharge showed non-pathogenic bacteria. A vaginal smear showed numerous bacilli under the microscope. The most likely organism is:

- A  *Escherichia coli*
- B  *Gardnerella vaginalis*
- C  *Lactobacillus* species
- D  *Proteus* species
- E  *Pseudomonas* species

microbiology

**4.5** **Which of the following structures is found in Gram-negative bacteria but not in Gram-positive bacteria?**

O A Capsule

O B Cell wall

O C Cytoplasmic membrane

O D Endospore

O E Outer membrane

**4.6** **A 26-year-old woman presents with a 2-month history of cough that has recently become productive, fatigue, night sweats and a recent weight loss of 5 lb. She has a history of intravenous drug abuse and has recently been diagnosed as HIV-positive. Sputum samples contain many acid-fast bacilli and her Mantoux test is positive. Which of the following is the most appropriate initial empirical therapy for this patient?**

O A Cefoxitin

O B Erythromycin

O C Clarithromycin + isoniazid

O D Rifampicin + isoniazid

O E Rifampicin + isoniazid + pyrazinamide + ethambutol

microbiology

**4.7** A week after undergoing sigmoid resection with diverting colostomy for ruptured sigmoid diverticulum, a 64-year-old man has a temperature of 39.7 °C and shaking chills. He received gentamicin and ampicillin therapy after the operation and his postoperative course had been uncomplicated until now. A blood culture grew Gram-negative bacilli. Which of the following is the most likely causative organism for this patient's present condition?

○ A *Bacteroides fragilis*

○ B *Brucella abortus*

○ C *Escherichia coli*

○ D *Proteus mirabilis*

○ E *Pseudomonas aeruginosa*

**4.8** Which of the following toxins continually stimulates adenylate cyclase to overproduce cAMP by catalysing the binding of ADP-ribose to the Gs protein, leading to severe fluid loss?

○ A *Bordetella pertussis* toxin

○ B Cholera toxin

○ C *Clostridium bolulinum* toxin

○ D Diphtheria toxin

○ E Tetanus toxin

microbiology

**4.9** **A 32-year-old man developed fatal food poisoning. Which of the following organisms is most likely to be associated with fatal food poisoning?**

   ○ A  *Bacillus cereus*
   ○ B  *Clostridium botulinum*
   ○ C  *Escherichia coli*
   ○ D  *Staphylococcus aureus*
   ○ E  *Vibrio cholerae*

**4.10** **A 26-year-old man has developed folliculitis. Which of the following organisms is most likely to be responsible for this condition?**

   ○ A  *Escherichia coli*
   ○ B  *Klebsiella* species
   ○ C  *Proteus* species
   ○ D  *Pseudomonas* species
   ○ E  *Staphylococcus aureus*

**4.11** **A 32-year-old man developed a high-grade fever with rusty-coloured sputum. His chest X-ray showed right-sided consolidation. The most accurate test for diagnosis in this case would be:**

   ○ A  Blood culture
   ○ B  Cold antibody titre
   ○ C  Lung biopsy
   ○ D  Sputum culture
   ○ E  Sputum Gram stain

microbiology

**4.12** **The drug of choice for treating pulmonary anthrax is:**

○ A Ceftriaxone
○ B Clindamycin
○ C Ciprofloxacin
○ D Metronidazole
○ E Tetracycline

**4.13** **A 21-year-old woman who had been feeling unwell since returning from a holiday trip to India presented to the emergency department on day 16 after the onset of fever. She had a positive Widal test. The most likely organism resposnsible for the fever is:**

○ A *Bacteroides fragilis*
○ B *Escherichia coli*
○ C *Klebsiella* species
○ D *Mycobacterium tuberculosis*
○ E *Salmonella typhi*

**4.14** **Which of the following is the most common portal of entry in *Blastomyces dermatitidis* infection?**

○ A Central nervous system
○ B Circulatory system
○ C Mouth
○ D Respiratory tract
○ E Skin

microbiology

**4.15**  **A 45-year-old hospital patient acquires a *Pseudomonas* infection. The most likely mechanism for pathogenesis in *Pseudomonas* infection is:**

○  A  Activation of cAMP

○  B  Activation of EF-2

○  C  Endotoxin

○  D  Exotoxin

○  E  Inhibition of cGMP

**4.16**  **A previously healthy, 24-year-old, male intravenous drug addict was admitted to hospital with complaints of fever and malaise over the past 5 days. Clinical examination suggested infective endocarditis, which was confirmed on echocardiography. From two sets of blood culture there was growth of Gram-positive cocci arranged in clusters. Which of the following organisms is most likely to be responsible for endocarditis in this patient?**

○  A  Enterococcus

○  B  *Escherichia colio*

○  C  *Pseudomonas aeruginosao*

○  D  *Staphylococcus aureuso*

○  E  *Streptococcus pneumoniae*

microbiology

**4.17** **A 28-year-old Asian woman with cervical lymphadenopathy is seen in a surgical outpatient clinic. An excision biopsy of one of the nodes is performed and sent for histopathology. This shows granulomatous inflammation. Which of the following histopathological features is most diagnostic for tuberculosis?**

- ○ A  Caseation necrosis
- ○ B  Liquefactive necrosis
- ○ C  The presence of fibroblasts
- ○ D  The presence of Gram positive cocci
- ○ E  The presence of neutrophils

**4.18** **The virulence of bacteria is related to:**

- ○ A  Toxin and enzyme production
- ○ B  The resistance of the patient
- ○ C  The number of bacteria
- ○ D  The age of the patient
- ○ E  The portal of entry

**4.19** **Brucellosis is transmitted by:**

- ○ A  Cats
- ○ B  Ticks
- ○ C  Flies
- ○ D  Mosquito bite
- ○ E  Unpasteurised milk

microbiology

**4.20 An abscess containing sulphur granules is a feature of:**

○ A Actinomycosis

○ B Amoebiasis

○ C Brucellosis

○ D Histoplasmosis

○ E *Staphylococcus aureus* infection

**4.21 A 6-year-old child is brought to the emergency department by his parents complaining of severe earache. On examination, there is greenish pus discharging from his right ear. Which of the following organisms is most likely to be responsible for this child's ear infection?**

○ A *Klebsiella* species

○ B *Pseudomonas aeruginosa*

○ C *Staphylococcus aureus*

○ D *Streptococcus pyogenes*

○ E *Streptococcus pneumoniae*

**4.22 A 38-year-old, HIV-positive, homosexual man presents in the emergency department complaining of weight loss associated with chronic, persistent, watery, non-bloody diarrhoea and loss of appetite. Numerous acid-fast cysts are found in his stool sample. Which of the following organisms is most likely to be responsible for this condition?**

○ A *Cryptosporidium parvum*

○ B *Entamoeba histolytica*

○ C *Giardia lamblia*

○ D *Mycobacterium avium-intracellulare complex*

○ E *Toxoplasma gondii*

microbiology

**4.23** **A 38-year-old woman with rheumatic mitral stenosis presented in the emergency department complaining of fever and malaise. Clinical examination and investigations suggested infective endocarditis. Which of the following bacteria is the most likely causative agent for infective endocarditis in this woman?**

○  A  *Escherichia coli*
○  B  *Haemophilus influenzae*
○  C  *Streptococcus pneumoniae*
○  D  *Streptococcus viridans*
○  E  *Staphylococcus aureus*

**4.24** **A 12-year-old boy is suffering from a parasitic infestation. Which type of anaemia is most likely to be seen in this boy?**

○  A  Aplastic anaemia
○  B  Anaemia of chronic disease
○  C  Folic acid deficiency anaemia
○  D  Haemolytic anaemia
○  E  Iron deficiency anaemia

**4.25** **A 22-year-old medical student presented in the emergency department with sore throat and lymphadenopathy. Her peripheral smear shows atypical lymphocytes. What is the most probable infectious cause for this patient's clinical condition?**

○  A  Cytomegalovirus
○  B  Epstein–Barr virus
○  C  Herpes simplex virus
○  D  Human immunodeficiency virus
○  E  *Mycobacterium tuberculosis*

microbiology

**4.26 A 63-year-old diabetic woman with septicaemia secondary to perforated appendix was commenced on meropenem. Which of the mechanisms given below describes the mechanism of action of meropenem?**

○ A  Acts as a competitive inhibitor of the enzyme dihydropteroate synthetase

○ B  Blockage of bacterial DNA replication

○ C  Inhibition of bacterial wall synthesis

○ D  Inhibition of translocation of peptides by binding to the 50S subunit of the bacterial ribosome

○ E  Prevents the amino-acyl t-RNA from binding to the A site of the ribosome

**4.27 A 73-year-old man with chronic prostatitis who declined surgery for benign prostatic hypertrophy was commenced on doxycycline after an acute exacerbation of prostatitis. Which of the mechanisms given below describes the mechanism of action of doxycycline?**

○ A  Acts as a competitive inhibitor of the enzyme dihydropteroate synthetase

○ B  Blockage of bacterial DNA replication

○ C  Inhibition of bacterial wall synthesis

○ D  Inhibition of translocation of peptides by binding to the 50S subunit of the bacterial ribosome

○ E  Prevents the amino-acyl t-RNA from binding to the A site of the ribosome

microbiology

**4.28 A 28-year-old woman developed Stevens–Johnson syndrome after taking an antibiotic. Stevens–Johnson syndrome is a recognised serious side-effect associated with which one of the following antibiotics?**

    A  Aztreonam

    B  Ceftriaxone

    C  Meropenem

    D  Sulphonamides

    E  Tetracycline

**4.29 A 53-year-old woman with infection with a resistant species of enterobacteria was commenced on oral ciprofloxacin. Which of the mechanisms given below describes the mechanism of action of ciprofloxacin?**

    A  Acts as a competitive inhibitor of the enzyme dihydropteroate synthetase

    B  Blockage of bacterial DNA replication

    C  Inhibition of bacterial wall synthesis

    D  Inhibition of translocation of peptides by binding to the 50S subunit of the bacterial ribosome

    E  Prevents the amino-acyl t-RNA from binding to the A site of the ribosome

microbiology

**4.30** **A 26-year-old man with cystic fibrosis was commenced on amikacin to treat pneumonia caused by a multidrug-resistant strain of *Pseudomonas aeruginosa*. Which of the mechanisms given below describes the mechanism of action of amikacin?**

○ A  Acts as a competitive inhibitor of the enzyme dihydropteroate synthetase

○ B  Blockage of bacterial DNA replication

○ C  Inhibition of bacterial wall synthesis

○ D  Inhibition of protein synthesis by binding to the 30S subunit of the bacterial ribosome

○ E  Prevents the amino-acyl t-RNA from binding to the A site of the ribosome

**4.31** **A 68-year-old man had a catheter placed in his urethra at the time of abdominal aortic aneurysm repair. The catheter had to be left in for longer than anticipated as this patient developed postoperative acute renal failure. One week later he experienced suprapubic and flank pain, with urinary urgency and frequency. He also had chills and fever. After examining him and evaluating the sediment of his centrifuged urine, he was informed by the intensive care consultant that he had acute ascending pyelonephritis. If the diagnosis is accurate and this man's urine is cultured, which of the following organisms is most likely to be isolated?**

○ A  *Clostridium difficile*

○ B  *Escherichia coli* with pili

○ C  *Pseudomonas aeruginosa*

○ D  *Staphylococcus aureus*

○ E  *Streptococcus pneumoniae*

microbiology

**4.32** **A 28-year-old man presented to his GP complaining of fatigue, night sweats and a dry unproductive cough 6 months after a holiday trip to South Africa. Until the past few months, he had apparently been in good health. A full blood count and differential blood count reveal that he is lymphopenic. X-ray examination reveals an interstitial pneumonia. Skin test reactions to a battery of materials are normal. Which of the following is the most appropriate next step in evaluating this patient's illness?**

○ A  $CH_{50}$ assay

○ B  Chemotaxis assay

○ C  Identification of the organism that is causing the pneumonia

○ D  Intracellular killing assay

○ E  Nitroblue tetrazolium reduction assay

**4.33** **A 12-year-old boy with recurrent pulmonary infections has been brought to the hospital with meningitis by his mother. Gram staining of the spinal fluid reveals numerous polymorphonuclear neutrophils and Gram-positive cocci in grape-like clusters. Which of the following will be the most appropriate empirical drug of choice to be employed until the antibiotic sensitivity report is received from the laboratory?**

○ A  Ampicillin

○ B  Chloramphenicol

○ C  Methicillin

○ D  Streptomycin

○ E  Penicillin

microbiology

75

**4.34** **A toddler is unprovokedly attacked and bitten on the shoulder by a stray dog and suffers a slight wound. In addition to flushing the wound, cleaning it surgically, and giving antitetanus prophylaxis and antibiotics as indicated, the physician should immediately:**

- ○ A  Observe the boy very carefully
- ○ B  Order a search for the attacking dog for autopsy
- ○ C  Report the incident to the local police
- ○ D  Start rabies vaccine
- ○ E  Start rabies vaccine and give antirabies serum

**4.35** **An FY2 doctor who had previously worked on the infectious diseases ward has been diagnosed as having tuberculosis. She has been ill for 10 months with symptoms that include a productive cough, intermittent fever, night sweats, and has lost nearly 6 kg in weight. Numerous acid-fast bacilli are seen in a sputum examination, and more than 50 colonies of organisms grow out in culture. In a situation such as this, those contacts who have a positive skin test but no other signs of disease should:**

- ○ A  Be checked periodically by chest X-ray
- ○ B  Be immunised with bacillus Calmette–Guérin (BCG) vaccine
- ○ C  Be vaccinated with purified protein derivative (PPD)
- ○ D  Receive a full course of isoniazid and ethambutol
- ○ E  Receive prophylactic isoniazid

**4.36 Certain surgical instruments are sterilized with ultraviolet light. Ultraviolet light is used as an antimicrobial physical agent because it:**

A Acts as an alkylating agent

B Causes the formation of pyrimidine dimers

C Disrupts the bacterial cell membrane

D Is a common protein denaturant

E Removes free sulphhydryl groups

**4.37 A 45-year-old patient who was receiving chemotherapy for cancer developed a disseminated varicella-zoster infection. The most likely reason for this viral infection is:**

A Deficiency in the third component of complement

B Hypogammaglobulinaemia

C Outgrowth of virus from varicella-zoster immunisation

D Synergism between varicella-zoster and chemotherapy

E T-cell deficiency

**4.38 A 2-year-old boy was brought to the emergency department with a suspected diagnosis of diphtheria. Which of the following modes of pathogenesis is most compatible with diphtheria?**

A Immune complex formation

B Lysis of natural killer T lymphocytes by bacterial envelope enzymes

C Possession of a capsule by the causative agent

D Production of an exotoxin by the causative agent

E Tumour necrosis factor production

microbiology

**4.39** **A laboratory test used to identify *Staphylococcus aureus* is based on the clotting of plasma. The microbial product that is responsible for this activity is:**

○ A  Coagulase

○ B  Coagulase reactive factor

○ C  Plasmin

○ D  Prothrombin

○ E  Thrombin

**4.40** **A 56-year-old diabetic patient in the intensive care unit was commenced on an antifungal agent that inhibits the biosynthesis of fungal ergosterol. Which of the following agents was most likely to have been given to the patient?**

○ A  Amphotericin B

○ B  Flucytosine

○ C  Griseofulvin

○ D  Ketoconazole

○ E  Nystatin

microbiology

# SECTION 5:
# DISORDERS OF FLUIDS AND ELECTROLYTES — QUESTIONS

For each question given below choose the ONE BEST option.

**5.1** **A 22-year-old woman was brought to the emergency department with profound nausea and vomiting for 24 hours. An arterial blood gas analysis was performed. Which of the following sets of values is most likely to be obtained?**

○ A pH 6.25, $p(CO_2)$ 28 mmHg, $HCO_3^-$ 15 mmol/l

○ B pH 7.20, $p(CO_2)$ 55 mmHg, $HCO_3^-$ 27 mmol/l

○ C pH 7.30, $p(CO_2)$ 40 mmHg, $HCO_3^-$ 24 mmol/l

○ D pH 7.35, $p(CO_2)$ 35 mmHg, $HCO_3^-$ 28 mmol/l

○ E pH 7.50, $p(CO_2)$ 47 mmHg, $HCO_3^-$ 35 mmol/l

**5.2** **A 26-year-old woman with nephrotic syndrome has developed generalised oedema. The most likely mechanism for oedema in this patient is:**

○ A Decreased colloid osmotic pressure

○ B Decreased protein synthesis

○ C Decreased protein intake

○ D Increased capillary hydrostatic pressure

○ E Lymphatic obstruction

fluids

**5.3** **A 26-year-old man with a 1-week history of severe diarrhoea feels dizzy when he stands up. His blood pressure (supine) is 112/76 mmHg with a pulse of 88/minute; blood pressure (on standing) is 80/60 mmHg with a pulse of 120/minute. In addition to controlling his diarrhoea, the most appropriate initial therapy is intravenous administration of:**

   ○  A  5% dextrose in water

   ○  B  Desmopressin

   ○  C  Fresh frozen plasma

   ○  D  Isotonic saline

   ○  E  Verapamil

**5.4** **A 28-year-old woman has presented in the emergency department with a 3-day history of vomiting and diarrhoea. She has postural hypotension and poor tissue turgor. Her serum sodium concentration is 130 mmol/l. Which of the following findings is most likely to be seen in this patient?**

   ○  A  Decreased serum aldosterone concentration

   ○  B  Increased serum atrial natriuretic peptide concentration

   ○  C  Increased effective circulating volume

   ○  D  Increased serum ADH (vasopressin) concentration

   ○  E  Urine osmolality less than the serum osmolality

fluids

**5.5** A 45-year-old diabetic woman was admitted to the emergency ward. Her electrolyte report showed: sodium 135 mmol/l, potassium 5 mmol/l, bicarbonate⁻ 10 mmol/l, chloride⁻ 102 mmol/l, pH 7.3, and $p(CO_2)$ 40 mmHg. The patient is most likely to have:

- A   Compensated respiratory acidosis
- B   Compensated metabolic alkalosis
- C   Compensated respiratory acidosis
- D   Respiratory alkalosis
- E   Wide anion gap metabolic acidosis

**5.6** One day after an emergency repair of a ruptured abdominal aortic aneurysm, a 64-year-old man has urine output of 40 ml over a 4-hour period. A Foley catheter is still in place. He received 14 units of blood during the operation. His temperature is 37.8 °C, blood pressure 100/50 mmHg, pulse 126/minute, and central venous pressure (CVP) 3 mmHg. Examination shows diffuse peripheral oedema. Heart sounds are normal. The lungs are clear to auscultation. The abdomen is soft. Laboratory studies show: haematocrit 34%, serum sodium 145 mmol/l, serum potassium 5.0 mmol/l, and urine sodium 6 mmol/l. Which of the following is the most likely cause of the oliguria?

- A   Heart failure
- B   Hypovolaemia
- C   Occluded Foley catheter
- D   Renal artery thrombosis
- E   Transfusion reaction

fluids

**5.7** A 48-year-old woman underwent surgery for an abdominal mass. While still in hospital, on the 6th postoperative day, she developed a cardiac problem. Her serum potassium was markedly elevated. What is the most likely cause for hyperkalaemia in this patient?

O  A  Prolonged dependency

O  B  Prolonged use of antibiotics

O  C  Multiple blood transfusions

O  D  Pulmonary embolism

O  E  Volume overload

**5.8** A blood gas analysis report of a 36-year-old patient admitted to hospital shows: pH 7.6, $p(O_2)$ 75 mmHg, $p(CO_2)$ 46 mmHg and bicarbonate 44 mmol/l. The most likely interpretation of this set of values is:

O  A  Metabolic acidosis

O  B  Metabolic alkalosis

O  C  Respiratory acidosis

O  D  Respiratory alkalosis

O  E  Respiratory failure

**5.9** A patient with renal failure has a serum potassium of 7 mmol/l. The most likely electrocardiographic manifestation of this abnormality will be:

O  A  Flattened T waves

O  B  Prolonged QT interval

O  C  ST depression

O  D  Tented T waves

O  E  U waves

fluids

**5.10** A semiconscious patient is brought to the emergency department with sweating, dehydration and weakness. Serum levels of which electrolyte are most likely to be low in this patient?

○ A $Ca^{2+}$

○ B $HCO_3^-$

○ C $K^+$

○ D $Na^+$

○ E $PO_4^-$

**5.11** The electrocardiogram (ECG) strip of a patient shows sagging of the ST segment, depression of the T wave, and elevation of the U wave. What is the most likely electrolyte abnormality responsible for these ECG findings?

○ A Hyperkalaemia

○ B Hypermagnesaemia

○ C Hypocalcaemia

○ D Hypokalaemia

○ E Hypomagnesaemia

**5.12** The serum electrolyte analysis of a patient shows hypokalaemia, with a serum potassium of 3.1 mmol/l. What is the most likely cause of this abnormality?

○ A Hyperglycaemia

○ B Liddle syndrome

○ C Metabolic acidosis

○ D Renal failure

○ E Rhabdomyolysis

fluids

**5.13** **The serum electrolyte analysis of a patient shows hyperkalaemia, with serum potassium of 6.5 mmol/l. Which of the following drugs could be responsible for this abnormality?**

○ A  Amphotericin B
○ B  Carbenicillin
○ C  Theophylline
○ D  Thiazide diuretic
○ E  Spironolactone

**5.14** **A 46-year-old-woman with chronic renal failure has hypermagnesaemia. Which of the following abnormalities is most likely to be seen in this patient?**

○ A  Anorexia
○ B  Generalised seizures
○ C  Respiratory depression
○ D  Tetany
○ E  Vomiting

**5.15** **The serum electrolyte analysis of a patient in the intensive care unit showed hyperphosphataemia, with a serum phosphate of more than 1.46 mmol/l. What is the most likely cause for this abnormality?**

○ A  Acute alcoholism
○ B  Hyperparathyroidism
○ C  Refeeding after prolonged malnutrition
○ D  Renal insufficiency
○ E  Severe chronic respiratory alkalosis

**5.16** **A 26-year-old woman has developed euvolaemic hyponatraemia. Which of the following conditions is most likely to be associated with this abnormality?**

O   A   Diuretic therapy
O   B   Pancreatitis
O   C   Protracted vomiting
O   D   Psychosis
O   E   Salt-losing nephropathy

**5.17** **A 56-year-old man has developed hypervolaemic hyponatraemia. Which of the following conditions is most likely to be associated with this abnormality?**

O   A   Cirrhosis
O   B   Diuretic therapy
O   C   Pancreatitis
O   D   Protracted vomiting
O   E   Salt-losing nephropathy

**5.18** **Extracellular fluid volume expansion is most likely to be seen in:**

O   A   Burns
O   B   Diarrhoea
O   C   Nephrotic syndrome
O   D   Sweating
O   E   Vomiting

fluids

**5.19** **A 26-year-old woman has hypocalcaemia. Which of the following conditions might be responsible for this electrolyte abnormality?**

O A Hypoparathyroidism

O B Primary hyperparathyroidism

O C Prolonged immobilisation

O D Secondaries in bone

O E Vitamin D toxicity

**5.20** **What percentage of calcium is available for buffering changes in Ca$^{2+}$ balance in the body?**

O A 1%

O B 10%

O C 20%

O D 50%

O E 99%

**5.21** **A 28-year-old patient was seen in the emergency department with metabolic acidosis and a decreased anion gap. What is the most likely cause for the decreased anion gap in this patient?**

O A Hypoalbuminaemia

O B Hypocalcaemia

O C Hypomagnesaemia

O D Lactic acidosis

O E Uraemia

fluids

**5.22** **A 36-year-old man was admitted to the emergency ward with metabolic acidosis and increased anion gap. What is the most likely cause for the increased anion gap in this patient?**

O  A  Halide (bromide or iodide) intoxication
O  B  Hypergammaglobulinaemia
O  C  Hyperviscosity
O  D  Lithium intoxication
O  E  Lactic acidosis

**5.23** **Which of the following conditions is associated with the generation of a metabolic alkalosis due to intracellular shifting of hydrogen ions?**

O  A  Chloride diarrhoea
O  B  Hypokalaemia
O  C  Loop diuretic therapy
O  D  Nasogastric suction
O  E  Vomiting

**5.24** **A 28-year-old woman was admitted through the emergency department with profuse vomiting. Arterial blood gas analysis suggested severe metabolic alkalosis. In this patient:**

O  A  Ammonia production is decreased
O  B  Cerebral perfusion is decreased
O  C  Coronary blood flow is increased
O  D  Diffuse arteriolar vasodilatation increases tissue perfusion
O  E  Serum concentration of ionised calcium is increased

fluids

**5.25** **A 63-year-old woman on long-term total parenteral nutrition was noticed to have hypophosphataemia. What is the normal plasma level of phosphate in adults?**

○ A  0.5–0.75 mmol/l
○ B  0.8–1.45 mmol/l
○ C  1.50–3.0 mmol/l
○ D  10.0–12.5 mmol/l
○ E  15.0–17.5 mmol/l

**5.26** **A 36-year-old woman with an ileostomy was found to have hypomagnesaemia on an urgent blood sample sent to the biochemistry laboratory. Which of the clinical features below will have prompted the on-call SHO to check the serum magnesium level in this patient?**

○ A  Bradycardia
○ B  Dizziness
○ C  Nausea
○ D  Seizures
○ E  Vomiting

**5.27** **A 46-year-old woman with chronic renal insufficiency has hyperphosphataemia. Which of the following is the most likely complication of hyperphosphataemia?**

○ A  Depressed cardiac output
○ B  Impaired diaphragmatic contractility
○ C  Metastatic calcification
○ D  Osteomalacia
○ E  Respiratory insufficiency

fluids

**5.28** **Ammonia is an important urine-buffering system for secreted hydrogen ions. Which of the following electrolyte abnormalities is associated with increased synthesis of ammonia in the kidneys?**

O   A   Hypercalcaemia
O   B   Hyperkalaemia
O   C   Hypernatraemia
O   D   Hypokalaemia
O   E   Hyponatraemia

**5.29** **A 52-year-old woman was admitted into the surgical intensive care unit after a prolonged and complex cardiac surgical operation. Her tissue perfusion was poor in the immediate postoperative period and arterial blood gas analysis showed lactic acidosis. What type of lactic acidosis did this woman have in the immediate postoperative period?**

O   A   Type A
O   B   Type B1
O   C   Type B2
O   D   Type B3
O   E   Type C

**5.30** **Which of the following conditions is most likely to cause hypervolaemic hypernatraemia?**

O   A   Burns
O   B   Central diabetes insipidus
O   C   Diarrhoea
O   D   Hyperalimentation
O   E   Nephrogenic diabetes insipidus

fluids

# SECTION 6: BLEEDING AND HAEMOSTASIS — QUESTIONS

For each question given below choose the ONE BEST option.

**6.1** After an abortion, a 32-year-old woman was brought to the emergency department in acute distress with multiple ecchymoses of the skin that had developed over the past 48 hours. Her prothrombin time (PT) was 38 seconds and her partial thromboplastin time (PTT) was 55 seconds. A full blood count showed a white blood cell count of $5.3 \times 10^9$/l, haemoglobin 8.1 g/dl, haematocrit 24.9%, mean corpuscular volume (MCV) 99 fl, and platelet count $16.3 \times 10^9$/l. Her D-dimer test was very high. She most likely had:

○   A   Afibrinogenaemia
○   B   Disseminated intravascular coagulopathy
○   C   Haemophilia A
○   D   Vitamin K deficiency
○   E   von Willebrand's disease

**6.2** A 26-year-old woman was informed by the haematologist that she had a quantitative as well as qualitative platelet defect. Which of the following is typically associated with a qualitative or quantitative platelet defect?

○   A   Epistaxis
○   B   Haemarthroses
○   C   Normal bleeding time
○   D   Prolonged partial thromboplastin time
○   E   Soft tissue haemorrhages

**6.3** **A 16-year-old girl was seen by the haematologist because she had developed skin and mucosal petechiae. Her prothrombin time (PT), partial thromboplastin time (PTT), platelet count and bleeding time were all normal. What would explain skin and mucosal petechiae in the presence of a normal PT, PTT, platelet count and bleeding time?**

- A Aspirin ingestion
- B Chronic alcoholism
- C Scurvy
- D Uraemia
- E vonWillebrand's disease

**6.4** **A 10-year-old boy was referred to the haematologist because he had a bleeding disorder characterised by haemarthrosis. On investigation, his prothrombin time was normal, but the partial thromboplastin time was quite elevated. His platelet count was normal. Which of the following statements regarding his clinical condition is correct?**

- A He has an underlying liver disease
- B He has had episodes of mucocutaneous bleeding
- C His sisters are affected as well
- D There is typically no family history in this condition
- E Transfusion of factor VIII concentrate is helpful

bleeding

**6.5** A 55-year-old man had a preoperative full blood count (FBC) performed prior to elective right hemicolectomy for a malignant growth in the ascending colon. The FBC revealed: haemoglobin 12.1 g/dl, haematocrit 35.8%, mean corpuscular volume (MCV) 90 fl, white blood cell count 13.5 × 10⁹/l, platelet count of 1000 × 10⁹/l. These findings are most indicative of:

○ A A myeloproliferative disorder
○ B Chronic liver disease
○ C Hereditary spherocytosis
○ D Postoperative haemorrhage
○ E von Willebrand's disease

**6.6** A 26-year-old man who has had multiple episodes of deep venous thrombosis presented in the emergency department with a suspected pulmonary embolism. Which of the following blood proteins is most likely to be deficient in this patient?

○ A Alpha-2-antiplasmin
○ B Alpha-2-macroglobulin
○ C Antithrombin III
○ D Factor V
○ E Fibrinogen

bleeding

**6.7** **An immunocompromised patient with sepsis due to Gram-negative bacteria had a prothrombin time of 34 seconds and a partial thromboplastin time of 59 seconds. His platelet count was 11 × 10⁹/l, he had elevated D-dimer. Which of the following statements regarding his condition is most appropriate?**

- A  It may result from endothelial cell injury
- B  The fibrinogen is increased
- C  There is an increase in factor VIII levels
- D  The prothrombin time (PT) is normal
- E  Venous thrombosis is more common than bleeding

**6.8** **A 28-year-old patient admitted for elective thyroidectomy is known to have von Willebrand's disease. Which of the following conditions is an unlikely complication in this patient?**

- A  Easy bruising
- B  Epistaxis
- C  Excessive bleeding from wounds
- D  Haemarthrosis
- E  Menorrhagia

bleeding

**6.9** A 25-year-old man admitted for elective hydrocoele repair had a full blood count that showed: haemoglobin 14.8 g/dl, haematocrit 45%, mean corpuscular volume 96 fl, white blood cell count $8.5 \times 10^9/l$ and platelet count $275 \times 10^9/l$. His prothrombin time was normal, but the partial thromboplastin time was prolonged to 210 seconds. A deficiency of which of the following is most likely to be associated with these findings?

    A  Antithrombin III

    B  Factor XII

    C  Protein C

    D  Protein S

    E  Vitamin C

**6.10** A 46-year-old alcoholic with sepsis was admitted into the intensive care unit for management of coagulopathy. Which of the following laboratory tests best distinguishes the coagulopathy of liver disease from disseminated intravascular coagulopathy (DIC)?

    A  D-Dimer test

    B  Factor XIII assay

    C  Partial thromboplastin time

    D  Platelet count

    E  Prothrombin time

bleeding

**6.11** **A 36-year-old woman was admitted through the emergency department with fever and neurological abnormalities. She had a full blood count which showed: white blood cell count 9.6 × 10⁹/l, haemoglobin 8.4 g/dl, haematocrit 25.9%, mean corpuscular volume 100 fl, platelet count 10.0 × 10⁹/l. Her serum haptoglobin was markedly decreased. Her serum total bilirubin was 5.5 mg/dl, with a direct bilirubin of 5.1 mg/ dl. The on-call consultant decided to perform a plasmapheresis on this woman but she died despite plasmapheresis. At autopsy, hyaline thrombi were observed in the small arteries of the kidney, heart and brain. Which of the following diseases did she probably have?**

- A  Alcoholic liver disease
- B  Malaria
- C  Systemic lupus erythematosus (SLE)
- D  Thrombotic thrombocytopenic purpura (TTP)
- E  von Willebrand's disease (vWD)

**6.12** **A 12-year-old boy was seen in the orthopaedics outpatient clinic with recurrent spontaneous joint haemorrhages. Which of the following laboratory findings are most likely to be seen in this patient?**

- A  Factor V deficiency
- B  Factor VIII deficiency
- C  Platelet count of 100,000
- D  Positive protamine sulphate test
- E  Prothrombin time twice normal control

bleeding

**6.13** In a patient who is to undergo elective surgery, the presence of which of the following findings on preoperative investigations is most often associated with clinical bleeding?

○ A  Factor IX deficiency

○ B  Factor XII deficiency

○ C  High-molecular-weight kininogen deficiency

○ D  Lupus anticoagulant

○ E  Prekallikrein deficiency

**6.14** A 28-year-old man experienced excessive bleeding following extraction of a decayed tooth. There is a family history of similar problems: his mother had menorrhagia; his sister has frequent nosebleeds. Laboratory tests show that he has a normal prothrombin time, normal partial thromboplastin time and normal platelet count. Which of the following should be considered in this patient?

○ A  Antiphospholipid antibody

○ B  von Willebrand's disease

○ C  Vitamin K deficiency

○ D  Haemophilia B

○ E  Protein C deficiency

bleeding

**6.15**  **A 55-year-old man undergoes an elective direct inguinal hernia repair. During this procedure there is significant loss of blood, with oozing from small vessels. Preoperative coagulation tests would have shown a normal prothrombin time, normal partial thromboplastin time and normal platelet count, but a prolonged bleeding time. What over-the-counter drug was the probable cause for these findings?**

O  A  Acetaminophen

O  B  Acetylsalicylic acid

O  C  Codeine

O  D  Ephedrine

O  E  Phenylpropanolamine

**6.16**  **Which of the following factors initiates coagulation in vivo?**

O  A  Factor VII

O  B  Factor VIII

O  C  Factor XIII

O  D  Fibrinogen

O  E  Tissue factor

**6.17** A 65-year-old woman was admitted into the intensive care unit with sepsis originating from an *Escherichi coli* urinary tract infection. A full blood count performed on admission showed: white blood cell count 17.7 × 10⁹/l, haemoglobin 10.5 g/dl, haematocrit 29.7%, mean corpuscular volume (MCV) 96 fl, platelet count 45 × 10⁹/l. On the peripheral blood smear, it was noted that schistocytes were present. The haematologist phoned the on-call intensive care unit SHO and asked her to send some more blood for a further investigation. Which of the following tests is the haematologist most likely to perform for this patient?

- A   D-Dimer
- B   Factor VIII
- C   Reticulocyte count
- D   Serum ceruloplasmin
- E   Serum ferritin

**6.18** A 56-year-old man complaining of vague abdominal pain in the right hypochondrium had an abdominal ultrasound scan that revealed a small, nodular liver. His routine blood investigations revealed only a prolonged prothrombin time. This isolated coagulation abnormality is most likely to be due to:

- A   Abnormal fibrinolysis
- B   A myeloproliferative disorder
- C   Factor VII deficiency
- D   von Willebrand's disease
- E   Thrombocytopenia

bleeding

**6.19** **A 68-year-old woman who was ambulated 10 days after an abdominoperineal resection complained of sudden onset of dyspnoea and left-sided chest pain on inspiration. A pulmonary embolism was suspected and the diagnosis was confirmed by emergency computed tomography. The best INITIAL therapy for this condition is:**

○ A  A fibrinolytic agent
○ B  Aspirin
○ C  Heparin (intravenous)
○ D  Prednisone
○ E  Warfarin

**6.20** **Warfarin is prescribed for a 40-year-old man who underwent aortic valve replacement with a mechanical prosthesis as treatment for infective endocarditis of his native aortic valve. Which of the following statements regarding the use of this medication is correct?**

○ A  His anticoagulation should be monitored with the partial thromboplastin time

○ B  If he also takes aspirin, the dosage of warfarin must be decreased

○ C  Renal disease will affect the response to warfarin

○ D  The action of warfarin is immediate after ingestion

○ E  Warfarin acts by inhibiting factor XII

bleeding

**6.21** **Which of the following laboratory profiles best describes a patient with haemophilia A (PT, prothrombin time; PTT, partial thromboplastin time; AHF, antihaemophilic factor; vWFAg, von Willebrand factor antigen)?**

○ A Increased PT, normal PTT, low factor VIII AHF, decreased vWFAg

○ B Increased PT, increased PTT, low factor VIII AHF, normal vWFAg

○ C Normal PT, increased PTT, low factor VIII AHF, normal vWFAg

○ D Normal PT, increased PTT, low factor IX, normal vWFAg

○ E Normal PT, increased PTT, low factor VIII AHF, decreased vWFAg

**6.22** **A 72-year-old man with an enlarged prostate and type 2 diabetes has a history of urinary tract infections. Recently, one of these episodes was complicated by acute pyelonephritis. He became septic, and a blood culture grew *Escherichia coli*. He developed severe hypotension, with purpuric areas on his skin. A stool for occult blood was positive. He had a prothrombin time of 50 seconds (control 12 seconds), a partial thromboplastin time of 100 seconds (control 25 seconds), a platelet count of $20 \times 10^9/l$ and a D-dimer level of $4 \mu g/ml$. These findings are most characteristic of which of the following conditions?**

○ A Acute fulminant hepatitis

○ B Antiphospholipid syndrome

○ C Disseminated intravascular coagulation

○ D Haemophilia A

○ E von Willebrand's disease

bleeding

**6.23** **A 23-year-old man experienced recurrent episodes of deep venous thrombosis and underwent two femoral arterial embolectomy procedures. Investigations revealed a normal prothrombin time, a normal partial thromboplastin time, a platelet count of 250 × 10⁹/l, and the presence of lupus anticoagulant. These findings are most characteristic of which of the following hypercoagulable states?**

○ A Antiphospholipid syndrome

○ B Elevated factor VIII

○ C Factor V Leiden mutation

○ D Paraneoplastic syndrome

○ E Protein C deficiency

**6.24** **A previously healthy, 38-year-old woman presented in the emergency department complaining of easy bruising. Physical examination revealed purpuric patches of variable size over her trunk and extremities, but no swelling, warmth or erythema. The peripheral pulses were all palpable and full. Laboratory findings included: lactate dehydrogenase (LDH) 300 U/l, total protein 6.9 g/dl, albumin 5.3 g/dl, alkaline phosphatase 50 U/l, aspartate aminotransferase (AST) 40 U/l and alanine aminotransferase (ALT) 20 U/l. Which of the following additional laboratory findings is most likely to be present in this patient?**

○ A Hypercholesterolaemia

○ B Hyperglycaemia

○ C Hypoprothrombinaemia

○ D Lactic acidosis

○ E Thrombocytopenia

bleeding

102

**6.25** **A 26-year-old man has undergone aortic valve replacement on cardiopulmonary bypass and is now actively bleeding. He has a full blood count that shows: white blood cell count 4.5 × 10⁹/l, haemoglobin 7.6 g/dl, haematocrit 23.9%, mean corpuscular volume (MCV) 98 fl, platelet count 120 × 10⁹/l. His prothrombin time is 30 seconds and his partial thromboplastin time is 63 seconds. Which of the following blood products is the most appropriate treatment in this situation?**

- A Cryoprecipitate
- B Fresh frozen plasma (FFP)
- C Granulocytes
- D Whole blood
- E Packed red blood cells

**6.26** **A 46-year-old patient admitted for elective cholecystectomy was noted to have a prolonged prothrombin time. Which of the following is the most likely cause for this abnormality?**

- A Antiphospholipid antibody
- B Factor XII deficiency
- C Haemophilia A
- D Heparin infusion
- E Liver damage

**6.27** **A 42-year-old woman who was admitted for elective subtotal thyroidectomy gave a history of a bleeding disorder. Preoperative evaluation showed a prolonged thrombin clotting time. What is the most likely cause for this abnormality?**

○ A Factor VIII deficiency

○ B Factor XII deficiency

○ C Hypofibrinogenaemia

○ D von Willebrand factor deficiency

○ E Warfarin therapy

**6.28** **A 27-year-old man has a deficiency of a coagulation factor which forms a complex with tissue factor to activate factors IX and X. Which of the following coagulation factors is most likely to be deficient in this patient?**

○ A Prothrombin

○ B Fibrinogen

○ C Factor VII

○ D Factor XI

○ E Factor XII

**6.29** **A 36-year-old woman who was commenced on warfarin following mechanical aortic valve replacement for a congenital bicuspid valve developed skin necrosis. Deficiency of which of the following proteins could be responsible for this disorder?**

○ A Heparin cofactor II

○ B Plasmin

○ C Protein C

○ D Protein S

○ E Protein Z

bleeding

**6.30** **A 22-year-old woman with repeated episodes of deep venous thrombosis was diagnosed with protein S deficiency. What is the normal role of protein S in the body?**

- A  It activates plasmin
- B  It activates thrombin
- C  It functions as a cofactor to protein C
- D  It inhibits heparin cofactor II
- E  It inhibits protein C

**6.31** **A 26-year-old woman who bled excessively after a therapeutic abortion was diagnosed as having a rare coagulation defect characterised by deficiency of an enzyme of the coagulation cascade that cross-links fibrin. Which of the following factors was deficient in this patient?**

- A  Factor II
- B  Factor VII
- C  Factor VIII
- D  Factor XII
- E  Factor XIII

**6.32** **A 26-year-old patient who bled excessively after excision of a thyroglossal cyst was investigated and found to have deficiency of a glycoprotein coagulation factor. Which of the following factors was deficient in this patient?**

- A  Factor II
- B  Factor V
- C  Factor IX
- D  Factor XII
- E  Factor XIII

bleeding

**6.33** **A 35-year-old woman has been diagnosed with deficiency of a protein that functions as a cofactor in the thrombin-induced activation of protein C in the anticoagulant pathway. Which of the following proteins was deficient in this patient?**

    A  Alpha-2-antiplasmin

    B  Fibronectin

    C  High-molecular-weight kininogen

    D  Prekallikrein

    E  Thrombomodulin

**6.34** **Heparin is a naturally occurring anticoagulant. Which of the following cell types produces heparin?**

    A  Endothelial cells

    B  Eosinophils

    C  Hepatocytes

    D  Mast cells

    E  Platelets

**6.35** **A 48-year-old woman with a mechanical mitral valve who was on long-term warfarin therapy was started on intravenous heparin prior to undergoing an elective cholecystectomy. What is the mechanism of action of heparin?**

    A  Activation of antithrombin III

    B  Activation of protein C

    C  Activation of protein S

    D  Inhibition of fibrinogen degradation

    E  Inhibition of synthesis of vitamin K-dependent clotting factors

bleeding

**6.36** **A 36-year-old pregnant woman with deep venous thrombosis was prescribed a low-molecular-weight heparin (LMWH) as an outpatient. What is the mechanism of action of LMWHs?**

○ A Inhibition of antithrombin III
○ B Inhibition of factor Xa
○ C Inhibition of fibrinogen degradation
○ D Inhibition of protein C
○ E Inhibition of synthesis of vitamin K-dependent clotting factors

**6.37** **After extensive investigation, a 26-year-old woman with epistaxis, haemarthrosis and rectal bleeding was diagnosed with a deficiency of a coagulation factor that acts by cleaving prothrombin in two places to yield active thrombin. Which of the following coagulation factors was deficient in this patient?**

○ A Factor VII
○ B Factor VIII
○ C Factor IX
○ D Factor X
○ E Factor XII

**6.38** **A 45-year-old Ashkenazi Jewish man was admitted for elective cholecystectomy and told the SHO that he suffers from haemophilia C. Which of the following coagulation factors is deficient in haemophilia C?**

○ A Factor VIII
○ B Factor IX
○ C Factor X
○ D Factor XI
○ E Factor XII

bleeding

**6.39** **A 35-year-old woman admitted for elective excision of a preauricular dermoid cyst told the SHO clerking her that she has a coagulation defect. This is known to be due to deficiency of a coagulation factor which is activated by factor XIIa and is produced in the liver. Which coagulation factor is deficient in this woman?**

○ A Factor VIII

○ B Factor IX

○ C Factor X

○ D Factor XI

○ E Factor XIII

**6.40** **A 22-year-old patient with a bleeding tendency was investigated and diagnosed with grey platelet syndrome. Which of the following components is deficient in this patients's platelets?**

○ A Alpha granules

○ B Canalicular system

○ C Dense bodies

○ D Lysosomes

○ E Mitochondria

# SECTION 7: CARDIOVASCULAR PATHOLOGY — QUESTIONS

For each question given below choose the ONE BEST option.

**7.1** A 32-year-old man was seen in the emergency department after a road traffic accident in which he sustained fracture to the mid-shaft of the right femur and an unstable fracture of the pelvis. On arrival in the department, his blood pressure is 80/45 mmHg and his pulse is 184/minute. What type of shock is this patient likely to be in?

- A  Anaphylactic shock
- B  Cardiogenic shock
- C  Hypovolaemic shock
- D  Neurogenic shock
- E  Septic shock

**7.2** A 15-year-old girl with a mitral valve that was repaired in infancy because she had a congenital mitral cleft was seen in the emergency department 1 month after an attack of acute pharyngitis. She had a severe febrile illness, prominent and changing heart murmurs and petechiae. She was diagnosed with infective endocarditis. In this patient the most likely pathogenic organism will be:

- A  *Chlamydia*
- B  *Haemophilus influenzae*
- C  *Staphylococcus aureus*
- D  *Streptococcus faecalis*
- E  *Streptococcus viridans*

**7.3** **Histological examination of a biopsy specimen from a 55-year-old man with vasculitis revealed giant-cell arteritis. The patient most likely has:**

○ A Hypersensitivity vasculitis

○ B Polyarteritis nodosa

○ C Takayasu's arteritis

○ D Temporal arteritis

○ E Wegener's granulomatosis

**7.4** **A 42-year-old woman presented in the emergency department complaining of palpitations. On examination, she had an irregularly irregular pulse and on electrocardiography there were no P waves. However, the QRS complexes were normal. The patient most likely had:**

○ A Atrial ectopic beats

○ B Atrial fibrillation

○ C Atrial flutter

○ D Wolff–Parkinson–White syndrome

○ E Ventricular tachycardia

**7.5** **A 55-year-old man presented in the emergency department complaining of crushing chest pain of 30 minutes' duration. Which of the following ECG changes will confirm the diagnosis of acute myocardial infarction as the cause of chest pain in this man?**

○ A Absent P waves

○ B Q wave

○ C ST-segment elevation

○ D Tented T waves

○ E U wave

**7.6**  **A 65-year-old bedridden man with paraplegia developed acute shortness of breath and a heart rate of 120/minute. He died suddenly and an autopsy is performed to determine the cause of death. His right lung showed an embolus completely obstructing the right pulmonary artery. Which of the following is the underlying factor most likely to be responsible for this patient's death?**

○  A  Hypercoagulable state
○  B  Injury to the vascular endothelium
○  C  Release of endotoxin
○  D  Stasis of blood
○  E  Turbulent blood flow

**7.7**  **A 32-year-old pregnant woman in her third trimester was severely injured in a road traffic accident, with a left-sided femoral shaft fracture and a right-sided tibial shaft fracture. On arrival in the emergency department she deteriorated and died suddenly. The most likely cause of her sudden death was:**

○  A  Amniotic fluid embolism
○  B  Anaphylaxis
○  C  Antepartum haemorrhage
○  D  Fat embolism
○  E  Spinal cord compression

**7.8** **A 55-year-old man dies from metastatic stomach carcinoma. At autopsy, small vegetations are found along the line of closure of the mitral valve. Which of the following is the most likely diagnosis?**

A  Acute infectious endocarditis

B  Calcific valvular disease

C  Carcinoid heart disease

D  Marantic endocarditis

E  Small mural thrombi

**7.9** **A 36-year-old man who has been a smoker for the last 20 years develops gangrenous toes on his left foot. His blood pressure is 118/76 mmHg. His serum cholesterol level is 3.5 mmol/l and his serum glucose is 4.9 mmol/l. The left anterior tibial artery is biopsied, which shows luminal thrombus and vasculitis. The most likely cause for this patient's clinical presentation is:**

A  Giant-cell arteritis

B  Kawasaki's disease

C  Monckeberg's arteriosclerosis

D  Severe atherosclerosis

E  Thromboangiitis obliterans

**7.10** An asymptomatic 40-year-old woman has hypertension. Urinary excretion of catecholamines is increased. Computed tomography shows a suprarenal mass. Which of the following is the most likely cause for her hypertension?

○ A Benign neoplasm of the adrenal cortex
○ B Benign neoplasm of the adrenal medulla
○ C Malignant neoplasm of the adrenal cortex
○ D Malignant neoplasm of the adrenal medulla
○ E Diffuse hyperplasia of the adrenal cortex

**7.11** A 48-year-old man in the surgical intensive care unit develops sudden onset of chest pain, cough, dyspnoea, tachypnoea and marked anxiety. Two days ago, he underwent a right hemicolectomy for cancer of the ascending colon. An accentuated pulmonary $S_2$ is heard on auscultation. An electrocardiogram shows non-specific ST-segment and T-wave changes. The leukocyte count is $12 \times 10^9$/l. An X-ray film of the chest shows no pulmonary infiltrates and no pleural effusions. Arterial blood gas analysis on room air shows an arterial $p(CO_2)$ of 30 mmHg and an arterial $p(O_2)$ of 55 mmHg. Which of the following conditions is most likely to be responsible for causing the symptoms experienced by this man?

○ A Acute pericarditis
○ B Pericardial tamponade
○ C Pleuritis
○ D Pulmonary embolism
○ E Spontaneous pneumothorax

**7.12** A 52-year-old man with long-standing hypertension was brought to the emergency department 30 minutes after the sudden onset of severe chest pain that radiated to his back and arms. On arrival, his blood pressure was 180/80 mmHg in his right arm, with no pressure reading obtainable from the left arm. Cardiac examination elicited a murmur of aortic insufficiency. Which of the following is the most likely diagnosis?

A  Acute aortic dissection

B  Acute myocardial infarction

C  Embolus to the right subclavian artery

D  Pulmonary embolism

E  Spontaneous pneumothorax

**7.13** A 57-year-old man was brought to the emergency department because he had had blood-tinged sputum for 2 weeks. He had a 6-month history of exertional dyspnoea, especially when walking uphill or climbing stairs. He takes no medications and does not smoke cigarettes. He is allergic to penicillin. On examination, his blood pressure is 120/80 mmHg, pulse 88/minute and respiratory rate 16/minute. There are crackles at both lung bases and a diastolic murmur can be heard at the cardiac apex. Electrocardiography shows a broad, notched P wave in the limb leads. An X-ray film of the chest shows pulmonary vascular redistribution to the upper lobes of the lungs. Which of the following is the most appropriate next step in diagnosis?

A  Bronchoscopy

B  Coronary angiography

C  Echocardiography

D  Magnetic resonance imaging

E  Pulmonary artery catheterisation

**7.14** An obese 68-year-old man underwent transvesical prostatectomy. While still in hospital he developed pain and swelling of his right leg. The leg is found to be tender and tense. Which of the following investigations will be most helpful to confirm the diagnosis?

O   A   Chest computed tomography
O   B   Duplex scan
O   C   Pelvic ultrasound
O   D   Venography
O   E   Urine test for fibrin products

**7.15** A previously healthy, 21-year-old man comes to the emergency department 12 hours after the onset of chest pain in the precordial area. He has had an upper respiratory tract infection for 9 days. A friction rub is heard over the precordium. An electrocardiogram shows an increase in the J point of all leads except aVR and $V_1$. After administration of aspirin, the pain subsides. Which of the following conditions is most likely to be responsible for this patient's symptoms?

O   A   Acute pericarditis
O   B   Cardiac tamponade
O   C   Cardiogenic shock
O   D   Mitral valve disease
O   E   Myocarditis

**7.16** **A 65-year-old diabetic man presents to the emergency department with a history of chest pain of 12 hours' duration. This pain has been getting worse for several hours. It is a substernal, 'crushing' type of pain that radiates down the left arm. Which of the following laboratory tests would it be most important to perform at the time of presentation?**

- A  Antinuclear antibody test
- B  Creatine kinase-MB
- C  Erythrocyte sedimentation rate
- D  Glucose
- E  White blood cell count

**7.17** **Five years after a cardiac transplant for dilated cardiomyopathy, a 42-year-old woman develops worsening congestive heart failure. She has had multiple episodes of rejection, but a recent endomyocardial biopsy shows no evidence of rejection this time. The most likely cause of her worsening cardiac function is:**

- A  Amyloidosis
- B  Constrictive pericarditis
- C  Coronary atherosclerosis
- D  Ciclosporin toxicity
- E  Cytomegalovirus myocarditis

**7.18** **A baby was born with complete failure of development of the spiral septum in the heart. He is most likely to have:**

○   A   Aortic arch interruption

○   B   Atrioventricular septal defect

○   C   Overriding aorta

○   D   Persistent truncus arteriosus

○   E   Transposition of the great vessels

**7.19** **A patient was admitted with a mycotic aneurysm. Which of the following conditions is most likely to be associated with a mycotic aneurysm?**

○   A   Disseminated aspergillosis

○   B   Endocarditis with *Staphylococcus aureus*

○   C   Marfan syndrome

○   D   Metastatic adenocarcinoma

○   E   Polyarteritis nodosa

**7.20** **A 10-year-old boy was born with a large ventricular septal defect (VSD) that was never surgically corrected. Now he has increasing dyspnoea with hypoxia and cyanosis. The reason for these symptoms is:**

○   A   Acute myocardial infarction

○   B   Endocardial fibroelastosis

○   C   Left atrial thrombosis

○   D   Natural closure of the VSD

○   E   Reversal of the shunt

cardiovascular

# SECTION 8:
# PULMONARY PATHOLOGY —
# QUESTIONS

For each question given below choose the ONE BEST option.

**8.1**   **A 15-year-old boy was was found in infancy to have an elevated sweat chloride, indicative of cystic fibrosis. This puts him at a greater risk for development of:**

○   A   Adenocarcinoma of the lung
○   B   Bronchiectasis
○   C   Lymphangiectasis
○   D   Pleural plaques
○   E   *Pneumocystis carinii* pneumonia


**8.2**   **A patient was admitted through the emergency department with lobar pneumonia. Which of the following sets of characteristics is most often associated with lobar pneumonia?**

○   A   Community-acquired, *Mycoplasma* infection, Hodgkin's disease
○   B   Community-acquired, *Streptococcus pneumoniae* infection, alcoholism
○   C   Congenital, *Escherichia coli* infection, premature rupture of membranes
○   D   Hospital-acquired, *Staphylococcus aureus* infection, AIDS
○   E   Hospital-acquired, *Klebsiella* infection, postoperative

**8.3** **You are asked to review the chest X-ray of an asymptomatic 9-year-old child. The X-ray shows a subpleural nodule in the right mid-lung field and enlarged mediastinal lymph nodes. After looking at the X-ray you feel that the child most probably has:**

○ A  Aspergillosis
○ B  Coccidiodomycosis
○ C  Primary tuberculosis
○ D  Secondary tuberculosis
○ E  Miliary tuberculosis

**8.4** **You are informed by the nurse in charge of the surgical high dependency unit that a 68-year-old woman on postoperative day 10 walked to the bathroom, but on returning to bed became extremely dyspnoeic and diaphoretic. You should strongly suspect:**

○ A  Pleural effusion
○ B  Pneumonia
○ C  Postoperative atelectasis
○ D  Pulmonary embolus
○ E  Pulmonary oedema

**8.5** **A 55-year-old man is diagnosed with pan-lobular pulmonary emphysema. He also has cirrhosis of the liver. Which of the following conditions could relate pan-lobular pulmonary emphysema with cirrhosis of the liver in this man?**

○ A  Alcoholism
○ B  Alpha$_1$-antitrypsin deficiency
○ C  Budd–Chiari syndrome
○ D  Cystic fibrosis
○ E  Wilson's disease

**8.6**    While doing a ward round in the intensive care unit you are asked to review a chest X-ray of a 78-year-old man who was admitted unconscious 3 days ago after a stroke. The X-ray shows a 4-cm-diameter mass lesion with an air–fluid level in the right lung. The left lung is normal. The chest X-ray appearance is most strongly suggestive of:

○    A    Lung abscess
○    B    Bronchiectasis
○    C    Bronchopulmonary sequestration
○    D    Septicaemia
○    E    Squamous cell carcinoma

**8.7**    While doing the surgical outpatient clinic you come across a 68-year-old man who is complaining of increasing dyspnoea over the past year. He has never smoked. On further enquiry, he divulges that he worked for 5 years in a shipyard in the 1950s. His chest X-ray reveals diaphragmatic pleural plaques and interstitial lung disease. The clinical picture is suggestive of:

○    A    Asbestosis
○    B    Berylliosis
○    C    Byssinosis
○    D    Silicosis
○    E    Siderosis

pulmonary

**8.8** A 56-year-old male smoker complaining of persistent dry cough had a chest X-ray which showed a 1.5-cm mass lesion in the left upper lung. Bronchoscopy revealed this mass lesion to be involving the left superior segmental bronchus. Biopsies of the mass were sent for histopathological examination. The histopathology report described polygonal pink cells with dark, angular nuclei. The most likely diagnosis is:

○ A   Adenocarcinoma

○ B   Bronchial carcinoid

○ C   Mesothelioma

○ D   Small cell anaplastic carcinoma

○ E   Squamous cell carcinoma

**8.9** A 35- year-old man who had been involved in a serious road traffic accident had a large flail segment involving his right chest. He was intubated and placed on a ventilator in the intensive care unit. He required multiple blood transfusions and external fixation of his right femur and pelvis. On day 5 he became increasingly difficult to oxygenate despite ventilation with positive end-expiratory pressure (PEEP) and an Fi(O$_2$) of 100%. He remained afebrile. His chest X-ray revealed bilateral fluffy deposits. He died several days later. At autopsy, the lung showed hyaline membranes, thickened alveolar walls, and type II pneumocyte proliferation. This man had:

○ A   Adult respiratory distress syndrome

○ B   Bronchopneumonia

○ C   Bronchiectasis

○ D   Chronic bronchitis

○ E   Viral pneumonia

**8.10** **A 58-year-old man with a persistent cough has a pneumonia-like area of consolidation in the left lower lobe that does not respond to antibiotic therapy. A bronchoalveolar lavage yields atypical cells. The most likely diagnosis is:**

○ A  Bronchoalveolar carcinoma
○ B  *Mycoplasma* pneumonia
○ C  Pulmonary infarction
○ D  Sarcoidosis
○ E  Silicosis

**8.11** **A 35-year-old woman with fever, weight loss and progressively increasing shortness of breath of 6 weeks' duration had a chest X-ray which showed prominent hilar lymphadenopathy and diffuse pulmonary interstitial disease. She had a video-assisted thoracoscopic lung biopsy. Microscopic examination of the lung biopsy showed non-caseating granulomas. She is most likely to have:**

○ A  Asbestosis
○ B  Interstitial pneumonitis
○ C  Sarcoidosis
○ D  Silicosis
○ E  Tuberculosis

pulmonary

**8.12** **A 65-year-old man, a heavy smoker, presented with chronic cough, weight loss and two episodes of haemoptysis over the last 2 months. He has developed truncal obesity, easy bruising and osteoporosis. Which of the following pulmonary diseases is most likely to be the cause of these findings?**

- ○ A Bronchial carcinoid
- ○ B Bronchioloalveolar carcinoma
- ○ C Large-cell anaplastic carcinoma
- ○ D Small-cell anaplastic carcinoma
- ○ E Squamous cell carcinoma

**8.13** **Of the neoplasms that involve the lung, the most common are:**

- ○ A Bronchial adenomas
- ○ B Pulmonary metastases
- ○ C Peripheral adenocarcinomas in non-smokers
- ○ D Small-cell anaplastic carcinomas in smokers
- ○ E Squamous cell carcinomas in smokers

**8.14** **A 55-year-old man has a serous pleural effusion. Which of the following conditions is most likely to be associated with a serous pleural effusion?**

- ○ A Bronchogenic carcinoma
- ○ B Congestive heart failure
- ○ C Metastatic carcinoma
- ○ D Pulmonary infarction
- ○ E Tuberculosis

**8.15** **The most probable cause for a chylothorax in an adult is:**

○ A Congestive heart failure
○ B Mediastinal malignant lymphoma
○ C Penetrating chest trauma
○ D Systemic lupus erythematosus
○ E Tuberculosis

**8.16** **A 55-year-old man has smoked two packs of cigarettes a day for many years. He has had a worsening cough for the past few months. In the past couple of weeks he has occasionally noted blood-tinged sputum. Otherwise, he has no major health problems. Which of the following procedures should be done first to begin the investigation of his disease?**

○ A Sputum cytology
○ B Bronchoalveolar lavage
○ C Fine-needle aspiration
○ D Pleural fluid cytology
○ E Arterial blood gases

pulmonary

**8.17** **A 50-year-old heart transplant recipient has recently been treated with increasing dosages of imunosuppressive medications because an endomyocardial biopsy demonstrated moderate acute rejection. About 1 month later, he is diagnosed with a chronic abscessing pneumonia that is involving the right middle lobe. Which of the following organisms is most likely to be causing this?**

A *Candida albicans*

B Cytomegalovirus

C *Nocardia asteroides*

D *Pneumocystis carinii*

E *Streptococcus pneumoniae*

**8.18** **While obtaining informed consent for a fine-needle aspiration of the right lung to obtain a tissue diagnosis of a lower-lobe mass in a 58-year-old man, the radiologist tells you that the most common problem associated with this procedure is:**

A Chronic pain after the procedure

B Empyema

C Haemothorax

D Inability to determine the cell type of a malignancy

E Pneumothorax

**8.19** **A bronchogram in a 35-year-old, non-smoking woman reveals an area of localised bronchiectasis in the left mid-lung, starting in a first segmental bronchus. Which of the following conditions is most likely to be associated with the bronchogram finding in this woman?**

○ A   Bronchial carcinoid

○ B   Mesothelioma

○ C   Metastatic adenocarcinoma

○ D   Large-cell undifferentiated carcinoma

○ E   Pulmonary hamartoma

**8.20** **A chest X-ray reveals a 3-cm, right upper lobe peripheral coin lesion in a healthy, asymptomatic 44-year-old male non-smoker. Which of the following conditions is most likely to be responsible for this radiographic appearance?**

○ A   Bronchial carcinoid

○ B   Mesothelioma

○ C   Metastatic adenocarcinoma

○ D   Large-cell undifferentiated carcinoma

○ E   Pulmonary hamartoma

pulmonary

# SECTION 9:
# RENAL PATHOLOGY —
# QUESTIONS

For each question given below choose the ONE BEST option.

**9.1    A 52-year-old man with a long history of smoking
        has atypical epithelial cells in a urinalysis
        specimen, but cystoscopy is negative. Which
        of the following conditions is most likely to be
        associated with these findings?**

○    A    Acute interstitial nephritis
○    B    Adenocarcinoma of prostate
○    C    Nodular glomerulosclerosis
○    D    Squamous cell carcinoma of penis
○    E    Transitional cell carcinoma of renal pelvis

**9.2    A 60 year-old-man is diagnosed with chronic
        renal failure. The findings from urine dipstick
        testing show no protein, blood, glucose, nitrite
        or ketones. However, the semi-quantitative
        sulphosalicylic acid test for urine protein is
        positive. Which of the following conditions is
        most likely to have caused the chronic renal
        failure in this patient?**

○    A    Diabetes mellitus
○    B    Membranous glomerulonephritis
○    C    Minimal-change disease
○    D    Multiple myeloma
○    E    Systemic lupus erythematosus

**9.3** **Which of the following is lacking in the renal cortex and medulla if you are looking at a slide of kidney under the microscope?**

○ A  Capillaries

○ B  Fenestrated endothelium

○ C  Henle's loop

○ D  Squamous epithelium

○ E  Type IV collagen in glomerular basement membrane

**9.4** **Which of the following findings will enable you to make a definite diagnosis of nephrotic syndrome?**

○ A  Haematuria, with >10 red blood cells/high-power field

○ B  Lipiduria in association with hypercholesterolaemia

○ C  No evidence of inflammation in a urinalysis specimen

○ D  Proteinuria of >3 g/24 hours

○ E  Renal tubular epithelial cells and casts

**9.5** **Which of the following renal functions will be assessed if you are measuring the urine specific gravity?**

○ A  Blood flow

○ B  Concentration

○ C  Filtration

○ D  Reabsorbtion

○ E  Secretion

renal

**9.6** **Which of the following patients is most likely to have a hyperplastic arteriolosclerosis with fibrinoid necrosis, petechial haemorrhages, and microinfarcts in the kidneys, in conjunction with a markedly elevated plasma renin?**

○ A A 56-year-old man with an acute myocardial infarction
○ B A 6-year-old boy with albuminuria
○ C A 62-year-old woman with end-stage renal disease
○ D A 15-year-old man with recent streptococcal infection
○ E A 45-year-old woman with scleroderma

**9.7** **A patient had nephrectomy for a neoplasm involving his right kidney. Microscopically, the tumour resembled an embryonic nephrogenic zone and the pathologist suggested that it might have resulted from a lack of a tumour suppressor gene on chromosome 11. Which of the following neoplasms was the pathologist most likely to be suggesting?**

○ A Angiomyolipoma
○ B Medullary fibroma
○ C Renal cell carcinoma
○ D Transitional cell carcinoma
○ E Wilms' tumour

renal

**9.8** **A 9-year-old girl is noted by her mother to have been lethargic for several weeks, and she appears to have some puffiness around her eyes. Dipstick urinalysis reveals no glucose, ketones or blood, but she has 4+ of protein. Microscopic urinalysis reveals no casts, but oval fat bodies are seen. Which of the following conditions is most likely to be responsible for this child's clinical features?**

- A  Berger's disease
- B  Goodpasture syndrome
- C  Focal segmental glomerulosclerosis
- D  Membranoproliferative glomerulonephritis
- E  Minimal-change disease

**9.9** **A 46-year-old man with a history of chronic alcoholism was admitted in the emergency department after drinking a litre of antifreeze solution containing ethylene glycol. Which of the following conditions is he most likely to develop?**

- A  Acute interstitial nephritis
- B  Acute pyelonephritis
- C  Acute tubular necrosis
- D  Chronic interstitial nephritis
- E  Rapidly progressive glomerulonephritis

renal

**9.10** **If you are an SHO on the renal unit and are asked to do a percutaneous needle biopsy of the kidney, which of the following situations do you think will be most appropriate for performing this investigation?**

○ A  Fever with suspected acute pyelonephritis
○ B  Prostatic hyperplasia with suspected hydronephrosis
○ C  Suspected polycystic kidney disease
○ D  Suspected renal cyst
○ E  Systemic lupus erythematosus and acute renal failure

**9.11** **Which of the following malignancies has a multicentric origin?**

○ A  Adenocarcinoma of prostate
○ B  Renal cell carcinoma
○ C  Squamous cell carcinoma of penis
○ D  Transitional cell carcinoma
○ E  Wilms' tumour of the kidney

**9.12** **A 36-year-old man has been diagnosed with rapidly progressive glomerulonephritis. Which of the following features is most characteristic of this condition?**

○ A  Glomerular crescents
○ B  IgA deposited in glomerular capillaries
○ C  Lipiduria
○ D  Polymorphonuclear infiltrates
○ E  Widened proximal tubules

renal

**9.13** **A 45-year-old man visits his GP after feeling generally unwell and lethargic for a couple of weeks. His clinical examination was normal, except for a blood pressure of 150/95 mmHg. Dipstick urinalysis showed no glucose, blood, ketones, nitrite or urobilinogen, but he had 4+ of proteinuria, and a 24-hour urine protein was 3.8 g. Microscopic urinalysis showed no casts. Which of the following conditions is most likely to be responsible for these findings?**

- A Amyloidosis
- B Membranous glomerulonephritis
- C Minimal-change disease
- D Post-streptococcal glomerulonephitis
- E Systemic lupus erythematosus

**9.14** **A 62-year-old man was admitted to the intensive care unit after a prolonged operation to repair an abdominal aortic aneurysm. He had been hypotensive throughout the operation and for several hours afterwards. His serum urea and creatinine were noted to be increasing. Granular and hyaline casts were present on microscopic urinalysis. Which of the following renal lesions is most likely to be present in this patient?**

- A Acute tubular necrosis
- B Chronic pyelonephritis
- C Minimal-change disease
- D Nodular glomerulosclerosis
- E Renal vein thrombosis

**9.15**  A 68-year-old man who had been feeling unwell and pyrexial for 10 days was seen in the emergency department. He described dull pain on palpation of his left lower back. He had burning dysuria. A full blood count revealed an elevated white blood cell count with a left shift. Which of the following urinalysis findings would be most diagnostic for his renal condition?

○  A  Broad renal casts
○  B  Oval fat bodies
○  C  Proteinuria
○  D  Renal tubular epithelial cells
○  E  White blood cell casts

**9.16**  A 38-year-old man had sudden-onset, severe, right flank pain that came in waves all night long. When he was seen in the emergency department (after waiting for 2 hours) he was exhausted. His urine specimen was examined by dipstick and this revealed no ketones, glucose, protein, nitrite or urobilinogen; the urine contained blood, but few white blood cells. The specific gravity of the urine was 1.015 and the pH was 5.5. The most likely diagnosis is:

○  A  Benign prostatic hyperplasia
○  B  Membranous glomerulonephritis
○  C  Renal angiomyolipoma
○  D  Transitional cell carcinoma of bladder
○  E  Ureteric calculus

renal

**9.17** **Which of the following congenital anomalies of the urinary tract carries the greatest significance in terms of morbidity?**

    A  Bilateral ureteral duplication

    B  Bladder exstrophy

    C  Horseshoe kidney

    D  Medullary sponge kidney

    E  Unilateral renal agenesis

**9.18** **Which of the following organisms is most frequently responsible for non-gonoccocal urethritis in a young, sexually active male?**

    A  *Chlamydia*

    B  *Haemophilus*

    C  Herpes simplex virus

    D  Human papilloma virus

    E  *Treponema*

**9.19** **A patient with renal problems had a urinalysis which showed oval fat bodies. Which of the following conditions is most likely to be associated with presence of oval fat bodies on urinalysis?**

    A  Ascending pyelonephritis

    B  Nephritic syndrome

    C  Nephrotic syndrome

    D  Obstructive uropathy

    E  Renal infarction

renal

**9.20** **A young man was admitted through the emergency department after passing blood-stained urine. The urine dipstick test for blood was positive but no red blood cells were seen on urine sediment microscopy. Which of the following conditions is most likely to be associated with these findings?**

○ A  Myoglobinuria

○ B  Post-streptococcal glomerulonephritis

○ C  Renal infarction

○ D  Renal papillary necrosis

○ E  Ureteric lithiasis

renal

# SECTION 10: GASTROINTESTINAL AND HEPATOBILIARY PATHOLOGY — QUESTIONS

For each question given below choose the ONE BEST option.

**10.1** An SHO working in a surgical ward developed hepatitis, which resolved in 2 weeks. His blood tests showed that he had hepatitis A. Six months after this episode a liver biopsy is performed for this SHO. What is it most likely to show?

- ○ A Central necrosis
- ○ B Chronic septal fibrosis
- ○ C Lobular fibrosis
- ○ D Normal architecture
- ○ E Periportal fibrosis

**10.2** A histopathology report of a liver biopsy taken from a patient mentions the presence of Mallory bodies. Mallory bodies are characteristically present in:

- ○ A Alcoholic hepatitis
- ○ B Alcoholic fatty liver
- ○ C Hepatitis B
- ○ D Hepatocellular carcinoma
- ○ E Primary biliary cirrhosis

**10.3** A 25-year-old woman presented in the emergency department with a 1-week history of right lower quadrant pain and fever. She described the pain as dull, constant and non-radiating. Over the past several months she had noticed passing an increasing number of stools and occasionally had had bloody diarrhoea. She denied any recent travel history. Clinical examination revealed right lower quadrant tenderness. Stool cultures were negative. A lower gastrointestinal endoscopic biopsy taken 5 cm proximal to the ileocaecal valve revealed transmural inflammation with hypertrophic lymphoid follicles, lymphoedema, lymphangiectasia, acute and chronic inflammatory cells and several granulomas. Acid-fast bacillus stain on the tissue section was negative. What is the most likely diagnosis?

- A  Coeliac sprue
- B  Crohn's disease
- C  Intestinal tuberculosis
- D  Ulcerative colitis
- E  Whipple's disease

**10.4** A 70-year-old man is suspected to have developed hepatocellular carcinoma. Elevated serum levels of which of the following susbtances would be most likely to help confirm the diagnosis?

- A  AFP
- B  Alkaline phosphatase
- C  CEA
- D  hCG
- E  AST

**10.5** A 16-year-old boy was brought to the emergency department complaining of pain in the abdomen that started from the umbilical region and later shifted to the right lower abdomen. He also had anorexia, nausea and fever. Which of the following findings is most likely to be present on investigation?

○ A   Anaemia

○ B   Gas shadow in the right iliac fossa on erect abdominal X-ray

○ C   Increased haematocrit

○ D   Leucocytosis

○ E   Microscopic haematuria

**10.6** A rectal polyp was excised from a patient and sent for biopsy. At the follow-up outpatient clinic appointment the surgeon told the patient: 'It has no tendency to turn malignant, and there is no need to do any further surgery.' What is the most likely type of polyp that was excised?

○ A   Adenomatous polyp

○ B   Hyperplastic polyp

○ C   Tubular adenoma

○ D   Tubulovillous adenoma

○ E   Villous adenoma

gastrointestinal

**10.7** A 2-week-old baby was brought to the emergency department by his mother. She reported that the infant has not passed stools for almost 4 days. Clinical examination revealed a crying baby with a distended and diffusely tender abdomen. Bowel sounds were absent. Abdominal X-ray showed a distended colon. A sigmoid colon biopsy was unremarkable except for a lack of mural ganglion cells. Which of the following is the most likely diagnosis?

- O  A  Chagas' disease
- O  B  Congenital pyloric stenosis
- O  C  Cystic fibrosis
- O  D  Hirschsprung's disease
- O  E  Rectal atresia

**10.8** A 25-year-old man with jaundice had laboratory investigations performed which showed: total bilirubin 7.0 mg/dl, direct bilirubin 1.2 mg/dl and anaemia. What is the most likely cause of his jaundice?

- O  A  Fibrosis of the common bile duct
- O  B  Haemolysis
- O  C  Hepatitis
- O  D  Sclerosing cholangitis
- O  E  Schistosomiasis

**10.9** A 48-year-old woman presented to her doctor complaining of increasing abdominal girth. Physical examination revealed an enlarged liver. Her serum alpha-fetoprotein is 40 times the upper limit of normal. Which of the following is the most likely diagnosis?

○ A Endometrial carcinoma
○ B Hepatocellular carcinoma
○ C Metastatic gastric adenocarcinoma
○ D Pancreatic carcinoma
○ E Serous papillary cystadenocarcinoma

**10.10** A 43-year-old man has developed sclerosing cholangitis and iron deficiency anaemia secondary to chronic bloody diarrhoea. A colonic biopsy would be most likely to show which of the following?

○ A Colonic adenocarcinoma
○ B Diverticulitis
○ C Granulomatous inflammation
○ D Pseudopolyps
○ E Villous adenoma

**10.11** A 58-year-old man had an adenocarcinoma of the colon that was surgically resected. Which of the following features of the tumour's growth most strongly suggest a poor prognosis?

○ A Circumferential growth
○ B Extension to the muscularis mucosa
○ C Extension to the serosa
○ D Polypoid growth
○ E Surface growth

gastrointestinal

**10.12** **A farm worker was seen in the surgical outpatient clinic complaining of right hypochondrial pain. Clinical examination revealed an enlarged liver with ascites. Analysis of the ascitic fluid revealed malignant cells. Hepatocellular carcinoma was diagnosed. Which of the following is the most likely cause of this tumour?**

○ A Aflatoxin
○ B Aromatic amines
○ C Hydrocarbons
○ D Oestrogens
○ E Saccharin

**10.13** **A 60-year-old man is noted to have mild jaundice and some weight loss. His alkaline phosphatase is very high. He has been passing very pale stools. The most likely diagnosis is:**

○ A Acute viral hepatitis
○ B Cirrhosis of liver
○ C Gilbert's syndrome
○ D Haemolysis secondary to G6PD deficiency
○ E Pancreatic carcinoma

**10.14** **A 42-year-old woman is complaining of pruritus. She has an elevated alkaline phosphatase level and positive antimitochondrial antibody. The most likely diagnosis is:**

○ A Haemochromatosis
○ B Hepatitis C
○ C Liver abscess
○ D Primary biliary cirrhosis
○ E Sclerosing cholangitis

gastrointestinal

**10.15** A 38-year-old man with ulcerative colitis develops pruritus and fatigue. His alkaline phosphatase is elevated. The biliary tree appears to have a 'beaded' appearance on barium radiography. Which of the following is the most likely diagnosis?

○ A Acute cholecystitis

○ B Chronic cholelithiasis

○ C Cholesterosis

○ D Gallstone ileus

○ E Sclerosing cholangitis

**10.16** You are asked to examine a 42-year-old man in the surgical outpatient clinic who gives a history of pain in the upper central abdomen that occurs 2–3 hours after meals. He also tells you that he often wakes up during the night with a similar pain. Based on this history, you feel that the most likely cause of the pain is:

○ A Duodenal ulcer

○ B Gastritis

○ C Gastric ulcer

○ D Pyloric stenosis

○ E Zollinger–Ellison syndrome

gastrointestinal

**10.17** A 44-year-old woman notes that her fingers turn blue on exposure to cold, and that this has been happening increasingly over the past 2 years. She also has difficulty with fine movement of her fingers because the skin has become increasingly taut. Her face has become mask-like, and she has been gradually losing weight. Laboratory findings include a positive anticentromere antibody, a negative antinuclear antibody and a negative rheumatoid factor. Which of the following pathological conditions is she most likely to have?

- ○ A  Acute pancreatitis
- ○ B  Chronic cholecystitis
- ○ C  Ischaemic enteritis
- ○ D  Micronodular cirrhosis
- ○ E  Oesophageal stricture

**10.18** A 48-year-old woman has noted increasing abdominal enlargement for several months. Physical examination reveals no abdominal tenderness, but a fluid thrill is present. A paracentesis is performed and 2 litres of clear, yellow ascitic fluid is removed. This fluid has a protein of 2.1 g/dl. Cytologically, the fluid contains a few mesothelial cells and a few mononuclear cells. Which of the following underlying conditions is she is most likely to have?

- ○ A  Acute pancreatitis
- ○ B  Colonic adenocarcinoma
- ○ C  Crohn's disease
- ○ D  Micronodular cirrhosis
- ○ E  Perforated gastric ulcer

gastrointestinal

**10.19** A 21-year-old man was seen in the surgical outpatient clinic complaining of lethargy and generalised weakness over a period of several weeks. Investigations showed: haemoglobin 9 g/dl, haematocrit 26.3%, mean corpuscular volume (MCV) 72 fl, platelet count 189 × 10⁹/l, and white blood cell count 7.5 × 10⁹/l. On physical examination, there was no tenderness and no masses; bowel sounds were present. His stool was positive for occult blood. A small-bowel series with barium enema revealed no masses or perforations, only a solitary, 2-cm outpouching in the ileum. The presence of which of the following is most likely to have led to these findings?

    A  Antiphospholipid antibody

    B  Elaboration of enterotoxin by *Escherichia coli*

    C  Inheritance of a faulty *APC* gene

    D  Proliferation of abnormal submucosal veins

    E  Ulceration of mucosa by ectopic gastric tissue

gastrointestinal

**10.20** You are examining a 55-year-old man in the emergency department who has presented with a 1-day history of increasing abdominal pain. He also has abdominal distension. While examining him you notice that he has diffuse abdominal pain. An old, right lower quadrant, 8-cm transverse scar is noted. Bowel sounds are high-pitched, faint and sporadic. A stool sample is negative for occult blood. A plain abdominal X-ray reveals dilated loops of bowel with air-fluid levels but no free air. Which of the following is the most likely predisposing factor with regard to his current condition?

- A   Adhesions from previous surgery
- B   Chronic persistent hepatitis
- C   *Entamoeba histolytica* infection
- D   Ileal adenocarcinoma
- E   Meckel's diverticulum

# SECTION 11: HAEMATOPATHOLOGY — QUESTIONS

For each question given below choose the ONE BEST option.

**11.1** **Histopathological examination of an enlarged lymph node demonstrated prominent, well-defined paracortical follicles with germinal centres. A lymph node excised from which of the following patients is most likely to show these features?**

○ A A 5-year-old boy with a sore throat and runny nose

○ B A 35-year-old woman who was scratched by her cat

○ C A 62-year-old woman with an infiltrating ductal carcinoma of breast and widespread metastases

○ D A 40-year-old man with peripheral basophilia noted on a peripheral blood smear

○ E A 58-year-old man with Bence Jones proteins in the urine

**11.2** **A 33-year-old woman presented with a 1-month history of cough. On physical examination, a few small lymph nodes were palpable in the axillae and the tip of the spleen was palpable. A full blood count showed: haemoglobin 10.2 g/dl, haematocrit 31.1%, mean corpuscular volume (MCV) 90 fl, white blood cell count 67 × 10⁹/l, and platelet count 36 × 10⁹/l. The peripheral blood smear showed blasts with Auer rods. Which of the following is the most likely diagnosis in this patient?**

- A  Acute lymphoblastic leukaemia
- B  Acute myelogenous leukaemia
- C  Plasma cell leukaemia
- D  Chronic lymphocytic leukaemia
- E  Leucoerythroblastosis

**11.3** **A 68-year-old man admitted for elective inguinal hernia repair was found to have the following haematology results: haemoglobin 12.8 g/dl, haematocrit 36.9%, mean corpuscular volume (MCV) 88 fl, platelet count 179 × 10⁹/l, and white blood cell count 30.5 × 10⁹/l. The peripheral blood smear showed numerous small, mature lymphocytes. He is most likely to have:**

- A  Acute lymphocytic leukaemia
- B  Chronic lymphocytic leukaemia
- C  Cytomegalovirus infection
- D  Infectious mononucleosis
- E  Leukaemoid reaction

haem

**11.4**  A 45-year-old woman who was admitted for elective cholecystectomy had a full blood count, with the following results: haemoglobin 9.5 g/dl, haematocrit 28.1%, mean corpuscular volume (MCV) 134 fl. The reticulocyte index was low. Hypersegmented polymorphonuclear neutrophils were seen on the peripheral blood smear. On further enquiry, she mentioned that she had been feeling tired for months. Which of the following tests should be ordered next?

○  A  Bone marrow biopsy
○  B  Haemoglobin electrophoresis
○  C  HIV antibody test
○  D  Serum vitamin $B_{12}$ and folate
○  E  Serum ferritin

**11.5**  An 18-year-old university student was seen in the emergency department with fever, lymphadenopathy and mild scleral icterus. He had a positive Monospot test. Which of the following will be the most characteristic peripheral blood finding in this patient?

○  A  Atypical lymphocytosis
○  B  Eosinophilia
○  C  Increased band neutrophils
○  D  Mild thrombocytopenia
○  E  Normocytic anaemia

haem

**11.6** A 72-year-old man has had chronic back pain for several months. He has lost some weight. He is not febrile. A full blood count is performed and shows a white blood cell count of $9.8 \times 10^9/l$, with a differential count of 63 polymorphonuclear leukocytes, 7 bands, 2 metamyelocytes, 2 myelocytes, 18 lymphocytes, 8 monocytes, and 4 nucleated red blood cells. The haemoglobin is 12.2 g/dl with a haematocrit of 37.1%, a mean corpuscular volume (MCV) of 84 fl, and a platelet count of $124 \times 10^9/l$. Which of the following conditions is most likely to be associated with these findings?

○ A Chronic lymphocytic leukaemia
○ B Haemolytic anaemia
○ C Metastatic carcinoma
○ D Previous splenectomy
○ E *Staphylococcus aureus* osteomyelitis

**11.7** In which of the following patients would you NOT be able to palpate the spleen tip?

○ A A 55-year-old man with chronic alcoholism
○ B A 39-year-old man with chronic myelogenous leukaemia
○ C A 6-year-old girl with Gaucher's disease
○ D A 20-year-old woman with hereditary spherocytosis
○ E A 15-year-old boy with haemoglobin SS disease

**11.8** A 42-year-old woman is seen in the surgical outpatient clinic with a mass in the left hypochondrium. On clinical examination, it is discovered that the mass is actually a palpable spleen tip. Her haematological investigations show: haemoglobin 22.3 g/dl, haematocrit 65.7%, mean corpuscular volume (MCV) 89 fl, mean cell haemoglobin concentration (MCHC) 33.9 g/dl, mean corpuscular haemoglobin (MCH) 34.2 pg, platelet count 445 × 10$^9$/l, and white blood cell count 13.5 × 10$^9$/l, with 80% polymorphonuclear leukocytes, 5% bands, 3% monocytes, and 7% lymphocytes. Which of the following is the most likely diagnosis?

- A  Chronic myelogenous leukaemia
- B  Dehydration
- C  Epstein–Barr virus infection
- D  Miliary tuberculosis
- E  Polycythaemia vera

**11.9** A lymph node biopsy was performed on a 24-year-old FY1 doctor who presented with low-grade fevers, night sweats and generalised malaise for a couple of months. He was found to have cervical and supraclavicular lymphadenopathy. The nodes were non-tender. The microscopic appearance at high magnification demonstrated the presence of Reed–Sternberg cells. Which of the following conditions is the most probable diagnosis in this doctor?

- A  Burkitt's lymphoma
- B  Cat scratch disease
- C  Hodgkin's lymphoma
- D  Multiple myeloma
- E  Mycosis fungoides

haem

**11.10** A 40-year-old patient admitted for elective thyroidectomy has a white blood cell count of $55 \times 10^9/l$ and 4% blasts. The leukocyte alkaline phosphatase (LAP) is elevated. This is most consistent with:

○ A  Acute myelogenous leukaemia
○ B  Chronic lymphocytic leukaemia
○ C  Chronic myelogenous leukaemia
○ D  Infectious mononucleosis
○ E  Leukaemoid reaction

**11.11** A 52-year-old woman with chronic abdominal pain was noticed to be pale at the time of assessment in the surgical outpatient clinic. Investigations showed that she had a decreased serum iron and total iron-binding capacity (TIBC) in association with an increased serum ferritin. These findings are most indicative of:

○ A  Anaemia of chronic disease
○ B  Autoimmune haemolytic anaemia
○ C  Chronic blood loss
○ D  Malabsorption
○ E  Vitamin $B_{12}$ deficiency

haem

**11.12** A 65-year-old woman has several non-tender, movable lymph nodes palpable in both the neck and axillae. Biopsy shows numerous crowded follicles of small, monomorphic lymphocytes without any Reed–Sternberg cells. This is most typical of:

○ A   Chronic lymphocytic leukaemia

○ B   Hodgkin's disease, lymphocyte predominance type

○ C   Infectious mononucleosis

○ D   Poorly differentiated lymphocytic lymphoma

○ E   Reactive hyperplasia

**11.13** A 36-year-old man is seen in the surgical outpatient clinic with massive splenomegaly (3000 g). Which of the following conditions is most likely to have caused the massive splenomegaly in this patient?

○ A   Haemochromatosis

○ B   Infectious mononucleosis

○ C   Myelofibrosis

○ D   Portal hypertension

○ E   Sickle cell anaemia

haem

**11.14** **A 42-year-old woman presented with a 1-week history of fever and mental confusion. Physical examination revealed widespread petechiae of the skin and mucosal surfaces. The urea and creatinine were elevated. She had marked thrombocytopenia, but deteriorated rapidly following platelet transfusion and died. At autopsy, pink hyaline thrombi were found in small myocardial arteries. Which of the following disorders is most likely to be responsible for this woman's condition?**

A   Disseminated intravascular coagulopathy

B   Idiopathic thrombocytopenic purpura

C   Thrombotic thrombocytopenic purpura

D   Trousseau syndrome

E   Warm autoimmune haemolytic anaemia

**11.15** **An 18-year-old man who was admitted for elective thyroglossal cyst excision was noted to have hypochromic anaemia in association with splenomegaly and haemochromatosis on preoperative evaluation. Which of the following conditions is he most likely to have?**

A   β-Thalassaemia

B   G6PD deficiency

C   Hereditary spherocytosis

D   Malaria

E   Sickle cell anaemia

haem

**11.16** **A 38-year-old woman has been diagnosed with atrophic gastritis. Which of the following findings is most likely to be found in this patient?**

○ A Decreased mean corpuscular volume in the red blood cells

○ B Decreased serum ferritin

○ C Decreased serum folate

○ D Increased neutrophil segmentation

○ E Increased reticulocyte count

**11.17** **A 65-year-old woman has bone pain, renal failure and pneumococcal pneumonia. In this setting, a bone marrow biopsy is most likely to show numerous:**

○ A Blasts

○ B Granulomas

○ C Plasma cells

○ D Reed–Sternberg cells

○ E Small mature lymphocytes

**11.18** **An abdominal ultrasound is performed on a 32-year-old woman who is complaining of vague abdominal symptoms. In which of the following conditions is the spleen most likely to be normal in size?**

○ A Haemolytic anaemia

○ B Idiopathic thrombocytopenic purpura

○ C Macronodular cirrhosis

○ D Myelofibrosis

○ E Sickle cell anemia

haem

**11.19** A 55-year-old man who is admitted for elective resection of a colonic carcinoma has a haemoglobin level of 9.2 g/dl, a white blood cell count of $1.5 \times 10^9$/l and a mean corpuscular volume (MCV) of 132 fl. Which of the following will be most prominent on this patient's peripheral blood smear?

- ○ A Blasts
- ○ B Hypersegmented neutrophils
- ○ C Hypochromic microcytic red blood cells
- ○ D Nucleated red blood cells
- ○ E Schistocytes

**11.20** A 52-year-old man has skin infiltration by neoplastic T lymphocytes. His condition is known as:

- ○ A Acute lymphocytic leukaemia
- ○ B Burkitt's lymphoma
- ○ C Hodgkin's disease
- ○ D Mycosis fungoides
- ○ E Hairy cell leukaemia

haem

# SECTION 12: ENDOCRINE PATHOLOGY — QUESTIONS

For each question given below choose the ONE BEST option.

**12.1** A 52-year-old woman who presented with a lump in her neck was seen in the surgical outpatient clinic. Examination of the lump revealed it to be a solitary nodule in the thyroid gland. A fine-needle aspiration of this lump was reported as medullary carcinoma. Which tumour-associated marker is most likely to be elevated in her serum?

○ A  Alpha-fetoprotein
○ B  CA15-3
○ C  CA-125
○ D  Calcitonin
○ E  Human chorionic gonadotrophin

**12.2** A 32-year-old woman with a solitary lump in the thyroid gland undergoes fine-needle aspiration of this lump, and the results were reported as papillary carcinoma. Which of the following conditions is most likely to be associated with papillary carcinoma of the thyroid gland?

○ A  Endemic goitrous area
○ B  Exposure to ionising radiation in childhood
○ C  Follicular adenoma
○ D  Hashimoto's thyroiditis
○ E  Riedel's thyroiditis

endocrine

**12.3** A 45-year-old man presented to the emergency department in congestive heart failure. His past medical history included intermittent hypertensive attacks precipitated by emotional stress. Physical examination revealed a right-sided abdominal mass. Computed tomography confirmed this mass to be retroperitoneal. A 24-hour urine specimen revealed raised metanephrine and vanillylmandelic acid levels. After he had been stabilised medically, surgery was performed to remove this right-sided retroperitoneal mass. Which of the following is the most likely diagnosis?

○ A  Malignant fibrous histiocytoma
○ B  Neuroblastoma
○ C  Neurofibroma
○ D  Phaeochromocytoma
○ E  Renal cell carcinoma

**12.4** A 36-year-old man with necrolytic migratory erythema was diagnosed with a rare tumour of the alpha cells of the islets of Langerhans. Which of the following would result from the excessive hormone secretion from this tumour?

○ A  Decreased plasma concentration of amino acids
○ B  Decreased blood glucose
○ C  Decreased hepatic gluconeogenesis
○ D  Decreased lipolysis
○ E  Decreased plasma concentration of insulin

endocrine

**12.5** A previously fit and healthy 32-year-old female lawyer consulted her GP because of nervousness, tremors, emotional lability and excessive sweating for 3 weeks. She told him that she had lost nearly 3 kg during this period in spite of having an increased appetite. Her blood pressure was 120/80 mmHg, pulse 95/minute and respiratory rate 12/minute. She had warm and moist skin, a fine tremor of the fingers and tongue and hyperreflexia. What is the most likely diagnosis?

- A  Alcohol withdrawl
- B  Hyperthyroidism
- C  Hypoglycaemia
- D  Major depressive disorder
- E  Phaeochromocytoma

**12.6** A 32-year-old woman with an unremarkable past medical history presented to her GP after noticing that she had had no menstrual periods for the past 6 months. She was not pregnant and had been taking no medications. She also mentioned that within the past week she had noted some milk production from her breasts. She had been bothered by headaches for the past 3 months and was also concerned that she was losing temporal vision. On physical examination, she was afebrile and normotensive. Which of the following laboratory test findings is most likely to be present in this woman?

- A  Hyperprolactinaemia
- B  Hyponatraemia
- C  Increased serum cortisol
- D  Increased serum alkaline phosphatase
- E  Lack of growth hormone suppression

endocrine

**12.7** A 45-year-old man was brought to the emergency department after a road traffic accident. He complained of tenderness in the right lower quadrant of the abdomen. On clinical examination, no injuries were noted externally and he had faint bowel sounds. Thinking of blunt abdominal trauma, the on-call consultant requested a computed tomographic scan of the chest, abdomen and pelvis, which was essentially normal except for a 1-cm left adrenal cortical mass. No other abnormality was detected on laboratory tests. A decision was made to leave the mass alone on this occasion because it was most likely to be a:

A  Haematoma

B  *Histoplasma* granuloma

C  Metastasis from a lung carcinoma

D  Non-functioning adrenal adenoma

E  Simple cyst

**12.8** A 52-year-old man with newly diagnosed hypertension was investigated by his GP. His routine laboratory investigations showed: sodium 145 mmol/l, potassium 2.9 mmol/l, chloride 107 mmol/l and bicarbonate 26 mmol/l. His blood glucose was 5.7 mmol/l. He felt fine otherwise and a physical examination revealed no abnormal findings. Which of the following conditions is most likely to be responsible for this patient's hypertension?

A  Congenital adrenal hyperplasia

B  Conn syndrome

C  Cushing syndrome

D  Multiple endocrine neoplasia, type IIA

E  Nelson syndrome

**12.9** **A 45-year-old woman has been diagnosed with subacute granulomatous thyroiditis. Which of the following statements would NOT be true of this condition?**

○ A An influenza virus infection of the lung preceded this lesion

○ B Psammoma bodies are a common histological feature

○ C The course of this disease can run for only 3 months

○ D The patient presented with an enlarged, painful thyroid

○ E The patient was hyperthyroid at the time of initial presentation

**12.10** **A 13-year-old girl with a 5-month history of headaches had a computed tomographic scan of the head that revealed a 4-cm suprasellar mass with calcifications that is eroding the bone of the surrounding sella turcica. No abnormal findings were present on physical examination. Which of the following is this lesion most likely to be:**

○ A ACTH-secreting pituitary adenoma

○ B Astrocytoma

○ C Craniopharyngioma

○ D Null cell adenoma

○ E Prolactinoma

endocrine

**12.11** A 15-year-old boy was brought into the emergency department with features suggestive of acute adrenocortical insufficiency. According to his parents, he had a high fever for only 24 hours prior to becoming unconscious. On clinical examination, his skin showed extensive purpura. The most likely cause of these clinical features is:

○ A  Amyloidosis

○ B  Idiopathic adrenalitis

○ C  Meningococcaemia

○ D  Tuberculosis

○ E  Adrenal cortex destruction by tumour

**12.12** A 42-year-old-man presented in the surgical outpatient clinic with enlargement of the anterior neck region. Fine-needle aspiration of the thyroid yielded cells that were consistent with a neoplasm. A chest X-ray was normal. He was euthyroid, but his serum ionised calcium was elevated. On clinical examination, he had a blood pressure of 165/105 mmHg. A thyroidectomy was performed, when frozen sections of several thyroid masses showed a malignant neoplasm composed of polygonal cells in nests. Immunoperoxidase staining of the permanent sections for calcitonin was positive, and the neoplasm had an amyloid stroma with Congo-red staining. Which of the following is the most likely diagnosis?

○ A  Multiple endocrine neoplasia type I

○ B  Multiple endocrine neoplasia type IIA

○ C  Papillary thyroid carcinoma type IIB

○ D  Parathyroid carcinoma

○ E  Thyroglossal duct cysts

**12.13** A 49-year-old man presented in the orthopaedic outpatient clinic with an X-ray that showed a compressed fracture at T10. He complained of increasing weakness over the past few months. Clinical examination revealed a blood pressure of 165/110 mmHg. Laboratory findings included a serum glucose of 8.6 mmol/l. He was mildly obese and had purplish striae on his thighs and abdomen. The pathological lesion most likely to explain these findings is:

○ A  Adrenal cortical carcinoma
○ B  Anaplastic thyroid carcinoma
○ C  Multinodular goitre
○ D  Parathyroid adenoma
○ E  Phaeochromocytoma

**12.14** You were asked to do the endocrine surgery outpatient clinic by your consultant and on that particular day you only saw patients with endocrine malignancies. Based on your knowledge about the natural history of various endocrine malignancies, which of the following neoplasms has the best prognosis?

○ A  Adrenal cortical carcinoma
○ B  Anaplastic carcinoma of the thyroid
○ C  Follicular carcinoma of the thyroid
○ D  Papillary carcinoma of the thyroid
○ E  Parathyroid carcinoma

endocrine

**12.15** A 25-year-old woman was seen in the emergency department complaining of vague abdominal pain and some pain in her extremities. On further enquiry she revealed that she had been feeling depressed for several months. Physical examination revealed no major findings. A chest X-ray was normal. Serum biochemistry revealed a calcium of 3.47 mmol/l, with a serum albumin of 3.8 g/dl and phosphate of 0.64 mmol/l. What is the most likely diagnosis in this patient?

- ○ A  Chronic renal failure
- ○ B  Metastatic carcinoma
- ○ C  Parathyroid adenoma
- ○ D  Pituitary adenoma
- ○ E  Thyroid carcinoma

**12.16** Which of the following conditions is most likely to develop over time in a 66-year-old man with type 2 diabetes and chronic renal failure?

- ○ A  Addison's disease
- ○ B  Cushing syndrome
- ○ C  Hypopituitarism
- ○ D  Primary hyperparathyroidism
- ○ E  Secondary hyperparathyroidism

**12.17** **A 45-year-old, full-time typist who is suffering from a constant headache consulted his GP. Clinical examination revealed a bitemporal hemianopia. Which of the following conditions is the most likely cause of his visual field defect?**

○ A Craniopharyngioma

○ B Empty sella syndrome

○ C Metastatic carcinoma

○ D Prolactinoma

○ E Sheehan syndrome

**12.18** **A 48-year-old male smoker presented to his GP complaining of chronic dry cough and backache. The GP noticed truncal obesity, muscular weakness, hypertension, purplish abdominal striae and tenderness in the region of the lower thoracic spine. The patient was taking no medications. Which of the following diseases is most likely to be the cause for these findings?**

○ A 21-hydroxylase enzyme deficiency

○ B Extra-adrenal paraganglioma

○ C Multiple endocrine neoplasia, type I

○ D Small-cell anaplastic (oat cell) carcinoma

○ E Tuberculosis

endocrine

**12.19** A 42-year-old woman has just been transferred from the operating theatre to the ward after a total thyroidectomy. If you were asked to write the postoperative orders for this patient, which of the following laboratory tests will you request in the early postoperative period (the first day) to help you to manage her?

- A  Antithyroglobulin antibody
- B  Serum calcium
- C  Free catecholamines
- D  Serum iodine
- E  Thyroid-stimulating hormone

**12.20** A 16-year-old girl presented in the surgical outpatient clinic with a mobile, 2-cm mass in the midline of her neck. A fine-needle aspiration of the mass yielded only clear, mucoid fluid. What is the most likely diagnosis?

- A  Follicular adenoma
- B  Lymph node metastasis of follicular carcinoma
- C  Nodule of a multinodular goitre
- D  Parathyroid cyst
- E  Thyroglossal duct cyst

endocrine

# SECTION 13:
# BREAST AND FEMALE
# REPRODUCIVE PATHOLOGY —
# QUESTIONS

For each question given below choose the ONE BEST option.

**13.1** **A 45-year-old woman underwent fine-needle aspiration biopsy of a suspicious area that was noticed on routine mammographic screening. The biopsy revealed cells suspicious for a malignancy. An excisional breast biopsy yielded a diagnosis of lobular carcinoma in situ of the breast. Which of the following statements regarding this woman's malignancy is correct?**

A   A family history of breast cancer is unlikely

B   Oestrogen receptor assay of this neoplasm will probably be negative

C   Paget's disease of the nipple probably preceded this lesion

D   This neoplasm will remain localised

E   The opposite breast might also be involved

**13.2** **While doing the breast clinic you see a 19-year-old female university student whose left breast has developed to be double the size of her right breast since puberty. Which of the following is the most likely cause for this?**

A   An ovarian tumour

B   Cystosarcoma phyllodes

C   Fibrocystic disease

D   Infiltrating ductal carcinoma

E   Virginal breast hypertrophy

**13.3** **A 25-year-old woman presented in the surgical outpatient clinic complaining that she had felt a lump in her right breast while showering. You examine her and discover that she does have a firm, rubbery, mobile, 1-cm mass in the upper outer quadrant of her right breast. No axillary lymph nodes are palpable. If mammography confirms that the lesion has no microcalcifications, and reveals no lesions of the opposite breast, then the most likely diagnosis is:**

- ○ A  Cystosarcoma phyllodes
- ○ B  Fibroadenoma
- ○ C  Focus of fat necrosis
- ○ D  Infiltrating ductal carcinoma
- ○ E  Intraductal papilloma

**13.4** **A 25-year-old lactating mother presented in the surgical outpatient clinic with a tender and swollen right breast 4 weeks after the delivery of a healthy baby boy. The most likely diagnosis is:**

- ○ A  Acute mastitis
- ○ B  Fat necrosis
- ○ C  Fibrocystic disease
- ○ D  Galactocele
- ○ E  Intraductal papilloma

**13.5**  A 32-year-old woman presented in the surgical outpatient clinic with a palpable lump in her right breast that has appeared recently. On enquiry she mentioned that she has been taking oral contraceptives for many years. Which of the following conditions is most likely to be associated with oral contraceptive use?

○  A  Acute mastitis
○  B  Cyst formation
○  C  Fat necrosis
○  D  Galactocele
○  E  Hypertrophy

**13.6**  A 48-year-old woman presented in the surgical outpatient clinic with a 10-cm, circumscribed mass in the left breast. The mass was biopsied and the histopathology report revealed that the lesion included a stromal component and an epithelial component. Which of the following lesions was most likely to have resulted in this biopsy report?

○  A  Fibroadenoma
○  B  Hamartoma
○  C  Medullary carcinoma of breast
○  D  Phyllodes tumour
○  E  Sclerosing adenosis

**13.7**  A 56-year-old woman with a leaking silicone breast implant is at an increased risk of:

○  A  Breast abscess
○  B  Cystosarcoma phyllodes
○  C  Infiltrating ductal carcinoma
○  D  Pain and contracture
○  E  Scleroderma

female

**13.8** **A 55-year-old woman with a palpable 1.5-cm lump in the upper outer quadrant of her right breast had a biopsy of the lump which suggested that the lump was a carcinoma. Which of the following features of her carcinoma would suggest a poor prognosis?**

○ A Axillary lymph node metastases

○ B Family history of breast carcinoma

○ C Lack of aneuploidy

○ D Oestrogen receptor positivity

○ E Presence of an in-situ component

**13.9** **A 22-year-old woman who is breastfeeding develops a tender 2-cm mass beneath the nipple in the right breast that shows several painful fissures. Which of the following pathological findings is most likely to be present in this breast?**

○ A Fat necrosis

○ B Infiltrating ductal carcinoma

○ C Numerous plasma cells

○ D Sclerosing adenosis

○ E *Staphylococcus aureus* infection

**13.10** A 40-year-old woman presented in the surgical outpatient clinic with a 1.5-cm eczematous area on the skin of the areola of the left breast, which she has had for nearly 6 months. Biopsy of the lesion revealed large cells at the dermal–epidermal junction that stained positively for mucin. Which of the following is the most likely diagnosis?

○ A  Dermatophyte infection
○ B  Inflammatory carcinoma
○ C  Intraductal carcinoma
○ D  Nipple discharge
○ E  Paget's disease of the breast

**13.11** A 35-year-old woman presented in the surgical outpatient clinic complaining of bloody nipple discharge that had been present for several weeks. No lump was palpable. Mammography did not show any obvious abnormality. Which of the following lesions is most likely to be responsible for these findings?

○ A  Fat necrosis
○ B  Infiltrating ductal carcinoma
○ C  Intraductal papilloma
○ D  Mastitis
○ E  Tuberculosis

female

**13.12** **A 43-year-old woman presented in the surgical outpatient clinic with a 6-cm, soft, fleshy left breast lump. A biopsy of the lump revealed lymphoid stroma with little fibrosis, surrounding sheets of large vesicular cells with frequent mitoses. The most likely diagnosis is:**

- A  Cystosarcoma phyllodes
- B  Infiltrating ductal carcinoma
- C  Lobular carcinoma
- D  Medullary carcinoma of breast
- E  Paget's disease of the breast

**13.13** **A 52-year-old man presented in the surgical outpatient clinic with bilateral gynaecomastia. Which of the following conditions is he most likely to have?**

- A  Hepatic failure
- B  History of antidepressant drug therapy
- C  Increased risk of breast carcinoma
- D  Increased testosterone levels
- E  Seminoma of the testis

**13.14** A 35-year-old woman who had been on oral contraceptives for nearly 3 years presented in the gynaecology outpatient clinic with abnormal vaginal bleeding. On speculum examination, an endocervical polypoid mass was discovered, which was biopsied and sent for histopathology reporting. Which of the following will be reported by the histopasthologist?

- O A Clear cell adenocarcinoma
- O B Ectopic pregnancy
- O C Endocervical adenocarcinoma
- O D Microglandular hyperplasia
- O E Sarcoma botryoides

**13.15** Endometrial biopsy of a woman revealed endometrial hyperplasia. Which of the following neoplasms is most likely to be associated with endometrial hyperplasia?

- O A Choriocarcinoma
- O B Fibrothecoma
- O C Krukenberg tumour
- O D Mature cystic teratoma
- O E Sertoli–Leydig cell tumour

female

**13.16** **A 28-year-old woman has been diagnosed with endometriosis. Which of the following statements regarding endometriosis is correct?**

○ A It causes amenorrhoea

○ B It causes dyspareunia

○ C It develops through metaplasia of the peritoneal mesothelium

○ D It transforms into well-differentiated adenocarcinoma

○ E Obesity is a risk factor

**13.17** **A 48-year-old woman with a large abdominal mass underwent laparotomy. The mass was found to be an ovarian tumour involving the right ovary. There was also some free ascitic fluid in the peritoneal cavity. The tumour was excised and cytological examination of fluid from this unilocular cystic tumour revealed clusters of malignant epithelial cells surrounding psammoma bodies. What is the most likely diagnosis?**

○ A Adenocarcinoma of Fallopian tube

○ B Endometrial adenocarcinoma

○ C Mesothelioma

○ D Ovarian mature cystic teratoma

○ E Ovarian serous cystadenocarcinoma

**13.18** **A 35-year-old woman had a Pap test which showed cervical intraepithelial neoplasia (CIN). The presence of CIN on biopsy is most strongly associated with:**

○ A Epstein–Barr virus infection

○ B Herpes simplex virus infection

○ C HLA DR5

○ D Human papillomavirus infection

○ E Previous pregnancy

female

**13.19** A 23-year-old woman passed grape-like masses of tissue per vagina in week 16 of her pregnancy. A dilation and curettage was then performed, and the microscopic appearance of the tissue obtained showed large avascular villi with trophoblastic proliferation. Which of the following is the best investigation to use for her follow-up?

○  A  Chest X-ray
○  B  Endometrial biopsy
○  C  Pap smear
○  D  Pelvic ultrasound
○  E  Serum β-hCG

**13.20** A 13-year-old girl is seen in the gynaecology outpatient clinic with haematocolpos. Which of the following conditions is most likely to be associated with haematocolpos?

○  A  Cervical condyloma
○  B  Cervical gonorrhoea
○  E  Endometriosis
○  D  Imperforate hymen
○  E  Ruptured Bartholin's cyst

female

# SECTION 14:
# MALE REPRODUCTIVE
# PATHOLOGY — QUESTIONS

For each question given below choose the ONE BEST option.

**14.1** **A young man presented in the emergency department complaining of swelling of the penis. On clinical examination, the penis was uncircumcised, with erythema and oedema of the glans penis. It was not possible to retract the foreskin over the glans penis. Which of the following infectious agents is most likely to be associated with these findings?**

○ A Herpes simplex virus

○ B Human papillomavirus

○ C *Sarcoptes scabiei*

○ D *Staphylococcus aureus*

○ E *Treponema pallidum*

**14.2** **A 32-year-old man with an uncircumcised penis presented in the emergency department complaining that he could not fully retract the foreskin. This condition is known as:**

○ A Cryptorchidism

○ B Epispadias

○ C Exstrophy

○ D Hypospadias

○ E Phimosis

**14.3** **While performing the initial clinical examination of a newborn baby boy, the paediatrician noted that the baby had an abnormal opening of the urethra onto the ventral surface of the penis. This is known as:**

○ A  Cryptorchidism

○ B  Epispadias

○ C  Exstrophy

○ D  Hypospadias

○ E  Phimosis

**14.4** **A 26-year-old man presented in the venereal diseases clinic complaining of an ulcer on the glans penis and enlarged inguinal lymph nodes. The examining doctor suspected primary syphilis. Which of the following would be the best test for diagnosing primary syphilis in this patient?**

○ A  Cytological smear

○ B  Dark-field microscopic examination of exudate or secretions

○ C  ELISA performed on exudate or secretions

○ D  Microbiological culture

○ E  Tissue biopsy

male

**14.5** A 25-year-old man with an enlarged right testis was diagnosed with a testicular tumour. He underwent inguinal orchidectomy and the histopathology report described the tumour as a germ cell tumour. Which of the following tumours was most likely to have been excised?

○ A  Embryonal carcinoma
○ B  Gonadoblastoma
○ C  Lymphoma
○ D  Leydig cell tumour
○ E  Sertoli cell tumour

**14.6** A 35-year-old man presented in the surgical outpatient clinic complaining of a left scrotal swelling. On examination, he had a painless, transilluminant swelling at the upper pole of the left testis. No cough impulse was visible or palpable. What is the most likely diagnosis?

○ A  Haematocoele
○ B  Inguinal hernia
○ C  Pyocoele
○ D  Spermatocoele
○ E  Varicocoele

male

**14.7** **A 25-year-old man presented in the surgical outpatient clinic complaining of a mass in his left scrotum. On examination, he had a non-tender, twisted mass along the spermatic cord. The mass was more prominent when the patient was standing and felt like a bag of worms. The left testis was smaller than the right testis. What is the most likely diagnosis?**

A  Haematocoele

B  Inguinal hernia

C  Pyocoele

D  Spermatocoele

E  Varicocoele

**14.8** **A 72-year-old man with complaint of urinary retention had a digital rectal examination which suggested that he had an enlarged prostate with a nodular feel to it. Biopsy of the prostatic nodule suggested a malignant lesion. Which of the following is the most common malignant lesion involving the prostate gland?**

A  Adenocarcinoma

B  Ductal transitional carcinoma

C  Prostatic intraepithelial neoplasia

D  Squamous cell carcinoma

E  Undifferentiated carcinoma

male

**14.9** A 46-year-old man with painful erections presented in the surgical outpatient clinic. On further enquiry, he told the consultant that his penis deviates to the right side when it is erect. What is the most likely diagnosis?

○ A   Balanitis

○ B   Orchitis

○ C   Peyronie's disease

○ D   Posthitis

○ E   Priapism

**14.10** A 25-year-old man is diagnosed with a germ cell tumour of the testis. Which of the following histological subtypes is most likely to be found on histopathological examination of the involved testis after orchidectomy?

○ A   Choriocarcinoma

○ B   Embryonal carcinoma

○ C   Seminoma

○ D   Teratocarcinoma

○ E   Teratoma

**14.11** A 40-year-old man with a seminoma of the left testis had a staging computed tomographic scan which demonstrated retroperitoneal lymph nodes that were larger than 2 cm but smaller than 5 cm in size. What is the nodal stage of this tumour?

○ A   N0

○ B   N1

○ C   N2

○ D   N3

○ E   N4

male

**14.12** **A 42-year-old man has been diagnosed with a seminoma of the right testis that is involving the tunica vaginalis. What is the tumour stage of this primary testicular tumour?**

○ A Tis

○ B T1

○ C T2

○ D T3

○ E T4

**14.13** **A 40-year-old man was diagnosed with a testicular seminoma. His serum tumour marker levels were: lactate dehydrogenase (LDH) less than 1.5 times the reference range, beta-human chorionic gonadotrophin (β-hCG) <5000 mIU/ml and alpha-fetoprotein (AFP) <1000 ng/ml. What is the serum tumour marker stage of this tumour?**

○ A S0

○ B S1

○ C S2

○ D S3

○ E S4

male

**14.14** A 40-year-old man was diagnosed with a testicular seminoma that was extending through the tunica albuginea, with involvement of the tunica vaginalis, retroperitoneal lymph nodes greater than 5 cm in greatest dimension, no distant metastasis, a serum lactate dehdrogenase (LDH) less than 1.5 times the reference range, beta-human chorionic gonadotrophin (β-hCG) <5000 mIU/ml and alpha-fetoprotein (AFP) <1000 ng/ml. What is the clinical stage of this tumour?

- A  Stage IA
- B  Stage IB
- C  Stage IIA
- D  Stage IIB
- E  Stage IIC

**14.15** A patient with prostatic adenocarcinoma has very high serum levels of prostate-specific antigen (PSA). What is the normal function of PSA?

- A  It converts testosterone to dihydrotestosterone in the prostate
- B  It increases FSH secretion from the anterior pituitary gland
- C  It inhibits the action of 5-alpha reductase
- D  It inhibits testosterone secretion
- E  It liquifies gelatinous semen after ejaculation

male

**14.16** A 72-year-old man with an elevated serum prostate-specific antigen (PSA) level was diagnosed with prostatic cancer on needle biopsy. What is the stage of this primary prostatic tumour?

- A  T1a
- B  T1b
- C  T1c
- D  T2a
- E  T2b

**14.17** A 78-year-old man with an elevated prostate-specific antigen level had a tumour palpable in both lobes of the prostate gland, with no nodal involvement or distant metastases. After a radical prostatectomy the tumour was reported as histological grade G2. What is the overall stage of the prostatic cancer?

- A  Stage 0
- B  Stage I
- C  Stage II
- D  Stage III
- E  Stage IV

**14.18** A 72-year-old man was prescribed finasteride as treatment for benign prostatic hyperplasia. What is the mechanism of action of finasteride?

- A  It blocks the action of FSH on prostate
- B  It enhances the activity of dihydrotestosterone
- C  It increases serum levels of testosterone-binding protein
- D  It is a 5-alpha-reductase inhibitor
- E  It is an anti-oestrogen

male

**14.19** A 68-year-old man presented in the urology outpatient clinic with a tumour that was invading the subepithelial connective tissue of the penis. What is the stage of this primary penile cancer?

○ A Ta

○ B T1

○ C T2

○ D T3

○ E T4

**14.20** A 5-year-old boy was brought to the urology outpatient clinic after his mother noted that his left testis was larger than the right. Investigations confirmed the presence of a tumour, which was later excised. The histopathology report described the presence of elements similar to skin and its appendages in the excised tumour. What is the most likely diagnosis?

○ A Choriocarcinoma

○ B Embryonal carcinoma

○ C Juvenile granulosa cell tumour

○ D Seminoma

○ E Teratoma

male

# SECTION 15:
# BONE AND JOINT PATHOLOGY — QUESTIONS

For each question given below choose the ONE BEST option.

**15.1** A 46-year-old patient was seen in the orthopaedic outpatient clinic complaining of pain in the first metatarsophalangeal joint. On examination, the joint was swollen, red and tender. Synovial fluid analysis revealed needle-shaped, strongly negatively birefringent crystals. What is the most likely diagnosis?

- A  Gout
- B  Infectious arthritis
- C  Osteoarthritis
- D  Pseudogout
- E  Rheumatoid arthritis

**15.2** A 56-year-old man complaining of pain in his right tibia presented in the orthopaedic outpatient clinic. On clinical examination, bowing of the affected tibia was noticed. An X-ray revealed increased bone density, abnormal architecture with coarse cortical trabeculations, bowing and bony enlargement. Which of the following is the most likely diagnosis?

- A  Osteitis fibrosa cystica
- B  Osteopetrosis
- C  Osteoporosis
- D  Paget's disease of bone
- E  Tuberculous osteomyelitis

**15.3** **A 28-year-old man presented to the orthopaedic outpatient clinic complaining of pain in his left tibia for the past 8 months. He said that the pain was particularly severe at night and was relieved by non-steroidal anti-inflammatory drugs. An X-ray of the affected bone showed a small radiolucent zone surrounded by a larger sclerotic zone. Which of the following is the most likely cause of this patient's clinical problems?**

○   A   Chondrosarcoma
○   B   Ewing's sarcoma
○   C   Giant-cell tumour of bone
○   D   Osteoid osteoma
○   E   Primary osteogenic sarcoma

**15.4** **A 62-year-old woman was seen in the orthopaedic outpatient clinic complaining of severe pain and stiffness in her neck, shoulders and hips for 2 months. She said that her symptoms were most pronounced in the morning, shortly after awakening. She has had chronic fatigue and low-grade fevers during this period. On examination, the range of movement in the neck, shoulders and hips was normal. The muscles were minimally tender to palpation. Muscle strength, sensations and deep tendon reflexes were all normal. The serum creatine kinase activity was 40 U/l and the erythrocyte sedimentation rate (ESR) was 80 mm/hour. The serum rheumatoid factor and antinuclear antibody assays were negative. Which of the following is the most likely diagnosis?**

○   A   Fibromyositis
○   B   Osteoarthritis
○   C   Polymyalgia rheumatica
○   D   Polymyositis
○   E   Seronegative rheumatoid arthritis

bone and joint

**15.5** **A 28-year-old man presented in the orthopaedic outpatient clinic complaining of pain in his right tibia, with a palpable swelling. X-ray of the affected bone revealed a lytic lesion involving the epiphysis and extending into the soft tissues. What is the most likely diagnosis?**

○ A Benign giant-cell tumour

○ B Chondroblastoma

○ C Chondroma

○ D Chondromyxofibroma

○ E Osteoid osteoma

**15.6** **A 52-year-old man presented in the orthopaedic outpatient clinic complaining of increasing back pain and right hip pain over the past 2 years. He said that the pain was worst at the end of the day. He had an unremarkable past medical history. On clinical examination, he had bony enlargement of the distal interphalangeal joints. An X-ray of the spine revealed the presence of prominent osteophytes involving the vertebral bodies. A pelvic X-ray showed sclerosis with narrowing of the joint space at the right acetabulum. Which of the following conditions is most likely to be responsible for this patient's clinical features?**

○ A Gout

○ B Lyme disease

○ C Osteoarthritis

○ D Osteomyelitis

○ E Rheumatoid arthritis

bone and joint

**15.7** A 52-year-old man presented in the orthopaedic outpatient clinic complaining of left hip pain of several months' duration. Clinical examination elicited deep tenderness. An X-ray revealed a 9 cm × 12 cm mass involving the ischium of the pelvis. The mass had irregular borders and there were extensive areas of bony destruction, as well as some scattered calcifications. The lesion was resected, and grossly the mass had a bluish-white cut surface. Which of the following statements regarding this lesion is correct?

   A  It is associated with Paget's disease of bone

   B  It is more common in women

   C  It sometimes arises in benign cartilagenous tumours

   D  It is the most common primary tumour of bone

   E  It is usually seen in distal skeletal bones

**15.8** A 60-year-old woman presented in the orthopaedic outpatient clinic complaining of back pain. A full blood count showed: white blood cell count 3.7 × 10$^9$/l, haemoglobin 10.3 g/dl, haematocrit 31.1%, mean corpuscular volume (MCV) 85 fl, and platelet count 110 × 10$^9$/l. Her total serum protein was 8.5 g/dl, with an albumin of 4.1 g/dl. A chest X-ray showed no abnormalities in the heart or lung fields, but there were several lucencies in the vertebral bodies. The consultant surgeon performed a sternal bone marrow aspiration and aspirated dark-red, jelly-like material into the syringe. Which of the following cell types will be a prominent feature of the smear of the aspirate?

   A  Fibroblasts

   B  Giant cells

   C  Metastatic renal cell carcinoma cells

   D  Osteoblasts

   E  Plasma cells

bone and joint

**15.9** A 15-year-old boy presented in the orthopaedic outpatient clinic complaining of persistent pain in his right leg for over 2 months. He also had a low-grade fever. A radiograph of the affected leg revealed a mass in the diaphyseal region of the right femur with overlying cortical erosion and soft-tissue extension. A biopsy was performed and the lesion was seen on microscopy to be composed of numerous small, round, blue cells. What is the most probable diagnosis in this case?

○ A Chondroblastoma
○ B Ewing's sarcoma
○ C Medulloblastoma
○ D Neuroblastoma
○ E Osteoblastoma

**15.10** A 79-year-old man presented in the orthopaedic outpatient clinic complaining of persistent back pain of several months' duration which was unrelated to physical activity. He thinks that he has also lost some weight during this time. Laboratory findings included: white blood cell count 6.7 × 10$^9$/l, haemoglobin 11.2 g/dl, haematocrit 33.3%, mean corpuscular volume (MCV) 88 fl and platelet count 89 × 10$^9$/l. He had a peripheral leucoerythroblastic picture. The serum biochemistry profile was normal. A computed tomographic scan of the spine revealed scattered bright lesions of varying sizes in the vertebral bodies. Which of the following additional laboratory test findings is he most likely to have?

○ A Blood culture positive for *Neisseria gonorrhoeae*
○ B Serum calcium of 1.37 mmol/l
○ C Serum prostate-specific antigen of 35 ng/ml
○ D Parathyroid hormone, intact, of 100 pg/ml
○ E Positive serology for *Borrelia burgdorferi*

bone and joint

**15.11** A 16-year-old girl presented in the orthopaedic outpatient clinic complaining of pain and swelling of her left distal thigh that was associated with activity. She noticed tenderness after performing physical exercise. She had no history of trauma. Radiography of the affected thigh showed an expansile, eccentric, lytic lesion located in the metaphysis of the distal femur that was surrounded by a rim of reactive new bone. What is the most likely diagnosis?

○ A  Aneurysmal bone cyst
○ B  Chondrosarcoma
○ C  Ewing's sarcoma
○ D  Fibrous dysplasia
○ E  Osteosarcoma

**15.12** Which of the following bone diseases is most likely to be seen in a 48-year-old woman who has been on long-term corticosteroid therapy for the treatment of severe rheumatoid arthritis?

○ A  Osteochondritis
○ B  Osteomalacia
○ C  Osteoporosis
○ D  Paget's disease of bone
○ E  Rickets

**15.13** An 18-year-old professional footballer noted some minor discomfort over the lateral aspect of his right knee after a fall during a game. There was a palpable 'bump' in this region. He consulted an orthopaedic surgeon, who ordered an X-ray of the affected knee. The X-ray revealed a lateral projection from the metaphyseal region of his lower femur. There was no soft-tissue swelling. The lesion was excised and was found to be composed of a 3-cm stalk of bony cortex, capped by cartilage. Which of the following is the most probable diagnosis in his case:

- A   Aneurysmal bone cyst
- B   Enchondroma
- C   Giant-cell tumour
- D   Osteochondroma
- E   Osteoid osteoma

**15.14** A man who had been experiencing persistent lower back pain and stiffness that diminished with activity since his twenties was diagnosed with ankylosing spondylitis. In his thirties he also developed hip and shoulder arthritis and in his forties he was bothered by decreased lumbar spine mobility. Which of the following HLA alleles is he most likley to have?

- A   HLA-B3
- B   HLA-B27
- C   HLA-D4
- D   HLA-W6
- E   HLA-DR2

bone and joint

**15.15** **A 21-year-old professional tennis player consulted an orthopaedic surgeon after he noted increasing pain in his left shoulder after taking part in an international tennis tournament. He could hardly raise his left arm. The orthopaedic surgeon aspirated clear fluid from the subacromial region. This young man probably has:**

○ A Bursitis
○ B Costochondritis
○ C Ganglion cyst
○ D Pseudogout
○ E Tenosynovitis

**15.16** **A 26-year-old cricketer complained to his bowling coach that for the previous 5 days he had had backache, with muscle spasms, weakness and pain in his right hip which was radiating all the way down to his toes. He was examined by an orthopaedic specialist, who noticed that this bowler also had paraesthesiae in an L5 distribution and pain radiating down the leg on straight-leg raising. These findings are most likely to be due to:**

○ A Herniated nucleus pulposus
○ B Osteoporosis
○ C Spina bifida
○ D Spondylolisthesis
○ E Paget's disease of bone

**15.17** A 48-year-old man has noticed that he cannot completely extend the middle and little fingers of his left hand. In the palm of his hand, at the base of these fingers, ill-defined, tender, firm nodules are palpable. This man is a chronic alcoholic. What histological appearance will this mass be most likely to show?

○ A Dystrophic calcification

○ B Fibromatosis

○ C Giant-cell tumour of the tendon sheath

○ D Granulomatous inflammation

○ E Rhabdomyosarcoma

**15.18** A 35-year-old female typist in a busy legal firm notices that she develops tingling and numbness over the palmar surface of her thumb, index and middle fingers after several hours at her computer workstation. Pain in the same area often occurs at night as well. Which of the following conditions is most likely to be responsible for her symptoms?

○ A Carpal tunnnel syndrome

○ B Dupuytren's contracture

○ C Gout

○ D Hypertrophic osteoarthropathy

○ E Rheumatoid arthritis

bone and joint

**15.19** A 45-year-old woman can feel a firm, non-tender, rounded subcutaneous mass, 1 cm in diameter, along the extensor surface of the forearm. Microscopically, the nodule shows an area of central necrosis surrounded by palisading epithelioid cells. Which of the following laboratory test findings is most likely to be positive in this woman?

○ A  Acetylcholine receptor antibody
○ B  Anti-Jo-1 (anti-histidyl-tRNA synthetase)
○ C  Elevated antinuclear antibody
○ D  Monoclonal gammopathy
○ E  Positive rheumatoid factor

**15.20** A 76-year-old woman presented in the surgical outpatient clinic with a swollen and painful right knee joint. On enquiry, she reported that she has had this swelling for several months and that it occasionally bothers her as the joint becomes very painful. The orthopaedic consultant aspirated synovial fluid from the joint and subjected it to polarised light microscopy. Rhomboid or rod-shaped, weakly positively birefringent crystals were seen on polarised light microscopy. What is the most likely diagnosis?

○ A  Calcium oxalate crystal deposition disease
○ B  Gout
○ C  Osteoarthritis
○ D  Pseudogout
○ E  Rheumatoid arthritis

bone and joint

# SECTION 16:
# CENTRAL NERVOUS SYSTEM
# PATHOLOGY — QUESTIONS

For each question given below choose the ONE BEST option.

16.1 **A 65-year-old man with known mitral valve disease and atrial fibrillation suffered a massive stroke and died. At autopsy, a 5-cm-diameter area of softening in the region of the left middle cerebral artery distribution was noticed. This is most consistent with:**

○ A  Hypertension
○ B  Mycotic aneurysm
○ C  Thromboembolism
○ D  Vasculitis
○ E  Venous thrombosis

16.2 **A 52-year-old woman presented in the neurosurgical oupatient clinic complaining of right-sided headaches for 5 years, which she had been ignoring until recently when she noted mild weakness in her left hand. Computed tomography showed a well-circumscribed lateral mass that was compressing the right hemisphere at the frontal-parietal junction. This lesion is most likely to be:**

○ A  Glioblastoma multiforme
○ B  Medulloblastoma
○ C  Meningioma
○ D  Metastatic carcinoma
○ E  Schwannoma

**16.3** **A 65-year-old woman presented in the emergency department after having a grand mal seizure. She had been healthy prior to this event. A neurological examination revealed no focal abnormalities. Magnetic resonance imaging of the brain revealed a large, poorly demarcated mass with central necrosis in the right frontal lobe. The most likely diagnosis is:**

   ○  A  Choroid plexus tumour

   ○  B  Glioblastoma multiforme

   ○  C  Low-grade astrocytoma

   ○  D  Medulloblastoma

   ○  E  Meningioma

**16.4** **Which of the following histopathological findings are most likely to be found in the cerebrum of a 75-year-old woman who suffered a cerebral infarction 1 week ago?**

   ○  A  Caseous necrosis

   ○  B  Coagulative necrosis

   ○  C  Fat necrosis

   ○  D  Gangrenous necrosis

   ○  E  Liquefactive necrosis

**16.5** **Which of the following laboratory tests that are done in the second trimester will most strongly suggest the presence of a neural tube defect in a fetus?**

   ○  A  Decreased human chorionic gonadotrophin

   ○  B  Decreased serum folate

   ○  C  Hypochromic microcytic anaemia

   ○  D  Increased alpha-fetoprotein

   ○  E  Positive serological test for syphilis

CNS

**16.6** A 55-year-old man with a 1-week history of headaches and fever was brought to the emergency department in a confused state. Computed tomography revealed a 4-cm, ring-enhancing mass in the right parietal region. Biopsy of the mass revealed gliosis and fibrosis with necrosis, neutrophils and lymphocytes. These findings strongly suggest a diagnosis of:

○ A  Cerebral abscess
○ B  Glioblastoma multiforme
○ C  Herpes simplex type 2 encephalitis
○ D  Subacute infarction
○ E  Vascular malformation

**16.7** A 32-year-old woman presented in the emergency department complaining of abrupt onset of dizziness with nausea and vomiting. She also had right-sided headache. On examination, she had nystagmus towards the affected side. The on-call consultant reassured her by telling her that her symptoms would disappear in 7–10 days. She probably has:

○ A  Cerebral abscess
○ B  Cerebral oedema
○ C  Gullain–Barré syndrome
○ D  Schwannoma
○ E  Vestibular neuronitis

cns

**16.8** **A patient with an intracranial neoplasm was informed by the neurosurgeon that he had a tumour which has the best prognosis following surgery. Which of the following intracranial neoplasms is this patient most likely to have?**

    ○  A  Astrocytoma

    ○  B  Glioblastoma multiforme

    ○  C  Medulloblastoma

    ○  D  Schwannoma

    ○  E  Solitary metastasis

**16.9** **A 22-year-old cricketer was hit on the left side of his head by a fast and rising cricket ball. He fell to the ground and was immediately seen by the team physiotherapist. Only a minor scalp abrasion was present at the site of the impact, with minimal bleeding that stopped in a few minutes. He was initially alert after this accident, but then became unconcious about 30 minutes later. A head computed tomographic (CT) scan revealed a convex, lens-shaped area of haemorrhage centered over the left parietal region. This history and the CT features are most likely to be associated with:**

    ○  A  Brain concussion

    ○  B  Epidural haematoma

    ○  C  Intracerebral haematoma

    ○  D  Subdural haematoma

    ○  E  Subarachnoid haemorrhage

**16.10** A 22-year-old motorcyclist was brought to the emergency department in a decerebrate posture following an episode of severe head trauma suffered in a road traffic accident. Fundal examination revealed marked bilateral papilloedema. Computed tomography revealed marked diffuse cerebral oedema. This increase in brain volume, due to an increase in sodium and water content, is likely to be most severe in which of the following components of the brain?

   A  Dura
   B  Ependyma
   C  Meninges
   D  Neuronal cell bodies
   E  White matter

**16.11** A previously healthy 32-year-old corporate lawyer who was complaining of headache suddenly lost consciousness and was taken to hospital where an emergency head computed tomographic scan revealed extensive subarachnoid haemorrhage at the base of the brain. He was afebrile. Which of the following conditions do you strongly suspect?

   A  Acute bacterial meningitis
   B  Parkinson's disease
   C  Progressive multifocal leucoencephalitis
   D  Ruptured berry aneurysm
   E  Tay–Sachs disease

cns

**16.12** A 55-year-old man was found lying on the street outside a pub. An ambulance was called and paramedics arrived. They discovered a bruise on his posterior occiput, but no other signs of trauma. He was transported to the hospital in a stable condition, with vital signs showing: blood pressure 115/80 mmHg, temperature 36.5 °C, pulse 81/minute and respirations 20/minute. On arrival in the hospital he became progressively obtunded. His right pupil was 8 mm and the left 4 mm. A computed tomographic scan of the head revealed a collection of blood in the right subdural region. Damage to which of the following structures has resulted in these findings?

- A  Cavernous sinus
- B  Dural bridging vein
- C  Great vein of Galen
- D  Middle cerebral artery
- E  Middle meningeal artery

**16.13** A 42-year-old man was seen in the emergency department complaining of a worsening headache for the past week, along with fever and increasing obtundation. A computed tomographic scan of the head revealed a solitary, 4-cm-diameter lesion with ring enhancement in the right parietal lobe. A stereotactic biopsy was performed and a frozen section showed granulation tissue with adjacent collagenisation, gliosis and oedema. Which of the following is the most probable diagnosis?

- A  Aspergillosis
- B  Chronic brain abscess
- C  Glioblastoma
- D  Progressive multifocal leukoencephalopathy
- E  Rabies

**16.14** A previously fit and healthy 48-year-old man with sudden onset of a generalised seizure was referred for computed tomography (CT) of the brain. The CT scan revealed a 4-cm, solid mass lesion in the right cerebral hemisphere which was distorting the lateral ventricle. The patient had an urgent operation to excise the tumour. The histopathology report of the tumour noted the presence of glial fibrillary acidic protein (GFAP). Which of the following tumours was excised from this patient's right cerebral hemisphere?

- A   Acoustic neuroma
- B   Astrocytoma
- C   Ependymoma
- D   Meningioma
- E   Neuroblastoma

**16.15** A previously healthy, 26-year-old male office assistant was noticed by his colleagues to be a bit confused. He then had a seizure and was brought to the hospital. His vital signs showed: blood pressure 100/60 mmHg, temperature 37 °C, pulse 88/minute and respiratory rate 22/minute. A lumbar puncture revealed a normal opening pressure and clear, colourless cerebrospinal fluid was obtained with 1 red blood cell and 20 white blood cells (all lymphocytes), with normal glucose and protein. Magnetic resonance imaging revealed swelling of the right temporal lobe with haemorrhagic areas. Which of the following infectious agents is the most likely cause of these findings?

- A   *Haemophilus influenzae*
- B   Herpes simplex virus
- C   Influenza virus
- D   *Neisseria meningitidis*
- E   *Mycobacterium tuberculosis*

cns

**16.16** A 55-year-old man was brought to the emergency department complaining of headaches, becoming irritable, and acting strangely about 1 month after being involved in a road traffic accident in which he was a front-seat passenger. He struck his head against the dashboard of the car, but did not lose consciousness at that time or at any point thereafter. This history is most consistent with the development of:

    ○  A  Epidural haematoma

    ○  B  Chronic subdural haematoma

    ○  C  Cerebral contusion

    ○  D  Subarachnoid haemorrhage

    ○  E  Intracerebral haematoma

**16.17** A 33-year-old man developed a progressive, ascending motor weakness over several days. He was hospitalised and required intubation with mechanical ventilation. He remained afebrile during this episode. A lumbar puncture was performed, with a normal opening pressure, and yielded clear, colourless cerebrospinal fluid with normal glucose, increased protein, and a cell count of 5 per mm$^3$, all lymphocytes. He gradually recovered after 4 weeks. Which of the following conditions was most likely to have preceded the onset of his illness?

    ○  A  Epilepsy

    ○  B  Ketoacidosis

    ○  C  *Staphylococcus aureus* septicaemia

    ○  D  Viral pneumonia

    ○  E  Systemic lupus erythematosus

**16.18** A 55-year-old man was examined by an SHO in the neurology outpatient clinic because he had developed a distal, symmetric, primarily sensory polyneuropathy over a period of several months. He also had a non-healing ulcer on the ball of his right foot. He had had a myocardial infarction 1 year previously, but had recovered and was doing well on anti-anginal medication. Which of the following abnormal laboratory test findings would the SHO expect to find in this patient?

○ A Decreased glucose level in the cerebrospinal fluid (CSF) (20 mg/dl)

○ B Elevated serum glucose of 10.8 mmol/l

○ C Elevated protein in the CSF

○ D Multiple osteoblastic lesions on X-ray of the vertebral column

○ E Markedly increased blood lead level of 2.4 µmol/l

**16.19** A 59-year-old woman complaining of new-onset headaches was referred to the neurosurgical oupatient clinic by her GP. Her clinical examination was unremarkable except for a chronic cough. She had a smoking habit of two packs of cigarettes per day. Magnetic resonance imaging of the brain revealed a solitary, 2.5-cm-diameter lesion that was located at the grey–white junction in the posterior left frontal lobe. There was no ring enhancement. A stereotactic biopsy of this lesion is most likely to show:

○ A An organising abscess

○ B A plaque of demyelination

○ C Metastatic carcinoma

○ D Neuronal loss with gliosis

○ E Viral inclusions

CNS

**16.20** **A 50-year-old woman presented to the emergency department with a severe headache. She was afebrile but was found to have papilloedema on fundal examination. She died before any further investigations could be performed. At autopsy there were recent haemorrhages in the pons. No other haemorrhages were found in the central nervous system, and she did not have any haemorrhages elsewhere in the body. What other pathological finding is most likely to be reported by the pathologist performing the autopsy?**

○ A Cerebral oedema with uncal herniation

○ B Fracture of the right parietal bone

○ C Gram-negative rods in the cerebrospinal fluid

○ D Loss of pigmented neurones in the substantia nigra

○ E Severe thrombocytopenia

# SECTION 17: PHARMACOLOGY — QUESTIONS

For each question given below choose the ONE BEST option.

**17.1** **A 38-year-old patient with central abdominal pain was seen by an SHO in the surgical oupatient clinic. Enquiries about his current medication therapy revealed that the patient was taking cimetidine for duodenal ulcer. What is the mechanism of action of cimetidine?**

○ A Adsorbs bile salts
○ B Competitively inhibits $H_2$ receptors
○ C Dopamine antagonist
○ D Holds water in the stool
○ E Lowers the surface tension of the stool, facilitating penetration of water and fats

**17.2** **A 42-year-old woman who was receiving chemotherapy for breast cancer was prescribed ondansetron for chemotherapy-induced vomiting. What is the mechanism of action of ondansetron?**

○ A Competitively inhibits $H_2$ receptors
○ B Holds water in the stool
○ C Inactivates pepsin
○ D Opiate agonist
○ E Serotonin antagonist

pharmacology

**17.3** **A 45-year-old patient with non-infective diarrhoea is prescribed diphenoxylate. What is the mechanism of action of diphenoxylate?**

    A  Competitively inhibits $H_2$ receptors

    B  Holds water in the stool

    C  Irreversibly inhibits $H^+/K^+$-ATPase

    D  Opiate agonist

    E  Serotonin antagonist

**17.4** **A 74-year old man with chronic constipation and diverticulosis uses methylcellulose on a regular basis as it helps him to move his bowels. What is the mechanism of action of methylcellulose?**

    A  Adsorbs bile salts

    B  Holds water in the stool

    C  Irreversibly inhibits $H^+/K^+$-ATPase

    D  Lowers the surface tension of the stool, facilitating penetration of water and fats

    E  Neutralises gastric acid

**17.5** **A 68-year-old woman with diverticulosis uses psyllium on a daily basis. What is the mechanism of action of psyllium?**

    A  Competitively inhibits $H_2$ receptors

    B  Holds water in the stool

    C  Inactivates pepsin

    D  Lowers the surface tension of the stool, facilitating penetration of water and fats

    E  Opiate agonist

pharmacology

**17.6** **A 35-year-old patient with severe gastro-oesophageal reflux disease is prescribed lansoprazole. What is the mechanism of action of lansoprazole?**

○ A Competitively inhibits $H_2$ receptors

○ B Dopamine antagonist

○ C Holds water in the stool

○ D Irreversibly inhibits $H^+/K^+$-ATPase

○ E Neutralises gastric acid

**17.7** **An SHO prescribes metoclopramide for the treatment of nausea and vomiting in a patient on day 3 after closure of an ileostomy. What is the mechanism of action of metoclopramide?**

○ A Irreversibly inhibits $H^+/K^+$-ATPase

○ B Dopamine antagonist

○ C Neutralises gastric acid

○ D Serotonin antagonist

○ E Competitively inhibits $H_2$ receptors

**17.8** **A 42-year-old patient with constipation and haemorrhoids is prescribed docusate sodium (dioctyl sodium sulphosuccinate). What is the mechanism of action of docusate sodium?**

○ A Competitively inhibits $H_2$ receptors

○ B Holds water in the stool

○ C Inactivates pepsin

○ D Lowers the surface tension of the stool, facilitating penetration of water and fats

○ E Promotes release of acetylcholine

pharmacology

**17.9** **A 32-year-old patient with diarrhoea is prescribed loperamide. What is the mechanism of action of loperamide?**

- A Competitively inhibits $H_2$ receptors
- B Irreversibly inhibits $H^+/K^+$-ATPase
- C Inactivates pepsin
- D Lowers the surface tension of the stool, facilitating penetration of water and fats
- E Opiate agonist

**17.10** **An anaesthetist gave a trauma patient a shot of sufentanil prior to changing his wound dressings in the intensive care unit. What is the mechanism of action of sufentanil?**

- A Modulates the GABAergic system
- B Modulates the noradrenergic system
- C Modulates the serotonergic system
- D Opiate agonist
- E Promotes the release of acetylcholine

**17.11** **A 48-year old man complaining of pain in his thoracotomy wound was prescribed regular tramadol. What is the mechanism of action of tramadol?**

- A Competitively inhibits $H_2$ receptors
- B Inhibits synthesis of prostaglandins
- C Modulation of GABAergic, noradrenergic and serotonergic systems
- D Opiate antagonist
- E Promotes release of acetylcholine

pharmacology

**17.12** **A 58-year old man was prescribed atorvastatin after coronary artery bypass surgery. What is the mechanism of action of atorvastatin?**

   ○  A  Inhibits apoprotein synthesis

   ○  B  Inhibits cholesterol synthesis

   ○  C  Inhibits lipoprotein lipase

   ○  D  Inhibits reabsorption of bile acids

   ○  E  Inhibits VLDL synthesis

**17.13** **A 58-year-old patient with an acute, evolving myocardial infarction was administered streptokinase. He presented 2 months later in the emergency department with another acute myocardial infarction. The doctor attending him did not give him streptokinase on this occasion because of the risk of which of the following side-effects?**

   ○  A  Allergic reaction

   ○  B  Angina

   ○  C  Bronchodilation

   ○  D  Damage to endothelial membranes

   ○  E  Hypotension

**17.14** **Which of the following is an indication for carbachol?**

   ○  A  Angina

   ○  B  Cataract surgery

   ○  C  Congestive heart failure

   ○  D  Hypertriglyceridaemia

   ○  E  Paroxysmal atrial tachycardia provoked by emotion or exercise

pharmacology

**17.15** **A 36-year-old multiple trauma patient who had been in the intensive care unit for over 3 weeks was prescribed griseofulvin. What class of drugs does griseofulvin belong to?**

- A  Antifungal
- B  Antimycobacterial
- C  Autonomic nervous system drugs
- D  Beta-blockers
- E  Vasodilators

**17.16** **A 38-year-old patient in the intensive care unit is on mexiletine. Which of the following is a recognised indication for mexiletine?**

- A  Paroxysmal atrial tachycardia provoked by emotion or exercise
- B  Prophylaxis of *Mycobacterium avium* infection in patients with AIDS
- C  *Streptococcus pneumoniae* infection
- D  Thyrotoxicosis (preparation for surgery)
- E  Ventricular arrhythmias

**17.17** **A 52-year-old diabetic and hypertensive patient admitted for elective cholecystectomy was noted to be on nadolol. Which of the following statements regarding nadolol is correct?**

- A  It accelerates atrioventricular conduction
- B  It crosses the placenta and can cause neonatal respiratory distress syndrome
- C  It has low efficacy
- D  It is poorly lipid-soluble
- E  It has a substantial first-pass effect

pharmacology

**17.18** **A 65-year-old woman underwent a prolonged operation on cardiopulmonary bypass for repair of an ascending aortic aneurysm. She was started on desmopressin postoperatively. Which of the following is a mechanism of action of desmopressin?**

○ A It blocks sustained repetitive neuronal firing

○ B It competitively inhibits binding of plasmin and plasminogen to fibrin's lysine residues

○ C It induces the release of stored factor VIII and von Willebrand factor

○ D It inhibits hepatic gluconeogenesis

○ E It inhibits angiotensin-converting enzyme

**17.19** **A 63-year-old woman admitted for elective resection of a rectal carcinoma was noted to be on buspirone (prescribed by her GP). Buspirone acts as:**

○ A Anticonvulsant

○ B Antimycobacterial

○ C Anxiolytic

○ D Benzodiazepine

○ E Beta-blocker

**17.20** **A 36-year-old patient with folliculitis is taking dicloxacillin. Dicloxacillin is a:**

○ A Macrolide

○ B Penicillin

○ C Quinolone

○ D Sulphonamide

○ E Tetracycline

pharmacology

**17.21** **A 55-year-old patient was commenced on sodium nitroprusside infusion after undergoing repair of an abdominal aortic aneurysm. Which class of drugs does nitroprusside belong to?**

- A   Antidepressants
- B   Glucocorticoids
- C   Immunoglobulins
- D   Quinolones
- E   Vasodilators

**17.22** **A 56-year-old woman who was admitted for elective right hemicolectomy was noted to be on spironolactone. What class of drugs does spironolactone belong to?**

- A   Beta-lactamase inhibitors
- B   Hydantoins
- C   Lipid-lowering drugs
- D   Oral hypoglycaemics
- E   Potassium-sparing diuretics

**17.23** **Which of the following is a recognised indication for abciximab treatment?**

- A   Bleeding due to deficiency of factor VIII
- B   Generalised motor seizures
- C   Muscle relaxation
- D   *Neisseria gonorrhoeae* infection
- E   Prevention of re-stenosis after angioplasty

pharmacology

**17.24 A 45-year-old patient who had been in the intensive care unit for nearly 1 month was commenced on fluconazole. Which of the following is the correct mechanism of action of fluconazole?**

○ A Inhibits cytochrome P450
○ B Inhibits phospholipase C
○ C Inhibits transpeptidase
○ D Inhibits viral protease
○ E Inhibits viral DNA polymerase

**17.25 A 55-year-old man underwent emergency surgery for a perforated duodenal ulcer and was commenced on ceftriaxone. The subclass of antibiotics that ceftriaxone belongs to is:**

○ A First-generation cephalosporins
○ B Second-generation cephalosporins
○ C Third-generation cephalosporins
○ D Fluoroquinolones
○ E Macrolides

**17.26 Etoposide is a chemotherapeutic agent. Which of the following is the correct indication for this drug?**

○ A Breast cancer
○ B Colon cancer
○ C Hairy cell leukaemia
○ D Lung cancer
○ E Myxoma

pharmacology

**17.27** **A 46-year-old patient is receiving vincristine as a part of chemotherapy for Hodgkin's lymphoma. Which of the following is a recognised major side-effect of vincristine?**

○ A Hepatitis
○ B Myelosuppression
○ C Peripheral neuropathy
○ D Respiratory suppression
○ E Thrombocytopenia

**17.28** **Which of the following is the correct mechanism of action of trimethoprim?**

○ A Beta-antagonist
○ B Inhibits cholesterol synthesis
○ C Inhibits dihydrofolate reductase
○ D Mitotic spindle poison
○ E Potentiates glucose-mediated insulin secretion

**17.29** **The prescription of a patient in the intensive care unit includes tazobactam. What is the mechanism of action of tazobactam?**

○ A Inhibits beta-lactamase
○ B Inhibits CD3 receptor
○ C Inhibits calcineurin
○ D Inhibits translocase
○ E Opiate agonist

pharmacology

**17.30 Which of the following is a recognised indication for mithramycin?**

○ A Defect in vitamin D metabolism/activation

○ B Fever

○ C Hypercalcaemia of malignancy

○ D Organ transplantation

○ E Rickets

**17.31 What is the mechanism of action of methimazole?**

○ A Binds to the 30S subunit of bacterial ribosome

○ B Inhibits cholesterol synthesis

○ C Inhibits the addition of iodide to thyroglobulin

○ D Inhibits release of iodothyronines

○ E Irradiates and destroys the thyroid gland

**17.32 A 42-year-old man with lymphoma who was treated with cyclophosphamide 8 years ago is potentially at risk of developing cancer of which of the following organs?**

○ A Bone

○ B Colon

○ C Liver

○ D Oesophagus

○ E Urinary bladder

pharmacology

**17.33** A 68-year-old woman in an intensive care unit developed pneumonia caused by *Pseudomonas aeruginosa*. Which of the following antibiotics is most likely to be effective against this organism?

○ A  Ampicillin
○ B  Erythromycin
○ C  Piperacillin
○ D  Sulphonamide
○ E  Tetracycline

**17.34** A 68-year-old woman in an intensive care unit developed pneumonia caused by a strain of *Pseudomonas aeruginosa* that is sensitive to piperacillin and one other antibiotic. Which of the following antibiotics is most likely to be the other antibiotic that is effective against *Pseudomonas aeruginosa*?

○ A  Azlocillin
○ B  Benzylpenicillin
○ C  Clarithromycin
○ D  Sulphonamide
○ E  Tetracycline

**17.35** A 63-year-old man who is on broad-spectrum antibiotics and who has been in an intensive care unit for nearly 3 weeks developed *Clostridium difficile* infection. He was treated with oral metronidazole but the diarrhoea persisted. Which of the following antibiotics could be used to treat this infection?

○ A  Amoxicillin
○ B  Cetriaxone
○ C  Clindamycin
○ D  Ciprofloxacin
○ E  Oral vancomycin

**17.36** **A 35-year-old patient in the intensive care unit was commenced on linezolid. Which of the following organisms is most likely to be effectively treated by linezolid?**

○ A  *Entamoeba histolytica*

○ B  Methicillin-resistant *Staphylococcus aureus*

○ C  *Pseudomonas aeruginosa*

○ D  *Salmonella typhi*

○ E  *Vibrio cholerae*

**17.37** **A 39-year-old multiple trauma patient with a methicillin-resistant *Staphylococcus aureus* chest infection was commenced on linezolid because he was allergic to vancomycin. What is the mechanism of action of linezolid?**

○ A  Inhibits bacterial cell wall synthesis

○ B  Inhibits bacterial cholesterol synthesis

○ C  Inhibits dihydrofolate reductase

○ D  Inhibits initiation of bacterial protein synthesis

○ E  Mitotic spindle poison

**17.38** **A 25-year-old woman with suspected pneumonia was empirically started on a macrolide antibiotic by her GP because she was allergic to penicillins. Which of the following antibiotics is a macrolide antibiotic?**

○ A  Amikacin

○ B  Ciprofloxacin

○ C  Clindamycin

○ D  Erythromycin

○ E  Vancomycin

pharmacology

**17.39 A 26-year-old man with suspected pneumonia was empirically started on erythromycin by his GP because he was allergic to penicillins. What is the mechanism of action of erythromycin?**

○ A  Inhibits bacterial cell wall synthesis

○ B  Inhibits bacterial cholesterol synthesis

○ C  Inhibits dihydrofolate reductase

○ D  Inhibits initiation of bacterial protein synthesis

○ E  Inhibits translocation of peptides

**17.40 A 25-year-old man with pneumonia caused by a Gram-negative bacterium was prescribed ciprofloxacin, which is a quinolone antibiotic. What is the mechanism of action of quinolones?**

○ A  Inhibit bacterial cell wall synthesis

○ B  Inhibit bacterial cholesterol synthesis

○ C  Inhibit DNA replication and transcription

○ D  Inhibit initiation of bacterial protein synthesis

○ E  Inhibit translocation of peptides

**17.41 A 26-year-old woman with tuberculous meningitis was treated with rifampicin. Which of the following is the mechanism of action of rifampicin?**

○ A  Disrupts the bacterial DNA helical structure

○ B  Inhibits bacterial protein synthesis by binding to the 30S ribosomal subunit

○ C  Inhibits bacterial protein synthesis by binding to the 50S ribosomal subunit

○ D  Inhibits DNA-dependent RNA polymerase

○ E  Prevents the translocation of elongation factor G from the ribosome

pharmacology

**17.42 A 35-year-old man with a *Staphylococcus aureus* wound infection was commenced on fusidic acid. Which of the following is the mechanism of action of fusidic acid?**

O  A  Disrupts the bacterial DNA helical structure

O  B  Inhibits bacterial protein synthesis by binding to the 30S ribosomal subunit

O  C  Inhibits bacterial protein synthesis by binding to the 50S ribosomal subunit

O  D  Inhibits DNA-dependent RNA polymerase

O  E  Prevents the translocation of elongation factor G from the ribosome

**17.43 A 25-year-old man with tuberculous lymphadenitis was treated with ethambutol in combination with other antituberculosis drugs. Which of the following is the mechanism of action of ethambutol?**

O  A  Disrupts the bacterial DNA helical structure

O  B  Inhibits bacterial protein synthesis by binding to the 30S ribosomal subunit

O  C  Inhibits bacterial protein synthesis by binding to the 50S ribosomal subunit

O  D  Inhibits DNA-dependent RNA polymerase

O  E  Obstructs the formation of the bacterial cell wall

pharmacology

**17.44 A 25-year-old man with tuberculous lymphadenitis was treated with isoniazid in combination with other antituberculosis drugs. Which of the following is the mechanism of action of isoniazid?**

   ○  A  Disrupts the bacterial DNA helical structure

   ○  B  Inhibits bacterial protein synthesis by binding to the 30S ribosomal subunit

   ○  C  Inhibits bacterial protein synthesis by binding to the 50S ribosomal subunit

   ○  D  Inhibits DNA-dependent RNA polymerase

   ○  E  Inhibits mycolic acid synthesis in the bacterial cell wall

**17.45 A 58-year-old man with colorectal carcinoma who is receiving adjuvant chemotherapy is on folinic acid. Which of the following is a recognised therapeutic use of folinic acid in this setting?**

   ○  A  Enhances the effect of 5-fluorouracil

   ○  B  Prevents chemotherapy-induced vomiting

   ○  C  Preserves renal function

   ○  D  Rescues bone marrow

   ○  E  Reverses pre-existing methotrexate-induced nephrotoxicity

**17.46 Chemotherapy regimens are often known by their acronyms, identifying the combination of agents used. Which of the following chemotherapy regimens is used for treating colorectal cancer?**

   ○  A  ABVD

   ○  B  BEP

   ○  C  CHOP

   ○  D  COP

   ○  E  FOLFOX

pharmacology

**17.47** **Chemotherapy regimens are often known by their acronyms, identifying the combination of agents used. Which of the following chemotherapy regimens is used for treating Hodgkin's lymphoma?**

○ A ABVD
○ B BEP
○ C CHOP
○ D COP
○ E FOLFOX

**17.48** **Chemotherapy regimens are often known by their acronyms, identifying the combination of agents used. Which of the following chemotherapy regimens is used for treating non-Hodgkin's lymphoma?**

○ A ABVD
○ B BEP
○ C CHOP
○ D ECF
○ E FOLFOX

**17.49** **A 28-year-old woman with severe Crohn's disease was prescribed methotrexate. What is the mechanism of action of methotrexate in this condition?**

○ A Disruption of the DNA helical structure
○ B Inhibition of dihydrofolate reductase
○ C Inhibition of mast cells
○ D Inhibition of T-cell activation
○ E Mitotic spindle poison

pharmacology

**17.50 A 48-year-old man with small-cell lung cancer was given cisplatin chemotherapy. What is the mechanism of action of cisplatin?**

○ A Cross-linking of DNA

○ B Disruption of the DNA helical structure

○ C Inhibition of dihydrofolate reductase

○ D Inhibition of T-cell activation

○ E Mitotic spindle poison

pharmacology

# ANSWERS

# SECTION 1: CELL INJURY AND WOUND HEALING — ANSWERS

## 1.1

*Answer: E*    Liquefactive necrosis

Liquefactive necrosis is characteristic of focal bacterial or, occasionally, fungal infections, because microbes stimulate the accumulation of inflammatory cells. Hypoxic death of cells within the central nervous system often evokes liquefactive necrosis, though the reasons for this are obscure. Whatever the pathogenesis, liquefaction completely digests the dead cells. The end result is transformation of the tissue into a viscous liquid mass. If the process was initiated by acute inflammation the material is frequently creamy yellow in colour because of the presence of dead white cells and this is called 'pus'.

## 1.2

*Answer: A*    Caseous necrosis

Caseous necrosis, a distinctive form of coagulative necrosis, is encountered most often in foci of tuberculous infection. In this disease the characteristic lesion is called a 'granuloma' or a 'tubercle' and is classically characterised by the presence of central caseous necrosis. The term 'caseous' is derived from the cheesy white gross appearance of the area of necrosis. On microscopic examination, the necrotic focus appears as amorphous granular debris, seemingly composed of fragmented, coagulated cells and amorphous granular debris enclosed within a distinctive inflammatory border known as a 'granulomatous reaction'. Unlike coagulative necrosis, the tissue architecture is completely obliterated. In a granuloma, macrophages are transformed into epithelium-like cells surrounded by a collar of mononuclear leukocytes, principally lymphocytes and occasionally plasma cells. In the usual haematoxylin and eosin-stained tissue sections, the epithelioid cells have a pale pink granular cytoplasm with indistinct cell boundaries, and often appear to merge into one another. The nucleus is less dense than that of a lymphocyte, is oval or elongated in shape, and can show folding of the nuclear membrane. Older granulomas develop an enclosing rim of fibroblasts and connective tissue. Epithelioid cells often fuse to form giant cells in the periphery or sometimes in the centre of granulomas. These giant cells can attain diameters of 40–50 μm. They have a large mass of cytoplasm containing 20 or more small nuclei arranged either peripherally (Langhans-type giant cell) or haphazardly (foreign body-type giant cell). There is no known functional difference between these two types of giant cells. The chronic infective lesion in this scenario is most probably a tuberculous granuloma.

## 1.3

*Answer: C*    Cell size decreases

Atrophy is the shrinkage in the size of the cell due to loss of cell substance. It represents a form of adaptive response and can result in cell death. Involvement of a sufficient number of cells causes the entire tissue or organ to diminish in size or become atrophic. Atrophy can be physiological or pathological. Physiological atrophy is commonly seen during early development and is exemplified by atrophy of the notochord and the thyroglossal duct during foetal development. Another common example of physiological atrophy is the decrease in size of the uterus shortly after childbirth. Pathological atrophy can be local or generalised, depending on the underlying cause. The common causes of atrophy are the following:

- Ageing (senile atrophy). Ageing is associated with cell loss, typically seen in tissues containing permanent cells, particularly the brain and heart.

- Decreased workload (atrophy of disuse). This is best seen when a broken limb is immobilised in a plaster cast or when a patient is restricted to complete bed rest resulting in rapid skeletal muscle. The initial rapid decrease in cell size is reversible once activity is resumed. With more prolonged disuse, however, skeletal muscle fibres decrease in number as well as in size, and this atrophy can be accompanied by increased bone resorption, leading to osteoporosis of disuse.

- Diminished blood supply. A decrease in blood supply (ischaemia) to a tissue occurring as a result of occlusive arterial disease results in atrophy of tissue because of progressive cell loss. An example of this is seen in late adult life as the brain undergoes progressive atrophy due to reduced blood supply secondary to atherosclerosis.

- Inadequate nutrition. In profound protein-calorie malnutrition (marasmus) skeletal muscle is used as a source of energy after other reserves such as adipose stores have been depleted. This results in marked muscle wasting (cachexia). Cachexia is also seen in patients with chronic inflammatory diseases or cancer. In the former, chronic overproduction of the inflammatory cytokine, tumour necrosis factor (TNF) is thought to be responsible for appetite suppression and muscle atrophy.

- Loss of endocrine stimulation. Many endocrine glands, the breast, and the reproductive organs are dependent on endocrine stimulation for normal metabolism and function. The loss of oestrogen stimulation after the menopause results in physiological atrophy of the endometrium, vaginal epithelium, and breast.

- Loss of innervation (denervation atrophy). Normal function of skeletal muscle depends on its nerve supply. Damage to the nerves leads to rapid atrophy of the muscle fibres supplied by those nerves.

- Pressure. Compression of tissues for any length of time can lead to atrophy. An enlarging benign tumour can cause atrophy in the surrounding compressed tissues. Atrophy in this setting is probably the result of ischaemic changes caused by compromise of the blood supply to the surrounding tissues by the expanding mass.

cell injury

Atrophy is brought about by a reduction in the structural components of the cell with concomitant diminished function. For instance in atrophic muscle the cells contain fewer mitochondria and myofilaments and a reduced amount of endoplasmic reticulum. The fundamental cellular changes associated with atrophy are identical in all of the above settings and represent an adaptive response to ensure survival.

## 1.4

*Answer: E*  Stratified squamous metaplasia

Metaplasia is a reversible change in which one adult cell type (epithelial or mesenchymal) is replaced by another adult cell type. It can represent an adaptive substitution of cells that are sensitive to stress by cell types better able to withstand the adverse environment. The most common type of epithelial metaplasia is columnar to squamous, as occurs in the respiratory tract in response to chronic irritation. In the habitual cigarette smoker, the normal ciliated columnar epithelial cells of the trachea and bronchi are often replaced focally or widely by stratified squamous epithelial cells.

The more rugged stratified squamous epithelium is able to survive under circumstances in which the more fragile, specialised columnar epithelium would have succumbed. Although the metaplastic squamous cells in the respiratory tract are capable of surviving this environment, an important protective mechanism — mucus secretion — is lost. Epithelial metaplasia is therefore a two-edged sword and, in most circumstances, represents an undesirable change. Moreover, the influences that predispose to metaplasia, if persistent, can induce malignant transformation in metaplastic epithelium. A common form of cancer in the respiratory tract is therefore composed of squamous cells, which arise in areas of metaplasia of normal columnar epithelium into squamous epithelium.

## 1.5

*Answer: E*   Increase in cell size and in its organelles

Hypertrophy is caused by an increase in the size of cells, resulting in an increase in the size of the organ. The hypertrophied organ has no new cells, just larger cells. The increased size of the cells is due not to cellular swelling but to the synthesis of more structural components. Cells capable of division can respond to stress by undergoing both hyperplasia and hypertrophy, whereas in non-dividing cells (eg myocardial fibres), hypertrophy occurs. The nuclei in hypertrophied cells can have a higher DNA content than normal cells, probably because the cells arrest in the cell cycle without undergoing mitosis.

Hypertrophy can be physiological or pathological and is caused by increased functional demand or by specific hormonal stimulation. The striated muscle cells in both the heart and the skeletal muscles are capable of tremendous hypertrophy, perhaps because they cannot adapt adequately to increased metabolic demands by mitotic division and production of more cells to share the work. The most common stimulus for hypertrophy of muscle is increased workload. For example, the bulging muscles of bodybuilders engaged in 'pumping iron' result from an increase in size of the individual muscle fibres in response to increased demand. The workload is thus shared by a greater mass of cellular components, and each muscle fibre is spared excess work and so escapes injury. The enlarged muscle cell achieves a new equilibrium, permitting it to function at a higher level of activity. In the heart, the stimulus for hypertrophy is usually chronic haemodynamic overload, resulting from either hypertension or faulty valves. Synthesis of more proteins and filaments occurs, achieving a balance between the demand and the cell's functional capacity. The greater number of myofilaments per cell permits an increased workload with a level of metabolic activity per unit volume of cell not different from that borne by the normal cell.

The massive physiological growth of the uterus that occurs during pregnancy is a good example of a hormone-induced increase in the size of an organ that results from both hypertrophy and hyperplasia. The cellular hypertrophy is stimulated by oestrogenic hormones acting on smooth-muscle oestrogen receptors, eventually resulting

cell injury

in increased synthesis of smooth-muscle proteins and an increase in cell size. Similarly, prolactin and oestrogen cause hypertrophy of the breasts during lactation. These are examples of physiological hypertrophy induced by hormonal stimulation.

## 1.6

*Answer: B*  Chromatin condensation

Apoptosis is a pathway of cell death that is induced by a tightly regulated intracellular programme in which cells destined to die activate enzymes that degrade the cells' own nuclear DNA and nuclear and cytoplasmic proteins. The cell's plasma membrane remains intact, but its structure is altered in such a way that the apoptotic cell becomes an avid target for phagocytosis. The dead cell is rapidly cleared, before its contents have leaked out, and therefore cell death by this pathway does not elicit an inflammatory reaction in the host. Apoptosis is therefore fundamentally different from necrosis, which is characterised by loss of membrane integrity, enzymatic digestion of cells, and frequently a host reaction. However, apoptosis and necrosis sometimes coexist, and they can share some common features and mechanisms.

The following morphological features, some best seen with the electron microscope, characterise cells undergoing apoptosis:

- Cell shrinkage. The cell is smaller in size; the cytoplasm is dense; and the organelles, although relatively normal, are more tightly packed.

- Chromatin condensation. This is the most characteristic feature of apoptosis. The chromatin aggregates peripherally, under the nuclear membrane, into dense masses of various shapes and sizes. The nucleus itself can break up, producing two or more fragments.

- Formation of cytoplasmic blebs and apoptotic bodies. The apoptotic cell first shows extensive surface blebbing, then undergoes fragmentation into membrane-bound apoptotic bodies composed of cytoplasm and tightly packed organelles, with or without nuclear fragments.

- Phagocytosis of apoptotic cells or cell bodies, usually by macrophages. The apoptotic bodies are rapidly degraded within lysosomes, and the adjacent healthy cells migrate or proliferate to replace the space occupied by the now deleted apoptotic cell.

Plasma membranes are thought to remain intact during apoptosis, until the last stages, when they become permeable to solutes that are normally retained. This classic description is accurate with respect to apoptosis during physiological conditions such as embryogenesis and deletion of immune cells. However, forms of cell death with features of necrosis as well as of apoptosis are not uncommon in reaction to injurious stimuli. Under such conditions, the severity, rather than the specificity, of the stimulus determines the form in which death is expressed. If necrotic features are predominant, early plasma membrane damage occurs, and cell swelling, rather than shrinkage, is seen.

## 1.7

*Answer: D*   Trauma to the breast

Fat necrosis can be seen after trauma to the breast. It can present as a painless palpable mass, skin thickening or retraction, a mammographic density, or mammographic calcifications. The majority of women will give a history of trauma or prior surgery. The major clinical significance of the condition is its possible confusion with breast carcinoma when there is a palpable mass or mammographic calcifications.

Grossly, the lesion can consist of haemorrhage in the early stages and, later, central liquefactive necrosis of fat. Later still, it can appear as an ill-defined nodule of grey-white, firm tissue containing small foci of chalky-white or haemorrhagic debris. The central focus of necrotic fat cells is initially surrounded by macrophages and an intense neutrophilic infiltration. Then, during the next few days, progressive fibroblastic proliferation, increased vascularisation, and lymphocytic and histiocytic infiltration wall off the focus. Subsequently, foreign-body giant cells, calcifications, and haemosiderin make their appearance. Eventually, the focus is replaced by scar tissue or is encysted and walled off by collagenous tissue.

cell injury

## 1.8

*Answer: A*    Decrease in the number of muscle fibres

Shrinkage in the size of the cell by loss of cell substance is known as 'atrophy'. It represents a form of adaptive response and can culminate in cell death. When a sufficient number of cells are involved, the entire tissue or organ diminishes in size, or becomes atrophic. When a broken limb is immobilised in a plaster cast or when a patient is restricted to complete bed rest, skeletal muscle atrophy rapidly ensues. The initial rapid decrease in cell size is reversible once activity is resumed. With more prolonged disuse, however, skeletal muscle fibres decrease in number as well as in size; this atrophy can be accompanied by increased bone resorption, leading to osteoporosis of disuse (see also *Answer* to **1.3**).

## 1.9

*Answer: C*    Mobilisation of fat stores

The metabolic response to injury is an important part of the stress reaction in that it improves the individual organism's chances of surviving under adverse circumstances or when injured. The metabolic response to trauma includes:

- Acid–base disturbance — usually a metabolic alkalosis or acidosis
- Early reduced urine output and increased urine osmolality
- Early reduction in metabolic rate
- Gluconeogenesis via amino acid breakdown
- Hyponatraemia due to impaired sodium pump action
- Hypoxia and coagulopathy
- Immunosuppression
- Increased extracellular fluid volume volume and hypovolaemia
- Increased vascular permeability and oedema

- Late diuresis and increased sodium loss
- Late increased metabolism, negative nitrogen balance and weight loss
- Mobilisation of fat stores, lipolysis and ketosis
- Pyrexia in the absence of infection
- Reduced 'free' water clearance
- Reduced serum albumin.

## 1.10

*Answer: C*    Free radical formation

Cells generate energy by reducing molecular oxygen to water. During this process small amounts of partially reduced reactive oxygen forms are produced as an unavoidable byproduct of mitochondrial respiration. Some of these forms are free radicals that can damage lipids, proteins and nucleic acids. They are referred to as 'reactive oxygen species'. Cells have defence systems for preventing injury caused by these products. An imbalance between free radical-generating and free radical-scavenging systems results in oxidative stress, a condition that has been associated with the cell injury seen in many pathological conditions. Free radical-mediated damage contributes to such varied processes as chemical and radiation injury, ischaemia-reperfusion injury (induced by restoration of blood flow in ischaemic tissue), cellular ageing and microbial killing by phagocytes.

## 1.11

*Answer: B*    Cholesterol crystals

In haemophiliac joints the lipid from the red cell membranes is broken down and cholesterol crystals form. Accumulation of lipofuscin is not a feature of haemorrhage. Russell bodies are intracellular accumulations of immunoglobulins in plasma cells. Neutrophils suggest acute inflammation. Anthracotic pigment is an exogenous carbon pigment from dusts in the air that accumulate in lung.

## 1.12

*Answer: E*   Metaplasia

Metaplasia is the substitution of one tissue type normally found at a site for another. The epithelium undergoes metaplasia in response to ongoing inflammation from reflux of gastric contents. It is common in the lower oesophagus with gastro-oesophageal reflux disease. The growth of the epithelial cells must become disordered in order to be dysplastic. Hyperplasia can occur with inflammation, as the number of cells increases, but hyperplasia does not explain the presence of the columnar cells. Carcinoma is characterised by cellular atypia with hyperchromatism and pleomorphism. Goblet cells would not be seen. Ischaemia would be unusual at this site and would be marked by coagulative necrosis.

## 1.13

*Answer: E*   Liquefactive necrosis

The brain undergoes liquefactive necrosis with infarction. As it resolves, a cystic area forms in the region of infarction. Atrophy would be a more generalised process, whereas a single cystic area in the brain suggests a remote infarction. Coagulative necrosis is more typical of parenchymal organs such as the kidney or spleen, which do not have as high a lipid content as the brain. Caseous necrosis is more typical of granulomatous inflammation with *Mycobacterium tuberculosis*. Apoptosis is single-cell necrosis that does not result in a grossly visible cystic area (see also *Answer* to **1.1**).

## 1.14

*Answer: C*   Lobular hyperplasia

There is an increase in lobules under hormonal influence to provide for lactation. Lobular hyperplasia would allow this woman to nurse the infant. The stroma of the breast consists of connective tissue, which provides structural support but does not have cells that produce milk. Dysplasia in epithelia is a premalignant change and not a normal physiological event. With poor nutrition and weight loss, steatocytes can decrease in size. Metaplasia is the exchange of normal epithelium for another type in response to chronic irritation. Metaplasia is not a normal physiological process.

## 1.15

*Answer: E*    Lipochrome, from 'wear and tear'

Lipochrome is a very common finding in older people, but it has little effect on cardiac function. Lipochrome is also known as 'lipofuscin'. Haemosiderosis is not a complication of ageing. Glycogen storage diseases are inherited conditions that appear early in life. Glycogen does not appear pigmented in haematoxylin and eosin-stained tissue sections. Cholesterol accumulates in atheromatous plaques in the arteries, not in the myocardium. Calcium deposits appear as irregular, dark-blue areas and are not associated with ageing of the myocardium.

## 1.16

*Answer: B*    Confirmation that a neoplasm is a carcinoma

Malignant tumours of diverse origin often resemble one another because they are poorly differentiated. These tumours are often quite difficult to distinguish on the basis of routine haematoxylin and eosin- (H&E-) stained tissue sections. For example, certain anaplastic carcinomas, malignant lymphomas, melanomas and sarcomas can look quite similar, but they must be accurately identified because their treatment and prognosis are different. Antibodies against intermediate filaments have proved to be of value in such cases because tumour cells often contain intermediate filaments characteristic of their cell of origin. For example, the presence of cytokeratins, detected immunohistochemically, points to an epithelial origin (carcinoma), whereas desmin is specific for neoplasms of muscle cell origin. Cytoskeletal alterations occur with ischaemia, but are not a useful marker for such an event. Many cell types contain intermediate filaments. Mallory's alcoholic hyaline can be observed by H&E staining. However, it is not entirely specific for alcoholism. Metaplasia and dysplasia are assessed using their light-microscopic appearances after H&E staining.

cell injury

**cell injury**

## 1.17

*Answer: D*  Hypertrophy

In this patient the pressure load of hypertension led to myocardial fibre hypertrophy and a heart twice normal size. Fat in the heart does not increase in response to the increase in workload from hypertension. Myocardial fibres do not undergo hyperplasia. Fatty degeneration of the myocardium is typically the result of a toxic or hypoxic injury. Myocardial oedema is not a characteristic feature of myocardial injury or increased workload. However, heart failure could lead to peripheral oedema (see also *Answer* to **1.5**).

## 1.18

*Answer: E*  Tyrosine

The tanning process in skin is stimulated by ultraviolet light exposure. Melanocytes have the enzyme tyrosinase to oxidize tyrosine to dihydroxyphenylalanine in the pathway for melanin production. Haem as part of haemosiderin from breakdown of red blood cells can impart a brownish colour, but this is typically local from trauma or more global as part of an iron storage disease such as haemochromatosis. Lipochrome (lipofuscin) is a 'wear and tear' pigment that imparts a golden-brown appearance to granules in cells (such as myocytes or hepatocytes), but this is not a feature of skin. Homogentisic acid can be part of the process of the rare disease alkaptonuria, in which a black pigment is deposited in connective tissues. Glycogen in sufficient quantity is starch-like and imparts a paler colour to organs in which it is stored in excess. It does not involve the skin.

## 1.19

*Answer: E*  Vitamin A deficiency

Vitamin A is necessary to maintain epithelia, and squamous metaplasia of the respiratory tract can occur if there is a deficiency. Tanning of the skin is a physiological event resulting from the accumulation of melanin pigment — there is no change of one cell type to another involved. Lactation following pregnancy is a form of physiological hyperplasia of breast lobules that occurs as a result of hormonal influences. An acute myocardial infarction will lead to cardiac muscle fibre necrosis, which will heal with the production of fibrous scar tissue, but this is not a reversible metaplasia. The enlarged prostate represents primarily glandular hyperplasia.

## 1.20

*Answer: E*    Viral hepatitis

Viral infection leads to individual hepatocyte necrosis, which is characterised by the microscopic appearances of karyorrhexis and cell fragmentation. Brown atrophy of the heart results when there is marked lipofuscin deposition in the myocardium. Tissue destruction with transplant rejection is more widespread. Single cell necrosis is not evident in chronic alcoholic liver disease. Barbiturate overdose causes hypertrophy of smooth endoplasmic reticulum, not individual cell necrosis.

## 1.21

*Answer: E*    Wet gangrene

Small-intestinal infarction following sudden and total occlusion of mesenteric arterial blood flow can involve only a short segment, but more often involves a substantial portion. The splenic flexure of the colon is at greatest risk of ischaemic injury because it is the watershed between the distribution of the superior and inferior mesenteric arteries, but any portion of the colon can be affected. With mesenteric venous occlusion, anterograde and retrograde propagation of thrombus may lead to extensive involvement of the splanchnic bed. Regardless of whether the arterial or venous side is occluded, the infarction appears haemorrhagic because of blood reflow into the damaged area. In the early stages, the infarcted bowel appears intensely congested and dusky to purple-red, with foci of subserosal and submucosal ecchymotic discoloration. With time, the wall becomes oedematous, thickened, rubbery, and haemorrhagic. The lumen commonly contains sanguinous mucus or frank blood. In arterial occlusions the demarcation from normal bowel is usually sharply defined, but in venous occlusions the area

cell injury

of dusky cyanosis fades gradually into the adjacent normal bowel, having no clear-cut definition between viable and non-viable bowel. Histologically, there is obvious oedema, interstitial haemorrhage, and sloughing necrosis of the mucosa. Normal features of the mural musculature, particularly cellular nuclei, become indistinct. Within 1–4 days, intestinal bacteria produce outright wet gangrene and sometimes perforation of the bowel. There may be little inflammatory response.

## 1.22

*Answer: C*    Free radical injury

Free radicals are chemical species that have a single unpaired electron in an outer orbit. Energy created by this unstable configuration is released through reactions with adjacent molecules, such as inorganic or organic chemicals (proteins, lipids, carbohydrates), particularly with key molecules in membranes and nucleic acids. Moreover, free radicals initiate autocatalytic reactions, whereby molecules with which they react are themselves converted into free radicals to propagate the chain of damage. Absorption of radiant energy such as ultraviolet rays in sunlight can hydrolyse water into hydroxyl (OH) and hydrogen (H) free radicals, which cause sunburn. The free radicals induce cell injury by the following mechanisms:

- **Lipid peroxidation of membranes:** free radicals in the presence of oxygen can cause peroxidation of lipids within plasma and organellar membranes. Oxidative damage is initiated when the double bonds in unsaturated fatty acids of membrane lipids are attacked by oxygen-derived free radicals, particularly by OH. The lipid-free radical interactions yield peroxides, which are themselves unstable and reactive, and an autocatalytic chain reaction ensues (called 'propagation'), which can result in extensive membrane, organellar and cellular damage. Other more favorable termination options take place when the free radical is captured by a scavenger, such as vitamin E, embedded in the cell membrane.

- **Oxidative modification of proteins:** free radicals promote oxidation of amino acid residue side chains, formation of protein–protein cross-linkages (eg disulfide bonds), and oxidation of the protein backbone, resulting in protein fragmentation. Oxidative modification enhances degradation of critical proteins by the multicatalytic proteasome complex, causing havoc throughout the cell.

- **Lesions in DNA:** reactions with thymine in nuclear and mitochondrial DNA produce single-stranded breaks in DNA. This DNA damage has been implicated in cell ageing and in malignant transformation of cells.

## 1.23

*Answer: D*   Liver

Carbon tetrachloride ($CCl_4$) was once used widely in the dry-cleaning industry. The toxic effect of $CCl_4$ results from its conversion by P450 to the highly reactive toxic free radical, $CCl_3$ ($CCl_4 + e = CCl_3 + Cl^-$). The free radicals produced locally cause auto-oxidation of the polyenoic fatty acids present within the membrane phospholipids. There, oxidative decomposition of the lipid is initiated, and organic peroxides are formed after reacting with oxygen (lipid peroxidation). This reaction is autocatalytic in that new radicals are formed from the peroxide radicals themselves. Rapid breakdown of the structure and function of the endoplasmic reticulum is therefore due to decomposition of the lipid. It is no surprise, therefore, that $CCl_4$-induced liver cell injury is both severe and extremely rapid in onset. Within less than 30 minutes there is a decline in hepatic protein synthesis; within 2 hours there is swelling of smooth endoplasmic reticulum and dissociation of ribosomes from the rough endoplasmic reticulum. Lipid export from the hepatocytes is reduced because of their inability to synthesise apoprotein to complex with triglycerides and thereby facilitate lipoprotein secretion. The result is the fatty liver of $CCl_4$ poisoning. Mitochondrial injury then occurs, and this is followed by progressive swelling of the cells due to increased permeability of the plasma membrane. Plasma membrane damage is thought to be caused by relatively stable fatty aldehydes, which are produced by lipid peroxidation in the smooth endoplasmic reticulum but which are able to act at distant sites. This is followed by massive influx of calcium and cell death.

## 1.24

*Answer: E*    Increased unfolded protein response

ATP depletion and decreased ATP synthesis are frequently associated with both hypoxic and chemical (toxic) injury. High-energy phosphate in the form of ATP is required for many synthetic and degradative processes within the cell. These include membrane transport, protein synthesis, lipogenesis, and the deacylation-reacylation reactions necessary for phospholipid turnover. ATP is produced in two ways. The major pathway in mammalian cells is oxidative phosphorylation of adenosine diphosphate, in a reaction that results in reduction of oxygen by the electron transfer system of mitochondria. The second is the glycolytic pathway, which can generate ATP in the absence of oxygen using glucose derived either from body fluids or from the hydrolysis of glycogen. Tissues with greater glycolytic capacity (eg liver) therefore have an advantage when ATP levels are falling because of inhibition of oxidative metabolism by injury.

Depletion of ATP to < 5%–10% of normal levels has widespread effects on many critical cellular systems:

- The activity of the plasma membrane energy-dependent sodium pump (ouabain-sensitive $Na^+$, $K^+$-ATPase) is reduced. Failure of this active transport system, due to diminished ATP concentration and enhanced ATPase activity, causes sodium to accumulate intracellularly and potassium to diffuse out of the cell. The net gain of solute is accompanied by isosmotic gain of water, causing cell swelling, and dilatation of the endoplasmic reticulum.

- Cellular energy metabolism is altered. If the supply of oxygen to cells is reduced, as in ischaemia, oxidative phosphorylation ceases and cells rely on glycolysis for energy production. This switch to anaerobic metabolism is controlled by energy pathway metabolites acting on glycolytic enzymes. The decrease in cellular ATP and associated increase in adenosine monophosphate stimulate phosphofructokinase and phosphorylase activities. These result in an increased rate of anaerobic glycolysis that is designed to maintain the cell's energy sources by generating ATP through metabolism of glucose derived from glycogen. As a consequence, glycogen stores are rapidly depleted. Glycolysis results in the accumulation of lactic acid and inorganic phosphates from the hydrolysis of phosphate esters. This reduces the intracellular pH, resulting in decreased activity of many cellular enzymes.

- Failure of the calcium pump leads to influx of calcium ions, with damaging effects on numerous cellular components.

- With prolonged or worsening depletion of ATP, structural disruption of the protein synthetic apparatus occurs, manifest as detachment of ribosomes from the rough endoplasmic reticulum and dissociation of polysomes into monosomes, with a consequent reduction in protein synthesis. Ultimately, there is irreversible damage to mitochondrial and lysosomal membranes, and the cell undergoes necrosis.

- In cells that are deprived of oxygen or glucose, proteins can become misfolded, and misfolded proteins trigger a cellular reaction called the 'unfolded protein response' that can lead to cell injury and even death. Protein misfolding is also seen in cells exposed to stress, such as heat, and when proteins are damaged by enzymes such as calcium-responsive enzymes and free radicals.

## 1.25

*Answer: D*    Lipofuscin

Lipofuscin is an insoluble pigment, also known as 'lipochrome' and is a wear-and-tear or ageing pigment. Lipofuscin is composed of polymers of lipids and phospholipids complexed with protein, suggesting that it is derived through lipid peroxidation of polyunsaturated lipids of subcellular membranes. Lipofuscin is not injurious to the cell or its functions. Its importance lies in its being the tell-tale sign of free-radical injury and lipid peroxidation. The term is derived from the Latin (*fuscus,* brown), so it is brown lipid. In tissue sections it appears as a yellow-brown, finely granular intracytoplasmic, often perinuclear pigment. It is seen in cells undergoing slow, regressive changes and is particularly prominent in the liver and heart of ageing patients or patients with severe malnutrition and cancer cachexia. On electron microscopy the granules are highly electron-dense, often have membranous structures in their midst, and are usually in a perinuclear location.

## 1.26

*Answer: C*    Malignancy

Complications of wound healing can arise from abnormalities in any of the basic components of the repair process. These aberrations can be grouped into three general categories: (1) deficient scar formation, (2) excessive formation of the repair components, and (3) formation of contractures.

1.  Inadequate formation of granulation tissue or assembly of a scar can lead to two types of complications: wound dehiscence and ulceration. Dehiscence or rupture of a wound is most common after abdominal surgery and is due to increased abdominal pressure. This mechanical stress on the abdominal wound can be generated by vomiting, coughing or ileus. Wounds can ulcerate because of inadequate vascularisation during healing. For example, lower-extremity wounds in individuals with atherosclerotic peripheral vascular disease typically ulcerate. Non-healing wounds also form in areas devoid of sensation. These neuropathic ulcers are occasionally seen in patients with diabetic peripheral neuropathy.

2. Excessive formation of the components of the repair process can also complicate wound healing. Aberrations of growth can occur even in what may begin initially as normal wound healing. The accumulation of excessive amounts of collagen can give rise to a raised scar known as a 'hypertrophic scar'; if the scar tissue grows beyond the boundaries of the original wound and does not regress, it is called a 'keloid'. Keloid formation appears to be an individual predisposition, and for unknown reasons this aberration is somewhat more common in African Americans. The mechanisms of keloid formation are still unknown. Another deviation in wound healing is the formation of excessive amounts of granulation tissue, which protrudes above the level of the surrounding skin and blocks re-epithelialisation. This has been called 'exuberant granulation' (or, with more literary fervour, 'proud flesh'). Excessive granulation must be removed by cautery or surgical excision to permit restoration of the continuity of the epithelium. Finally (fortunately rarely), incisional scars or traumatic injuries can be followed by exuberant proliferation of fibroblasts and other connective tissue elements that can even recur after excision. Called 'desmoids', or 'aggressive fibromatoses', these lie in the interface between benign proliferations and malignant (though low-grade) tumours. The line between the benign hyperplasias characteristic of repair and neoplasia is frequently finely drawn.

3. Contraction in the size of a wound is an important part of the normal healing process. An exaggeration of this process is called a 'contracture' and results in deformities of the wound and the surrounding tissues. Contractures are particularly prone to develop on the palms, the soles, and the anterior aspect of the thorax. Contractures are commonly seen after serious burns and can compromise the movement of joints.

## 1.27

*Answer: D*    Vitamin A deficiency

Healing is modified by a number of known influences and some unknown ones, frequently impairing the quality and adequacy of both inflammation and repair. These influences include both systemic and local host factors.

**Local factors** include the following:

- Blood supply
- Denervation
- Local infection
- Foreign body
- Haematoma
- Mechanical stress
- Necrotic tissue
- Surgical techniques
- Protective dressings
- Type of tissue.

**Systemic factors** include the following:

- Nutrition has profound effects on wound healing. Protein deficiency, for example, and particularly vitamin C deficiency, inhibit collagen synthesis and retard healing. Similarly, deficiency of trace elements such as zinc affects wound healing. Vitamin A deficiency is not a recognised factor that retards wound healing.

- Metabolic status can affect wound healing. Diabetes mellitus, for example, is associated with delayed healing, as a consequence of the microangiopathy that is a frequent feature of this disease.

- Circulatory status can modulate wound healing. Inadequate blood supply, usually caused by arteriosclerosis or venous abnormalities (eg varicose veins) that retard venous drainage, also impairs healing.

- Hormones, such as glucocorticoids, have well-documented anti-inflammatory effects that influence various components of inflammation. These agents also inhibit collagen synthesis.

## 1.28

*Answer:* C    Presence of sutures

Although any foreign body will delay wound healing, the net effect of having sutures is to aid the process of healing more than to hinder it. Secondary wound infection is a serious postoperative complication. Diabetics and people with severe atherosclerosis with poor tissue perfusion have notoriously poor wound healing. Corticosteroids dampen the inflammatory response that contributes to healing. Poor nutrition, leading to hypoalbuminaemia, is a detrimental factor in wound healing (see also *Answer* to **1.27**).

## 1.29

*Answer:* E    Tyrosine kinase

Cell-surface growth-factor receptors recruit intracellular protein kinases such as tyrosine kinase that begin a sequence of events leading to cell division and growth. A tyrosine kinase is an enzyme that can transfer a phosphate group from adenosine triphosphate (ATP) to a tyrosine residue in a protein. Tyrosine kinases are a subgroup of the larger class of protein kinases. Phosphorylation of proteins by kinases is an important mechanism in signal transduction for regulation of enzyme activity.

Fibronectin acts in the extracellular matrix to bind macromolecules (such as proteoglycans) via integrin receptors to aid attachment and migration of cells. Laminin is an extracellular matrix component that is abundant in basement membranes. Hyaluronic acid is one of the proteoglycans in the extracellular matrix. Collagen fibres are part of the extracellular matrix that gives strength and stability to connective tissues.

## 1.30

*Answer: A*   Hageman factor

Hageman factor (factor XII in the intrinsic coagulation pathway) activates factor XI and prekallikrein. It is an enzyme of the serine protease (or serine endopeptidase) class. Hageman factor deficiency is a rare hereditary disorder with a prevalance of about one in a million, although it is a little more common among Asians. Deficiency does not cause excessive haemorrhage as the other coagulation factors make up for the deficiency of factor XII. It can increase the risk of thrombosis due to inadequate activation of the fibrinolytic pathway. The deficiency leads to activated partial thromboplastin times (PTT) greater than 200 seconds.

Thromboxane, a product of the cyclo-oxygenase pathway, promotes vasoconstriction and platelet aggregation. Plasmin, derived from plasminogen, is one of the anticoagulants generated to break down thrombi. Platelet activating factor promotes platelet aggregation and release. It is also chemotactic to neutrophils and causes them also to aggregate and adhere. Histamine functions as a vasodilator of arterioles and increases vascular permeability in venules.

## 1.31

*Answer: B*   Homogeneous, ground-glass, pink-staining
appearance of cells

Hyaline degeneration is a complex series of cellular events. It has a particular appearance microscopically, with its ground-glass, pink-staining appearance and intact cell membrane. The accumulation of lipids, the presence of calcium salts, or an amorphous appearance of the cell, with no discernable membranes (as seen in amyloid) are all distinctly different. The pyknotic nucleus is not a characteristic of hyaline degeneration.

## 1.32

*Answer: A*    A greater number of autophagic vacuoles

Autophagic vacuoles appear to form when breakdown of intracellular components and organelles occurs. Separation of damaged cell substances in the form of autophagic vacuoles appears to be an adaptive response in atrophy.

## 1.33

*Answer: C*    Erythrocyte

The erythrocyte is an end-stage cell that is not capable of futher division and regeneration. Hepatocytes, osteocytes, and acinar cells are stable cells that are capable of some regeneration under certain conditions. Colonic mucosal cells are labile cells.

## 1.34

*Answer: E*    Uterine growth during pregnancy

In uterine growth during pregnancy, both cell proliferation involving the endometrial glands and muscle enlargement of the uterine wall occur. These processes offer models of both hyperplasia and hypertrophy. When both are present, DNA synthesis is markedly accelerated. Hyperplasia is an increase in the number of cells, whereas hypertrophy is an increase in cell size, as is seen in cardiac muscle in response to volume overload or systemic hypertension. Breast tissue enlargement resulting from hormonal influences is due solely to an increase in cell numbers.

## 1.35

*Answer: C*   Coagulative necrosis

The process of necrosis results in the final rupture of the cell and release of its contents into the surrounding media. Cloudy swelling and hydropic change are reversible because the cell membrane remains viable. Pyknosis and apoptosis are nuclear events that are not reversible but in which the cell membrane remains intact and these are therefore distinctly different from coagulative necrosis.

## 1.36

*Answer: D*   Macrophages

Tuberculous granulomas are often called 'tubercles' and consist of round, plump, mononuclear phagocytes, Langhans cells, and epithelioid cells. The enlarged macrophages are called 'epithelioid cells' because of their abundant cytoplasm and their tendency to arrange themselves very closely together, which makes them resemble epithelial cells.

## 1.37

*Answer: C*   Hamartoma

A hamartoma is a conglomeration of tissues that are normal to the area but haphazardly arranged in an abnormal fashion. All of the neoplastic lesions listed contain a mixture of different cell types, but only in the hamartoma are the cells normal to that particular area. These are best regarded as developmental anomalies rather than true neoplasms, and they are never malignant so do not metastasise.

## 1.38

*Answer: C*   Organisation of the haematoma

New capillaries, fibroblasts, and collagen describe granulation tissue occurring at the periphery of a haematoma or collection of blood. Although lysis of the blood clot can occur as a result, the actual formation of this response is known as 'organisation' and is an attempt to heal the area and fill the defect with collagen or scar tissue. If this occurs within a blood vessel, recanalisation of the occluded lumen can take place subsequently and embolisation can be an eventual complication. Thrombosis describes clot formation in the vascular lumen but this has nothing to do with the process described.

## 1.39

*Answer: A* Diapedesis

Diapedesis is the movement of leukocytes across the endothelial lining of blood vessels into the interstitial fluid. The process is driven by chemotactic factors that serve to up-regulate expression of adhesion molecules on the endothelial cells of postcapillary venules adjacent to the site of infection. Neutrophils, monocytes and natural killer (NK) cells use 'roll-to-stop' kinetics in order to slow down and 'ooze through' (diapedesis) interendothelial spaces between endothelial cells and infiltrate the infected tissue.

On recognition of and activation by pathogens, resident macrophages in the infected tissue release cytokines such as interleukin 1 (IL-1), tumour necrosis factor (TNF) and chemokines. IL-1 and TNF cause the endothelial cells of blood vessels close to the site of infection to express adhesion molecules such as integrin receptors and selectin. Like Velcro, selectin ligands on the leukocyte bind selectin molecules on the inner wall of the vessel with marginal affinity in order to slow the leukocyte down near the infected tissue. This causes the leukocyte to slow down and begin rolling on the inner surface of the vessel wall. At the same time, chemokines released by macrophages activate the rolling leukocytes and cause their integrin molecules to switch from the default low-affinity state to a high-affinity state in which they can bind tightly to complementary integrin receptors that have been expressed on the endothelial cells. At this point, the integrin (VLA-4, LFA-1 or Mac-1) on the surface of the leukocytes is now able to produce the 'stopping' effect by binding the integrin receptors (VCAM-1 or ICAM-1) on the inner wall of the vessel with high affinity. This leads to immobilisation of leukocytes and the reorganisation of their cytoskeletons in such a way that they are 'spread out' over the endothelial cells. In this form, they are able to pass between gaps in the vessel's endothelial cells.

Diapedesis usually occurs when an area is injured or damaged and an inflammatory response is needed. This trafficking system is regulated by the background cytokine environment produced by the inflammatory response. In leukocyte adhesion deficiency (LAD) there is defective integrin and this impairs the ability of the leukocytes to stop and undergo diapedesis. Neutrophilia is a hallmark of LAD.

Euperiporesis describes the movement of lymphocytes through the cytoplasm of endothelial cells rather than between the cells. After the injury, neutrophils are attracted to the injured site (chemotaxis) from the blood vessels. The neutrophils marginate or 'pavement' on the inner walls of the vessel and then pass through the widened pores between the endothelial cells in a movement known as 'migration'. Foreign bodies (bacteria, antigen–antibody complexes, tissue debris) are engulfed by the neutrophils (phagocytosis) aided by serum opsonin. The lysosomal granules of the neutrophils empty their hydrolytic enzymes (proteases, esterases) into the phagocytic vacuole for digestion. The undigested residue might be deposited as lipofuscin residual body.

## 1.40

*Answer: E*    Several months

A week after myocardial infarction, little collagen has formed. At the end of 2 weeks, a cellular vascular scar is present, some collagen has been laid down in a disorderly fashion, and the scar has attained some strength. During the next 6 months, collage is laid down and rearranged to make the scar smaller. Most of the blood vessels are pinched off, leading to decreased cellularity in the scar. The end result of these processes is a mature scar. The slow healing of a myocardial infarct is the result of the decreased blood supply.

cell injury

# SECTION 2: INFLAMMATION AND IMMUNOLOGY — ANSWERS

## 2.1

*Answer: D*    Sinus histiocytosis

Sinus histiocytosis, also known as 'reticular hyperplasia' refers to distension and prominence of the lymphatic sinusoids. Although non-specific, this form of hyperplasia can be particularly prominent in lymph nodes draining cancers, such as carcinoma of the breast. The lining lymphatic endothelial cells are markedly hypertrophied, and macrophages are greatly increased in numbers, resulting in expansion and distension of the sinuses. In the setting of cancer, this pattern of reaction has been thought to represent a host immune response against the tumour or its products.

In this vignette there is no evidence that the patient has infection or another malignancy that could account for the enlargement of the lymph nodes. Paracortical lymphoid hyperplasia is caused by stimuli that trigger cellular immune responses. It is characterised by reactive changes within the T-cell regions of the lymph node that encroach on, and sometimes appear to efface, the B-cell follicles. Within interfollicular regions, activated T cells (immunoblasts) are observed. These cells are three to four times the size of resting lymphocytes and have round nuclei, open chromatin, several prominent nucleoli, and moderate amounts of pale cytoplasm. In addition, there is hypertrophy of sinusoidal and vascular endothelial cells and a mixed cellular infiltrate, principally of macrophages and sometimes of eosinophils. Such changes are encountered in immunological reactions induced by drugs (especially phenytoin), in acute viral infections, particularly infectious mononucleosis, and following vaccination against certain viral diseases. In florid reactions, immunoblasts can be so numerous that special studies are needed to exclude a lymphoid neoplasm.

## 2.2

*Answer: D*   Neutrophils

A reduction in the number of granulocytes in the peripheral blood (neutropenia) can be seen in a wide variety of circumstances. A marked reduction in neutrophil count, referred to as 'agranulocytosis', has serious consequences by making individuals susceptible to infections. A reduction in circulating granulocytes will occur if there is (1) reduced or ineffective production of neutrophils, or (2) accelerated removal of neutrophils from the circulating blood.

**Inadequate or ineffective granulopoiesis** is observed in the setting of:

- Suppression of myeloid stem cells, as occurs in aplastic anaemia and a variety of infiltrative marrow disorders (tumours, granulomatous diseases etc.). In these conditions, granulocytopenia is accompanied by anaemia and thrombocytopenia.

- Suppression of committed granulocytic precursors due to exposure to certain drugs (see below).

- Disease states associated with ineffective granulopoiesis, such as megaloblastic anaemias due to vitamin $B_{12}$ or folate deficiency and myelodysplastic syndromes, where defective precursors are susceptible to death in the marrow.

- Rare inherited conditions (such as Kostmann syndrome) in which genetic defects in specific genes result in impaired granulocytic differentiation.

**Accelerated removal or destruction of neutrophils** occurs with:

- Immunologically mediated injury to the neutrophils, which may be idiopathic, associated with a well-defined immunological disorder (such as systemic lupus erythematosus), or produced by exposure to drugs.

inflammation

- Splenic sequestration, in which excessive destruction occurs secondary to enlargement of the spleen, usually associated with increased destruction of red cells and platelets.

- Increased peripheral utilisation, as can occur in overwhelming bacterial, fungal or rickettsial infections.

## 2.3

*Answer: B*    Formation of IgG/IgM antibodies

Type II hypersensitivity is mediated by antibodies (mainly IgG or IgM) directed towards antigens present on cell surfaces or in the extracellular matrix. The antigenic determinants can be intrinsic to the cell membrane or matrix, or they can take the form of an exogenous antigen, such as a drug metabolite, that is adsorbed on a cell surface or matrix. In either case, the hypersensitivity reaction results from the binding of antibodies to normal or altered cell-surface antigens. Clinically, antibody-mediated cell destruction and phagocytosis occur in the following situations: (1) transfusion reactions, in which cells from an incompatible donor react with and are opsonised by preformed antibody in the host; (2) erythroblastosis fetalis, in which there is an antigenic difference between the mother and the fetus, and antibodies (of the IgG class) from the mother cross the placenta and cause destruction of fetal red cells; (3) autoimmune haemolytic anaemia, agranulocytosis, and thrombocytopenia, in which individuals produce antibodies to their own blood cells, which are then destroyed; and (4) certain drug reactions, in which antibodies are produced that react with the drug, which can be attached to the surface of erythrocytes or to other cells.

inflammation

## 2.4

*Answer: E*    Vasodilation

Inflammation is the first response of the immune system to infection or irritation. Inflammation is characterised by the following quintet: redness (*rubor*), heat (*calor*), swelling (*tumur*), pain (*dolor*) and dysfunction of the organs involved (*functio laesa*). The first four characteristics have been known since ancient times and are attributed to Celsus; *functio laesa* was added to the definition of inflammation by Rudolf Virchow in 1858.

Inflammation is not a synonym for infection. Even in cases when it is caused by infection it is incorrect to use the terms as synonyms — infection is caused by an outside agent, while inflammation is the body's response.

Inflammation has two main components, vascular (exudative) and cellular. The exudative component involves the movement of fluid, usually containing many important proteins such as fibrin and immunoglobulins (antibodies). Blood vessels are dilated upstream of an inflamed area (causing redness and heat) and constricted downstream, while capillary permeability to the affected tissue is increased, resulting in a net loss of blood plasma into the tissue, giving rise to oedema or swelling. The swelling distends the tissues, compresses nerve endings, and so causes pain.

The cellular component involves the movement of white blood cells from blood vessels into the inflamed tissue. The white blood cells, or leukocytes, take on an important role in inflammation: they extravasate (filter out) from the capillaries into tissue, and act as phagocytes, picking up bacteria and cellular debris. They may also aid by walling off an infection and preventing its spread.

If inflammation of the affected site persists, released cytokines, interleukin-1 (IL-1) and tumour necrosis factor (TNF) will activate endothelial cells to up-regulate receptors VCAM-1, ICAM-1, E-selectin, and L-selectin for various immune cells. Receptor up-regulation increases extravasation of neutrophils, monocytes, activated T-helper and T-cytotoxic cells, and memory T and B cells to the inflamed site.

Neutrophils are characteristic of inflammation in the early stages. They are the first cells to appear in an infected area, and any section

inflammation

of recently inflamed tissue (within a couple of days or so) viewed under a microscope will appear packed with them. They are easily identified by their multilobed nuclei and granular cytoplasm and perform many important functions, including phagocytosis and the release of extracellular chemical messengers. Neutrophils only live for a couple of days in these interstitial areas, so if the inflammation persists for any longer they are gradually replaced by longer-lived monocytes.

## 2.5

*Answer: B*    Leukocyte adhesion

ICAM-1 (intercellular adhesion molecule-1) is continuously present in low concentrations in the membranes of leukocytes and endothelial cells. On cytokine stimulation, the concentrations greatly increase. ICAM-1 can be induced by interleukin-1 (IL-1) and tumour necrosis factor alpha (TNF-$\alpha$) and is expressed by the vascular endothelium, macrophages and lymphocytes. ICAM-1 has been implicated in subarachnoid haemorrhage (SAH). Levels of ICAM-1 are shown to be significantly elevated in patients with SAH compared with control subjects in many studies. While ICAM-1 has not been shown to be directly correlated with cerebral vasospasm, a secondary insult which affects 70% of SAH patients, treatment with anti-ICAM-1 has been found to reduce the severity of vasospasm.

VCAM-1 (vascular cell adhesion molecule-1), also known as 'CD106', is a molecule with a considerable role in the human immune system. It contains six or seven immunoglobulin domains, and is expressed on both large and small vessels only after the endothelial cells are stimulated by cytokines. Up-regulation of VCAM-1 in endothelial cells by cytokines occurs as a result of increased gene transcription (eg in response to TNF-$\alpha$ and IL-1) and through stabilisation of mRNA (eg in response to IL-4). The promoter region of the *VCAM-1* gene contains functional tandem NF-$\kappa$B sites. The sustained expression of VCAM-1 lasts over 24 hours. Primarily, VCAM-1 is an endothelial ligand for VLA-4 (very late antigen-1 or $\alpha4\beta1$) of the $\beta1$ subfamily of integrins, and for integrin $\alpha4\beta7$. VCAM-1 expression has also been observed in other cell types (eg smooth muscle cells). VCAM-1 promotes the adhesion of lymphocytes, monocytes, eosinophils and basophils. Interestingly, certain melanoma cells can use VCAM-

1 to adhere to the endothelium, and VCAM-1 might participate in monocyte recruitment to atherosclerotic sites. As a result, VCAM-1 is a potential drug target.

## 2.6

*Answer:* C    Release of histamine from mast cells

Skin allergy testing is a method used for medical diagnosis of allergies. A microscopic amount of an allergen is introduced to a patient's skin by:

- pricking the skin with a needle or pin containing a small amount of the allergen ('prick testing' or 'scratch testing'); or by

- applying a patch to the skin, where the patch contains the allergen.

If an immune response is seen in the form of a rash, hives, urticaria or, much worse, anaphylaxis, it can be concluded that the patient has a hypersensitivity (or allergy) to that allergen. Further testing can be performed in order to identify the particular allergen. Release of histamine from mast cells produces the characteristic response in a skin test.

## 2.7

*Answer:* A    Activation of tyrosine kinase

Platelet-derived growth factor (PDGF) is one of the numerous growth factors, or proteins that regulate cell growth and division. In particular, it plays a significant role in angiogenesis, the growth of blood vessels from already existing blood vessel tissue. Uncontrolled angiogenesis is a characteristic of cancer. PDGF also plays a role in embryonic development, cell proliferation and cell migration. PDGF has also been linked to several diseases, including atherosclerosis, fibrosis and malignant diseases.

In addition, PDGF has demonstrated that not only is it a cell proliferator, but a required element in cellular division for fibroblasts. Specifically, fibroblasts have PDGF receptors on their plasma membranes that allow for their signal transductions from PDGFs. These plasma membrane receptors are called 'tyrosine kinases' and allow the signal transduction and inevitably the cell division stimulation to occur. In essence, the PDGFs allow a cell to skip the G1 checkpoints in order to divide.

## 2.8

*Answer: D*    Type III hypersensitivity

In type III hypersensitivity, soluble immune complexes (aggregations of antigens and IgG and IgM antibodies) form in the blood and are deposited in various tissues (typically the skin, kidney and joints), where they can trigger an immune response according to the classical pathway of complement activation. The reaction takes hours to days to develop. Some clinical examples include:

- Immune-complex glomerulonephritis

- Rheumatoid arthritis

- Serum sickness

- Subacute bacterial endocarditis

- Systemic lupus erythematosus

- Arthus reaction.

## 2.9

*Answer: B*    Type I hypersensitivity

Immediate, or type I hypersensitivity is a rapidly developing immunological reaction that occurs within minutes after the combination of an antigen with antibody bound to mast cells in individuals previously sensitised to the antigen. These reactions are often called 'allergy', and the antigens that elicit them are 'allergens'. Immediate hypersensitivity can occur as a systemic disorder or as a local reaction. The systemic reaction usually follows injection of an antigen to which the host has become sensitised. Often within minutes, a state of shock is produced, which is sometimes fatal. The nature of local reactions varies depending on the portal of

*inflammation*

entry of the allergen, and can take the form of localised cutaneous swellings (skin allergy, hives), nasal and conjunctival discharge (allergic rhinitis and conjunctivitis), hay fever, bronchial asthma or allergic gastroenteritis (food allergy).

Many local type I hypersensitivity reactions have two well-defined phases. The immediate, or initial response is characterised by vasodilation, vascular leakage and, depending on the location, smooth muscle spasm or glandular secretions. These changes usually become evident within 5–30 minutes after exposure to an allergen and tend to subside in 60 minutes. In many instances (eg allergic rhinitis, bronchial asthma), a second, late-phase reaction sets in, 2–24 hours later without additional exposure to antigen and can last for several days. This late-phase reaction is characterised by infiltration of tissues with eosinophils, neutrophils, basophils, monocytes and CD4+ Tcells, as well as tissue destruction, typically in the form of mucosal epithelial cell damage.

## 2.10

*Answer:* C    Type II hypersensitivity

In type II hypersensitivity the antibodies produced by the immune response bind to antigens on the patient's own cell surfaces. The antigens recognised in this way can either be intrinsic ('self' antigen, innately part of the patient's cells) or extrinsic (absorbed onto the cells during exposure to some foreign antigen, possibly as part of an infection with a pathogen, or a drug metabolite). Type II hypersensitivity diseases are mediated by:

- Opsonisation and phagocytosis of cells (antibody-dependent cell-mediated cytotoxicity). Opsonisation and phagocytosis of target cells in type II hypersensitivity occurs through the same mechanisms that are involved in the phagocytosis and destruction of micro-organisms. The process begins when target cells are coated with molecules such as IgG antibodies and activated complement protein, C3b (opsonisation). The phagocyte Fc receptor that is specific for heavy chains of IgG antibody and the C3b receptor then facilitate binding of the phagocyte to the target cell.

inflammation

This mechanism is responsible for the destruction of red blood cells in autoimmune haemolytic anaemia.

- Complement and Fc receptor-mediated inflammation and tissue damage. Activation of complement stimulates the release of complement peptides (C3a and C5a), which induce inflammation by binding to mast cells and inducing degranulation. C5a also stimulates the recruitment and activation of neutrophils, can directly cause increased permeability of vascular endothelial cells, and can promote neutrophil binding.

- Inappropriate hindering or stimulating of normal cellular processes. This mechanism does not involve tissue damage but occurs when IgG antibody acts as an analogue by binding to cell-surface receptors for hormones or neurotransmitters. This binding can cause non-specific stimulation of a cellular process or can inhibit a process by preventing normal ligand binding to the receptor. An example of this type of interference is seen in a form of insulin-resistant diabetes, where autoantibody bound to the insulin receptor initially mimics insulin activity but after prolonged exposure induces insulin resistance.

Some examples of type II hypersensitivity include:

- Autoimmune haemolytic anaemia
- Goodpasture syndrome
- Erythroblastosis fetalis
- Pemphigus
- Pernicious anaemia
- Immune thrombocytopenia
- Transfusion reactions
- Hashimoto's thyroiditis
- Graves' disease
- Myasthenia gravis

inflammation

- Farmer's lung

- Rheumatic fever

- Haemolytic disease of the newborn.

(See also *Answer* to **2.3**).

## 2.11

*Answer:* C    Gamma interferon

Interferon-gamma (IFN-γ) is the only member of the type II class of interferons. It is a dimerised soluble cytokine that was originally called 'macrophage-activating factor'. In human beings, the gene which codes for IFN-γ is located on chromosome 12. It is produced by a variety of immune cells. These include: T-helper cells, 0 and 1 types (CD4); cells with immunological memory (CD45PA); T-killer cells (CD8); natural killer (NK) cells (CD16, CD56); dendrite cells (CD23, CD35); and B lymphocytes (CD22, CD23). During secretion, IFN-γ influences the secreting cells (as well as the surrounding cells) through IFN-γ receptors. The first necessary step in the functioning of IFN-γ is the interaction of IFN-γ with receptors located on the surface of the cells. IFN-γ can stimulate defending or pathological effects. It can induce the differentiation process of myeloid cells in bone marrow, forming cells with high-affinity Fcγ receptors, which combine with IgG monomers. In contrast, in mature granulocytes, IFN-γ induces the expression of medium-affinity Fcγ receptors, which combine with only the aggregated IgG. IFN-γ also activates the antibody-dependent cytotoxins, implemented by the matured granulocytes.

IFN-γ activates macrophages and thus increases their anti-tumour activities. If the macrophages are infected by intracellular parasites, it activates macrophages which in turn destroy the parasites. Suppression of intracellular parasites under the influence of IFN-γ takes place in non-macrophage cells as well.

IFN-γ reinforces the anti-tumour activities of the cytotoxic lymphocytes. Together with lymphotoxins CD4 or CD8, produced by lymphocytes, it suppresses the growth of the tumour cells. IFN-γ induces expression of the receptors of lymphotoxins by acting in the nucleus of the target cells. It increases the non-specific activities of

NK cells. It is one of the factors that controls the differentiation of B cells. It can either increase or decrease B-cell immune responses. In the late stages, for example, IFN-γ increases the secretion of immunoglobins.

IFN-γ plays an very important role in increasing the expression of HLA class I and II molecules on the cell membranes. Moreover, IFN-γ induces the expresion of HLA-DR and HLA-DP molecules more quickly than the expression of HLA-DQ molecules. If the expression of HLA class I and II molecules on the pathological cells takes place more vigorously, then they become more readily recognised for the destructive process.

In the case of viral infections, IFN-γ can cause considerable changes on the surface of cell membrane which inhibit the adhesion and penetration of virus into the cells. IFN-γ promotes the synthesis of oligoadenylate synthetase in cells. The polymers of oligoadenylate activate the endogenous endonucleases, which promote the destruction of mRNA and rRNA, disturbing the intracellular synthesis in viral cells. IFN-γ also promotes the formation of ferment-proteinkinases, resulting in a decrease in protein synthesis. IFN-γ also activates osteoclasts, increasing the resorption of bone-tissue.

## 2.12

*Answer: E*    Prostaglandin and bradykinin

Prostaglandin and bradykinin production is associated with pain. Bradykinin, a product of the kinin-kallikrein system, is a physiologically and pharmacologically active peptide of the kinin group of proteins. It is composed of nine amino acids. It is produced by proteolytic cleavage of its kininogen precursor, high-molecular weight kininogen (HMWK), by the enzyme kallikrein. Bradykinin is a potent endothelium-dependent vasodilator, causes contraction of non-vascular smooth muscle, increases vascular permeability, and also is involved in the mechanism of pain. In some aspects, it has similar actions to those of histamine and, like histamine, is released from venules rather than from arterioles.

Bradykinin raises internal calcium levels in neocortical astrocytes, causing them to release glutamate. Bradykinin is also thought to be the cause of the dry cough experienced by some patients who are on angiotensin-converting enzyme (ACE) inhibitor drugs. This refractory cough is a common cause for stopping ACE-inhibitor therapy.

Aspirin, by inhibiting the cyclo-oxygenase pathway, can decrease prostaglandin synthesis. Complement C3b and IgG can act as opsonins. Interleukin-1 and tumour necrosis factor cause fever. Histamine and serotonin are vasodilators. Leukotriene and HPETE are products of the lipo-oxygenase pathway and promote chemotaxis.

## 2.13

*Answer: B*   Giant cell

The glass fragment is a foreign material and produces a foreign body reaction characterised by giant cells. Mast cells are not numerous in tissues and do not proliferate significantly as part of a foreign body inflammatory response. Eosinophils are typical of parasitic and allergic inflammatory responses, not of inflammatory responses to foreign bodies. A few neutrophils might be present, but giant cells are more specific for a foreign body inflammatory response. Plasma cells are more typical of chronic inflammation.

## 2.14

*Answer: A*   Hydrogen peroxide

Hydrogen peroxide is reduced by myeloperoxidase to form a powerful oxidant that kills bacteria. In chronic granulomatous disease, this system is not operative against many bacterial species. Platelet-activating factor leads to leukocyte aggregation, adhesion, and chemotaxis, but does not directly facilitate bacterial destruction. Prostaglandins potentiate vasodilation, but not neutrophil function. Kallikrein is released from neutrophil lysosomes and promotes bradykinin formation, leading to vasodilation. Leukotrienes promote vascular permeability, but not leukocyte function.

## 2.15

*Answer: E*    Release of growth factors by macrophages

This patient has developed interstitial lung disease over the course of several years. Growth factors are released from macrophages that have ingested silica crystals and these factors stimulate collagen production by fibroblasts. Leukotrienes are more important mediators in acute inflammation, leading to chemotaxis and increased vascular permeability, among other functions. Foreign body giant cells are not a significant feature of silicosis. Plasma cell proliferation is not a key feature of silicosis or of other pneumoconioses. Histamine release by mast cells is an acute inflammatory response.

## 2.16

*Answer: A*    Acute inflammation

The short course of 1 day and the purulent exudate are typical features of acute inflammation. The acute inflammatory response has three main functions:

- The affected area is occupied by a transient material called the 'acute inflammatory exudate'. The exudate carries proteins, fluid and cells from local blood vessels into the damaged area to mediate local defences.

- If an infective causative agent (eg bacteria) is present in the damaged area, it can be destroyed and eliminated by components of the exudate.

- The damaged tissue can be broken down and partially liquefied, and the debris removed from the site of damage.

Acute inflammation can result from physical damage, chemical substances, micro-organisms, or other agents. The inflammatory response consists of changes in blood flow, increased permeability of blood vessels, and escape of cells from the blood into the tissues. The changes are essentially the same whatever the cause and wherever the site.

Acute inflammation is short-lived, lasting only a few days. If inflammation lasts longer than this, it is referred to as 'chronic

inflammation

inflammation'. Examples of acute inflammation include sore throat, reactions in the skin to a scratch or a burn or insect bite, and acute hepatitis.

Granulomatous inflammation typically pursues a course lasting months to years. An abscess usually takes a bit longer to form than 1 day, and the purulent inflammation is localised to an abscess cavity. With resolution, the purulent exudate should be gone, and the course would probably be longer. Chronic inflammation pursues a course of weeks, and purulent exudate is not typical.

## 2.17

*Answer:* C    Macrophage

Epithelioid cells and giant cells are derived from macrophages and are important in the development of granulomatous inflammation, as seen in this patient with tuberculosis. The tuberculous granuloma (caseating tubercle) has central caseous necrosis bordered by giant multinucleated cells (Langhans cells), and surrounded by epithelioid cell aggregates, lymphocytes and fibroblasts. Granulomatous tubercles tend to become confluent. Multinucleated giant cells (mature, Langerhans-type) are 50–100 μm in diameter, with numerous small nuclei (over 20) lying peripherally in the cell (in a crown or horseshoe distribution). They have abundant eosinophilic cytoplasm. They are formed when activated macrophages merge. Epithelioid cells are activated macrophages that resemble epithelial cells. They are elongated, with finely granular, pale eosinophilic (pink) cytoplasm and a central, ovoid nucleus. They have indistinct shape and contour and form aggregates. At the periphery of the tubercle are the lymphocytes (T-cells) and rare plasma cells and fibroblasts. Caseous necrosis is a central area, amorphous, finely granular, and eosinophilic. If recent, it can contain nuclear fragments. The caseous material is the result of the accumulated destruction of giant cells and epithelioid cells.

Fibroblasts lay down collagen. Although collagen is laid down around a granuloma as part of the response, it is not the major component involved in granuloma formation. Although some neutrophils might be present in a granuloma, they are not the major contributors to granuloma formation. Mast cells are few in number. They are

inflammation

involved in the release of mediators that are primarily involved in acute inflammatory responses. Platelets are mainly involved in coagulation.

## 2.18

*Answer: B*    Complement C5a

C5a is a protein fragment released from complement component C5. It is chemotactic for neutrophils similar to tumour necrosis factor (TNF), leukotrienes, and bacterial products. In humans, the polypeptide contains 74 amino acids but is rapidly metabolised by a serum enzyme, carboxypeptidase B to a 73-amino-acid form, C5a des-Arg. C5a is an anaphylatoxin and causes the release of histamine from mast cells. C5a des-Arg is a much less potent anaphylatoxin. However, both forms are effective leukocyte chemoattractants, causing the accumulation of white blood cells, especially neutrophil granulocytes, at sites of complement activation.

C5a binds to a receptor protein on the surface of target cells, C5aR or CD88. This is a member of the G-protein-coupled receptor superfamily of proteins, predicted to have seven transmembrane helical domains of largely hydrophobic amino acid residues, forming three intracellular and three extracellular loops, with an extracellular N-terminus and an intracellular C-terminus. C5a binding to the receptor is a two-stage process: an interaction between basic residues in the helical core of C5a and acidic residues in the extracellular N-terminal domain allows the C-terminus of C5a to bind to residues in the receptor transmembrane domains. The latter interaction leads to receptor activation, and the transduction of the ligand binding signal across the cell plasma membrane to a cytoplasmic G protein.

Histamine increases vascular permeability and promotes vasodilation. Prostaglandin is more important as a mediator of inflammation in producing pain, vascular permeability, and vasodilation. Hageman factor is factor XII of the coagulation sequence and is activated by contact with collagen and basement membrane in damaged tissues. Bradykinin, a product of the kinin system and derived from high-molecular-weight kininogen, causes pain and promotes vasodilation and vascular permeability.

inflammation

**2.19**

*Answer: E*   Prostaglandin-mediated vasodilation

Prostaglandins are pain mediators produced via the cyclo-oxygenase pathway of arachidonic acid metabolism. Aspirin and non-steroidal anti-inflammatory drugs block the synthesis of prostaglandins, which can reduce pain. Aspirin suppresses the production of prostaglandins and thromboxanes through non-competitive and irreversible inhibition of the cyclo-oxygenase (COX) enzyme. Cyclo-oxygenase is required for prostaglandin and thromboxane synthesis. Aspirin acts as an acetylating agent, where an acetyl group is covalently attached to a serine residue in the active site of the COX enzyme. This makes aspirin different from other non-steroidal anti-inflammatory drugs (NSAIDs) such as diclofenac and ibuprofen, which are reversible inhibitors.

Prostaglandins are local hormones (paracrine) produced in the body and have diverse effects in the body, including but not limited to transmission of pain information to the brain, modulation of the hypothalamic thermostat, and inflammation. Thromboxanes are responsible for the aggregation of platelets and aspirin prevents platelet aggregation by blocking the synthesis of thromboxanes.

Aspirin has two additional modes of action, contributing to its strong analgesic, antipyretic and anti-inflammatory properties:

- It uncouples oxidative phosphorylation in cartilaginous (and hepatic) mitochondria, by diffusing from the inner membrane space as a proton carrier back into the mitochondrial matrix, where it ionises once again to release protons. In short, aspirin buffers and transports the protons. (Note that this effect in high doses of aspirin actually causes fever due to the heat released from the electron transport chain, in contrast to its normal antipyretic action).

- It induces the formation of NO-radicals in the body that enable the white blood cells (leukocytes) to fight infections more effectively.

More recent data suggest that salicylic acid and its derivatives will modulate NF-κB signalling. NF-κB is a transcription factor complex that plays a central role in many biological processes, including inflammation.

inflammation

Leukotriene B4 is generated through the lipo-oxygenase pathway of arachidonic acid metabolites, which is not affected by aspirin. Interleukin-1 is a cytokine that is not part of the arachidonic acid metabolic pathway. Aspirin has no direct effect on bradykinin generation. Aspirin does not affect Hageman factor. The anticoagulant effect of aspirin occurs through its action on platelets.

## 2.20

*Answer: A*  Complement C3b

The C3b is a protein fragment released from complement component C3. It serves as an effective opsonin. Soluble C3-convertase, also known as 'iC3Bb', catalyses the proteolytic cleavage of C3 complement component into C3a and C3b as part of the alternative complement system. C3b can then bind to microbial cell surfaces within an organism's body. This can lead to the production of surface-bound C3 convertase and so more C3b components. Also known as 'C3bBb', this convertase is similar to soluble C3-convertase, except that it is membrane bound. Alternatively, bound C3b can help in the opsonisation of the microbe by macrophages. Complement receptor-1 (CR1) on macrophages allows the engaging of C3b-covered microbes.

Glutathione peroxidase does not act as an opsonin, but is involved in scavenging free radicals. IgM does not act as an opsonin, although IgG does. Selectins aid in the initial binding of leukocytes to endothelial surfaces. NADPH oxidase in leukocytes aids in the killing of phagocytosed microbes.

## 2.21

*Answer: D*  Localised anaphylaxis

A food allergy is an allergic (type I hypersensitivity) reaction to a particular food. Food allergies are typically seen in 6%–8% of children and 2% of adults. Many different foods can cause allergic reactions. However, food allergies are most commonly triggered by certain nuts, peanuts, shellfish, fish, milk, eggs, wheat, and soybeans. Allergic reactions to food may be severe and sometimes include an

inflammation

anaphylactic reaction. There is currently no cure for food allergies. Treatment consists of avoidance diets, where the allergic person avoids any and all forms of the food to which they are allergic. For people who are extremely sensitive, this can involve the total avoidance of any exposure with the allergen, including touching or inhaling the problematic food as well as any surfaces that may have come into contact with it. Food allergy is distinct from food intolerance, which is not caused by an immune reaction.

Cell-mediation is a feature of type IV hypersensitivity. Release of complement C3b is a feature of type III hypersensitivity. Plasma cells are not involved in this clinical setting. Localised immune complexes occur in an Arthus reaction with type III hypersensitivity. Systemic immune complex deposition can occur in diseases such as systemic lupus erythematosus.

## 2.22

*Answer: A*    Antinuclear antibody test

These non-specific findings, put together, suggest the possibility of autoimmune disease. An antinuclear antibody (ANA) test is a good way to begin the investigations, then more specific tests can be ordered. The ANA test measures the pattern and amount of autoantibody, which can attack the body's tissues as if they were foreign material. Everyone has a small amount of autoantibody but in about 5% of the population this is raised, and about half of this 5% have an autoimmune disease. The test is used to aid in the diagnosis of systemic lupus erythematosus and drug-induced lupus, but may also be positive in cases of scleroderma, Sjögren's syndrome, Raynaud's disease, juvenile chronic arthritis, rheumatoid arthritis, antiphospholipid antibody syndrome, autoimmune hepatitis, and many other autoimmune and non-autoimmune diseases. A thorough medical history, physical examination and other tests are needed to confirm the presence of a suspected autoimmune disease.

The findings given in the scenario are non-specific and do not point to a septicaemia. A decreased CD4 lymphocyte count is more typical of AIDS (an immune deficiency) than of an immunologically mediated disease process such as systemic lupus erythematosus. Creatine phosphokinase (CPK) is more useful for diagnosis of acute

inflammation

disease (it is raised after myocardial infarction). CPK can be increased with myositis, but with the multiple manifestations in this patient, it is not the best screening test. The sedimentation rate is a very non-specific test that is elevated in many inflammatory conditions. The history here points more to an immunological disease.

## 2.23

*Answer: E*    X-linked agammaglobulinaemia

Recurrent bacterial infections suggest a lack of B-cell immune function, with lack of gamma globulin production. Once maternal antibody is gone, the disease manifests more severely. X-linked agammaglobulinaemia (also known as 'X-linked hypogammaglobulinaemia', 'XLA' or 'Bruton-type agammaglobulinaemia') is a rare X-linked genetic disorder that affects the body's ability to fight infection. XLA is classified with other inherited defects of the immune system in a group of disorders known as primary immunodeficiency disorders.

It results from mutations in a gene on the X chromosome that encodes the Bruton tyrosine kinase (Btk). Btk is essential for B-cell development and maturation; without it, there are no B-cells and no antibodies. People with XLA do not generate mature B-cells that are capable of manufacturing immunoglobulins.

Patients with untreated XLA are prone to develop serious and even fatal infections. Patients typically present in early childhood with recurrent infections, particularly with extracellular, encapsulated bacteria. XLA is an X-linked disorder, and therefore is almost always limited to males, with a frequency of about 1 in 100,000 male newborns, and shows no ethnic predisposition. XLA is treated by infusion of human gamma globulins. Treatment with pooled gamma globulins cannot restore a functional population of B-cells, but it is sufficient to reduce the severity and number of infections due to the passive immunity afforded by the exogenous antibodies.

Acute leukaemias can result in immune deficiency, but not so selective and not typically in infancy. DiGeorge syndrome is predominantly the result of a loss of T-cell function. This is pronounced in complete DiGeorge syndrome, but less severe in partial DiGeorge syndrome.

inflammation

There are often congenital anomalies. Epstein–Barr virus infection does not lead to immunodeficiency states. A selective IgA deficiency is seen in about 1 in 600 people and leads to mild diarrhoea and/or occasional respiratory tract infections, but is not life-threatening.

## 2.24

*Answer: C*    CD4 lymphocyte activation

The human leukocyte antigen (HLA) system, the major histocompatibility complex (MHC) in humans, is located on chromosome 6. It encodes cell surface molecules specialized to present antigenic peptides to the T-cell receptor (TCR) on T-cells. MHC molecules which present antigen are divided into 2 major classes: Class I and Class II. HLA were originally defined as cell-surface antigens that mediate graft-versus-host disease, which results in the rejection of tissue transplants in HLA mismatched donors. Identification of these antigens has led to greater success and longevity in organ transplant patients.

Class II HLA antigens are part of the process of CD4 lymphocyte activation. HLA-DR is a major histocompatibility complex, class II, cell surface receptor encoded by the human leukocyte antigen complex on chromosome 6, region 6p21.31. Receptor is frequently found with ligand, a peptide that is nine amino acids in length or longer, within the binding groove. The receptor/peptide complex is a ligand for the TCR. HLA-DR is also involved in several autoimmune conditions, disease susceptibility and disease resistance. It is also closely linked to HLA-DQ and this linkage often makes it difficult to elucidate the principle causative factor in diseases.

Amyloidosis is a complication of chronic inflammation that has lasted for many years or of multiple myeloma. Cell lysis by CD8 lymphocytes is a function of class I antigen recognition. Graft-versus-host disease is not a consequence of renal transplantation, and few if any donor lymphocytes are present in the allograft. Serum sickness is caused by antigen–antibody complexes.

## 2.25

*Answer:* C   Liver flukes

Parasitic infestations can be accompanied by a type I hypersensitivity reaction. Amyloid deposition does not result in an immune response. Some organic dusts can lead to a localised type III reaction. Natural immune mechanisms directed against neoplasia are not generally effective. Both cell-mediated and humoral immune mechanisms play a role in syphilis, but not specifically a type I hypersensitivity reaction.

## 2.26

*Answer:* E   Type IV hypersensitivity

Granuloma formation with reactivation or reinfection tuberculosis in an adult is a classic type IV hypersensitivity reaction. Type IV hypersensitivity is often called 'delayed-type hypersensitivity' because the reaction takes 2–3 days to develop. Unlike the other types, it is not antibody-mediated, but rather is a type of cell-mediated response. CD8 cytotoxic T-cells and CD4 helper T-cells recognise antigen in a complex with either type I or type II major histocompatibility complex. The antigen-presenting cells in this case are macrophages and they release interleukin-1, which stimulates the proliferation of further CD4 cells. These cells release interleukin-2 and interferon-gamma, further inducing the release of other type I cytokines, thus mediating the immune response. Activated CD8 cells destroy target cells on contact, while activated macrophages produce hydrolytic enzymes and, on presentation with certain intracellular pathogens, transform into multinucleated giant cells.

Graft-versus-host disease does not produce a granulomatous reaction. Granulomatous reactions are based mainly on cell-mediated immunity. Type I reactions are associated with allergy and anaphylaxis. Type II reactions are associated with complement-mediated immune reactions.

inflammation

## 2.27

*Answer: D*   It is an appetite suppressant

Tumour necrosis factor (TNF), which used to be known as 'tumour necrosis factor alpha', is a cytokine involved in systemic inflammation and is a member of a group of cytokines that all stimulate the acute phase reaction. TNF causes apoptotic cell death, cellular proliferation, differentiation, inflammation, tumorigenesis, and viral replication. TNF's primary role is in the regulation of immune cells. Dysregulation and, in particular, overproduction of TNF have been implicated in a variety of human diseases, including cancer.

TNF is primarily produced as a 212-amino-acid-long type II transmembrane protein, arranged in stable homotrimers. From this membrane-integrated form the soluble homotrimeric cytokine (sTNF) is released via proteolytic cleavage by the metalloprotease TNF-alpha-converting enzyme (TACE). The soluble 51-kDa trimeric sTNF tends to dissociate at concentrations below the nanomolar range, thereby losing its bioactivity.

The 17-kDa TNF protomers (185 amino acids long) are composed of two antiparallel β-pleated sheets with antiparallel β-strands, forming a Swiss roll β-structure, typical of the TNF family, but also found in viral capsid proteins.

TNF is mainly produced by macrophages, but also by a wide variety of other cell types, including lymphoid cells, mast cells, endothelial cells, cardiac myocytes, fibroblasts and neuronal tissue. Large amounts of sTNF are released in response to lipopolysaccharides, other bacterial products, and interleukin-1 (IL-1).

TNF has a number of actions on various organ systems, generally together with IL-1 and IL-6:

- Effects on the hypothalamus:
  - o  stimulates the hypothalamic-pituitary-adrenal axis by stimulating the release of corticotrophin-releasing hormone (CRH)
  - o  suppresses appetite
  - o  causes fever.

- Effects on the liver:

  o stimulates the acute phase response, leading to an increase in C-reactive protein and a number of other mediators

  o induces insulin resistance by promoting serine-phosphorylation of insulin receptor substrate-1 (IRS-1), which impairs insulin signalling.

- Effects on neutrophils:

  o attracts neutrophils very potently, helping them to stick to the endothelial cells for migration.

- Effects on macrophages:

  o stimulates phagocytosis and production of IL-1 oxidants and the inflammatory lipid, prostaglandin E2 ($PGE_2$).

- Effects on other tissues:

  o increases insulin resistance.

A locally increasing concentration of TNF will cause the cardinal signs of inflammation to occur: heat, swelling, redness and pain. High concentrations of TNF induce shock-like symptoms, whereas prolonged exposure to low concentrations of TNF can result in cachexia, a wasting syndrome. This can be found for example in patients with cancer.

## 2.28

*Answer: A*    It increases the expression of adhesion factors on endothelial cells

Interleukin-1 (IL-1) actually composed of two distinct proteins, IL-1α and IL-1β, is one of the first cytokines ever described. Its initial discovery was as a factor that could induce fever, control lymphocytes, increase the number of bone marrow cells and cause degeneration of bone joints. It is also known as 'endogenous pyrogen', 'lymphocyte-activating factor', 'haemopoetin-1' and 'mononuclear cell factor'. Both, IL-1α and IL-1β, belong to a family of cytokines known as the 'interleukin-1 superfamily'.

inflammation

The original members of the IL-1 superfamily are IL-1α, IL-1β and the IL-1 receptor antagonist (IL-1RA). IL-1α and IL-β are pro-inflammatory cytokines involved in immune defence against infection. IL-1RA is a molecule that competes for receptor binding with IL-1α and IL-1β, blocking their role in immune activation. Both IL-1α and IL-1β are produced by macrophages, monocytes and dendritic cells. They form an important part of the inflammatory response of the body against infection. These cytokines increase the expression of adhesion factors on endothelial cells, enabling transmigration of leukocytes to sites of infection and re-set the hypothalamic thermoregulatory centre, leading to an increased body temperature which expresses itself as fever. IL-1 is therefore called an 'endogenous pyrogen'. The increased body temperature helps the body's immune system to fight infection. IL-1 is also important in the regulation of haematopoiesis.

IL-1α and IL-1β are produced as precursor peptides which are then processed to release a shorter, active molecule, which is the 'mature' protein. Mature IL-1β, for instance, is released from Pro-IL-1β following cleavage by a member of the caspase family of proteins (caspase-1) or by the interleukin-1-converting enzyme (ICE). The three-dimensional structure of the mature forms of each member of the human IL-1 superfamily is composed of 12 to 14 β strands, producing a barrel-shaped protein.

## 2.29

*Answer: A*  It binds to a cytosolic protein (cyclophilin) of immunocompetent lymphocytes

Ciclosporin is an immunosuppressant drug that is widely used after allogeneic organ transplantation to reduce the activity of the patient's immune system and so the risk of organ rejection. It has been studied in transplants of skin, heart, kidney, lung, pancreas, bone marrow and small intestine. Ciclosporin is a cyclic nonribosomal peptide of 11 amino acids (an undecapeptide) produced by the fungus *Tolypocladium inflatum Gams* and was initially isolated from a Norwegian soil sample.

Ciclosporin is thought to bind to the cytosolic protein, cyclophilin (immunophilin) of immunocompetent lymphocytes, especially

inflammation

T lymphocytes. This complex of ciclosporin and cyclophylin inhibits calcineurin, which under normal circumstances is responsible for activating the transcription of interleukin-2. It also inhibits lymphokine production and interleukin release and therefore leads to a reduced function of effector T cells. It does not affect cytostatic activity. It also has an effect on mitochondria. Ciclosporin A prevents the mitochondrial permeability transition pore from opening, thus inhibiting cytochrome c release, a potent apoptotic stimulation factor. However, this is not the primary mode of action for clinical use but rather an important effect for the purposes of research on apoptosis.

Apart from its use in transplant medicine, ciclosporin is also used in psoriasis and infrequently in rheumatoid arthritis and related diseases, although it is only used in severe cases. It has been investigated for use in many other autoimmune disorders. Ciclosporin has also been used to help treat patients with ulcerative colitis who do not respond to treatment with steroids, and is also used to treat non-infective posterior or intermediate uveitis. Ciclosporin has been investigated as a possible neuroprotective agent in conditions such as traumatic brain injury, and has been shown in animal experiments to reduce brain damage associated with injury. As mentioned above, ciclosporin blocks the formation of the mitochondrial permeability transition pore, which has been found to cause much of the damage associated with head injury and neurodegenerative diseases.

Treatment with ciclosporin can be associated with a number of potentially serious adverse drug reactions and drug interactions. Ciclosporin interacts with a wide variety of other drugs and other substances, including grapefruit juice, although this interaction with grapefruit juice has been used beneficially to increase the blood level of ciclosporin in expermental studies.

Adverse drug reactions include gum hyperplasia, convulsions, peptic ulcers, pancreatitis, fever, vomiting, diarrhoea, confusion, breathing difficulties, numbness and tingling, pruritis, high blood pressure, potassium retention and possibly hyperkalaemia, nephrotoxicity and hepatotoxicity, and also an increased vulnerability to opportunistic fungal and viral infections. Cytokine release syndrome is seen after anti-thymocyte globulin administration.

inflammation

**2.30**

*Answer: C*    Is complement-mediated

Hyperacute rejection is a complement-mediated response in recipients with pre-existing antibodies to the donor (for example, ABO blood group antibodies). Hyperacute rejection occurs within minutes and the transplant must be immediately removed to prevent a severe systemic inflammatory response. Rapid coagulation of the blood occurs. This is a particular risk in kidney transplants, and so a prospective cytotoxic cross-match is performed prior to kidney transplantation to ensure that antibodies to the donor are not present. For other organs, hyperacute rejection is prevented by transplanting only ABO-compatible grafts. Hyperacute rejection is the likely outcome of xenotransplanted organs.

**2.31**

*Answer: B*    Lymphocytes

The lymphocyte and monocyte series are the characteristic cells seen in more prolonged forms of inflammation. The eosinophils and the neutrophils are usually associated with early or acute inflammatory responses. The mast cell is involved in liberating histamine in early inflammation. The platelets, although they may aggregate, are not characteristic of either type of inflammation.

**2.32**

*Answer: E*    Proliferation of new capillaries, with fibroblasts and
new collagen formation

Granulation tissue is the first phase of the healing process at the end of acute inflammation. New capillaries proliferate in the tissue, with fibroblasts and the first laying-down of new collagen, which eventually will become largely avascular scar tissue. It is not to be confused with granulomatous inflammation or granuloma, which is the hallmark of a form of chronic inflammation in which healing and the stimulation for damage occur concurrently. Granulation tissue is an abnormal response in the normal healing process.

During the proliferative phase of wound healing, granulation tissue is:

- Light red or dark-pink in colour, being perfused with new capillary loops or 'buds'

- Soft to the touch

- Moist

- Granular in appearance.

## 2.33

*Answer: A*    Chemotaxis

During the vascular stasis stage of hyperaemia, neutrophils and monocytes adhere to the vascular endothelium prior to migration into the extravascular space in a process known as 'margination'. Leukocytes emigrate (diapedesis) through gaps between the endothelial cells. Chemotaxis is the process by which leukocytes undergo unidirectional migration towards a specific target. Various chemotactic substances or factors influence the rate of movement of the cells. Several chemotactic factors have an apparently specific action on selected cell types.

## 2.34

*Answer: A*    Bone marrow

There is evidence that most, if not all macrophages originate from a committed bone marrow stem cell, which differentiates into a monoblast and then a promonocyte, which in turn matures into a monocyte in the circulating peripheral blood. When called upon, the circulating monocyte can enter into an organ or tissue bed as a tissue macrophage (previously called a 'histiocyte'). Examples of tissue macrophages are Kupffer cells (liver), alveolar macrophages (lung), osteoclasts (bone), Langerhans cells (skin), microglial cells (central nevous system), and possibly the dendritic immunocytes of the dermis, spleen and lymph nodes. The entire system, including the peripheral blood monocytes, constitutes the mononuclear phagocyte system.

inflammation

**2.35**

*Answer: B*    Granulomatous inflammation

Langhans giant cells are the hallmarks of granulomatous inflammation. They are formed by the fusion of epithelioid cells (macrophages) and contain nuclei arranged in a horseshoe-shaped pattern in the cell periphery.

**2.36**

*Answer: A*    Allograft

This type of graft is an allograft (ie the graft is transferred between two members of the same species). Because the donor and recipient are histo-incompatible (genetic differences exist in the human leukocyte antigen or HLA system; genetic differences are also likely in minor histocompatibility loci), rejection of the graft is likely but can be controlled with immunosuppressive therapy (eg with ciclosporin). 'Isograft' and 'syngraft' are synonymous terms. They refer to a graft transferred between genetically identical individuals (ie identical twins) or highly inbred laboratory animals. The donor and recipient are histocompatible and rejection will not occur. An autograft is performed by transferring cells or tissues from one part of the body to another part of the same individual. Autografting of skin and bone is performed quite commonly. Rejection will not occur after this kind of graft. A xenograft is tissue transferred from a member of one species to a member of another species (eg baboon to human). The donor and recipient are histo-incompatible. Rejection is highly likely without immunosuppressive therapy.

**2.37**

*Answer: A*    Acute rejection

The patient in this clinical scenario was most likely to be experiencing acute rejection. This type of rejection is primarily a cell-mediated attack against the transplanted organ. Antigen presentation can occur in at least two different ways. In the direct path, blood-borne cells within the graft (ie 'passenger' dendritic cells and monocytes expressing class I and class II major histocompatibility complex

[MHC] molecules) act as the antigen-presenting cells. In the indirect path, the recipient's antigen-presenting cells could be presenting allogeneic class I and class II molecules that have been shed by the graft. Peptides presented in the context of MHC class I molecules will activate CD8-positive T-cytotoxic lymphocytes, which can directly attack the graft. Peptides presented in the context of MHC class II molecules can activate CD4-positive T-helper cells, resulting in secretion of helper factors. This intensifies the rejection by expansion of antigen-specific cytotoxic T-cell clones and accumulation and activation of macrophages. Antilymphocyte globulin (anti-T-cell antibodies made in an animal) is the agent used to reverse acute rejection episodes. Without immunosuppression of the recipient, allograft rejection usually takes place in approximately 11–14 days.

Chronic rejection is a slow, smouldering phenomenon that is poorly understood. The mechanisms that are responsible can include monocyte secretion of interleukin-1 and release of platelet-derived growth factor (PDGF) from platelets and endothelial cells. If it is going to occur, it generally begins several months to years after the transplantation is performed. It is characterised by proliferation of endothelial cells of blood vessels feeding the graft and fibrotic changes within the vessel wall. Blockage of the vessels results in necrosis and demise of the graft. It is not reversed by antilymphocyte globulin.

In a graft-versus-host reaction, the cells of the graft attack the recipient, either directly or indirectly, by recruiting the recipient's cells to attack the host. This type of reaction is seen primarily in recipients of bone marrow grafts.

Hyperacute (accelerated or second-set) rejection is mediated by pre-existing antibodies in the recipient which can bind to the graft and activate complement (type II hypersensitivity). These antibodies may be present as the result of sensitisation by human antigens during pregnancy, previous blood transfusions or previous transplants. This type of rejection occurs within minutes to hours. It is virtually impossible to reverse. Organ recipients are screened for antibodies against donor HLA antigens prior to transplantation.

The case history does not mention reduction in drug dosage. Administration of antilymphocyte globulin will not reverse immunosuppressive drug toxicity.

inflammation

**2.38**

*Answer: C*    Anti-B isohaemagglutinin of the IgM class preformed in the recipient

In this scenario the husband, who has blood group A, has preformed immunoglobulin M (IgM) against the B antigen on the transfused erythrocytes. The IgM binds to the cells, activates complement, and lysis occurs (type II hypersensitivity). The antibody–antigen complexes on the erythrocyte surface also activate Hageman factor, which leads to production of kinins (vasoactive peptides that cause hypotension and shock by increasing capillary permeability). If the infusion of ABO-incompatible blood is not stopped promptly, kidney failure caused by renal vasoconstriction and intravascular thrombi can occur.

IgM isohaemagglutinins begin to appear shortly after birth, presumably because of colonisation of the gastrointestinal and respiratory tracts by normal flora, which have oligosaccharide antigenic determinants that are similar to those on the A and B antigens. However, an individual will produce antibodies only against those antigens that are different from self.

| Group | Antigen | Antibody |
|-------|---------|----------|
| A | A | anti-B |
| B | B | anti-A |
| O | — | anti-A + anti-B |
| AB | AB | — |

The term 'isohaemagglutinin' refers to antibodies in one species that are directed against major antigens on erythrocytes of other individuals of the same species.

**2.39**

*Answer: E*    Haemolytic disease of the newborn

The infant is at risk of developing haemolytic disease of the newborn. The mechanism involves passage of Rh-positive erythrocytes from

inflammation

the fetus into the blood circulation of a Rh-negative mother, which usually occurs near the time of delivery. The mother becomes sensitised and can begin producing anti-Rh antibodies. The firstborn child is generally not at great risk, because it is born before an appreciable level of immunoglobulin G (IgG) antibody is formed. However, in a subsequent pregnancy with an Rh-positive fetus, the mother can have a strong secondary immune response. Maternal anti-Rh antibody of the IgG isotype crosses the placenta and binds to the fetal red blood cells, which are removed by macrophages (type II hypersensitivity). IgG antibodies against the Rh antigen are the principal cause of haemolytic disease of the newborn.

## 2.40

*Answer: B*     Anti-Rh antibody (Rh immunoglobulin)

The intramuscular administration of high-titre anti-Rh antibodies, also known as 'anti-Rh immunoglobulins', into an Rh-negative mother within 72 hours after delivery is effective in preventing the development of haemolytic disease of the newborn. The mechanism of action of this prophylaxis is not entirely understood, but it is believed that the anti-Rh antibodies attach to the fetal Rh-positive cells in the mother's circulation and thus prevent sensitisation. This type of prophylaxis also is used for Rh-negative women after abortion or amniocentesis. Large doses of the antibody can also be used to suppress sensitisation following accidental tranfusion of Rh-positive blood into an Rh-negative recipient, if administered within 72 hours.

Infusion of Rh-positive red blood cells could further increase the risk of the mother producing anti-Rh antibodies. Plasma from randomly selected donors is useful in immunodeficiency diseases. Some preparations could conceivably contain anti-Rh antibodies, but this is not the best choice. Albumin from Rh-positive donors or platelet transfusion would not protect the infant against anti-Rh antibodies.

inflammation

**2.41**

*Answer: D*  Monocytes

A monocyte is a leukocyte that protects against blood-borne pathogens and moves quickly (in approximately 8–12 hours) to sites of infection in the tissues. Monocytes are usually identified in stained smears by their large bilobed nucleus.

Monocytes are produced by the bone marrow from haemopoietic stem cell precursors called 'monoblasts'. Monocytes circulate in the bloodstream for about 1–3 days and then typically move into tissues throughout the body. They comprise 3%–8% of the leukocytes in the blood. In the tissues, monocytes mature into different types of macrophages at different anatomical locations.

Monocytes are responsible for phagocytosis (ingestion) of foreign substances in the body. Monocytes can perform phagocytosis using intermediary (opsonising) proteins such as antibodies or complement that coat the pathogen, as well as by binding to the microbe directly via pattern-recognition receptors that recognise pathogens. Monocytes are also capable of killing infected host cells via antibody (antibody-mediated cellular cytotoxicity). A cell that has recently phagocytosed foreign matter can have a vacuolated appearance.

**2.42**

*Answer: E*  Neutrophils

Neutrophils are the most abundant type of white blood cell and form an integral part of the immune system. Their name is derived from the staining characteristics on haematoxylin and eosin histological preparations: whereas basophilic cellular components stain dark-blue and eosinophilic components stain bright-red, neutrophilic components stain a neutral pink. These phagocytes are normally found in the bloodstream. However, during the acute phase of inflammation, particularly as a result of bacterial infection, neutrophils leave the vasculature and migrate towards the site of inflammation in a process called 'chemotaxis'. They are the predominant cells in pus, accounting for its whitish appearance. Neutrophils react within an hour of tissue injury and are the hallmark of acute inflammation.

Neutrophil granulocytes have an average volume of 330 fl and a diameter of 12–15 μm in peripheral blood smears. Together with the eosinophil and the basophil, they form the class of polymorphonuclear cells, so-named because of the characteristic multilobulated shape of their nuclei (quite different from that of lymphocytes and monocytes, the other types of white cells). Neutrophils are the most abundant white blood cells, accounting for 70% of all white blood cells.

The stated normal range for blood counts varies between laboratories, but a neutrophil count of $2.5–7.5 \times 10^9/l$ is a standard normal range. People of African and Middle Eastern descent may have lower counts which are still normal.

## 2.43

*Answer: B*    Eosinophils

Eosinophils are white blood cells that are responsible for combating infection by parasites. They are also involved in the pathogenesis of allergy and asthma. They are granulocytes that develop in the bone marrow before migrating into blood. These cells are naturally transparent but appear brick-red when stained with eosin using Romanowsky's method; the red colour stains small granules within the cellular cytoplasm which contain chemical mediators such as histamine and proteins such as eosinophil peroxidase, RNase, DNases, lipase, plasminogen and major basic protein. These mediators are released by degranulation following activation of the eosinophil, and are toxic to both parasite and host tissues.

Eosinophils make up about 1%–5% of all white blood cells, and are about 10–12 μm in size. They are found in the medulla and the junction between the cortex and medulla of the thymus, and in the lower gastrointestinal tract, ovary, uterus, spleen and lymph nodes, but not in the lung, skin, oesophagus or some of the other internal organs under normal conditions. The presence of eosinophils in these latter organs is associated with disease. Eosinophils persist in the circulation for 6–12 hours, and can survive in tissue for an additional 2–3 days in the absence of stimulation.

inflammation

## 2.44

*Answer: D*   Interleukin-6

Interleukin-6 (IL-6) is a pro-inflammatory cytokine secreted by T cells and macrophages to stimulate the immune response to trauma, especially burns or other tissue damage leading to inflammation. IL-6 is also a 'myokine', a cytokine produced by muscle, and is elevated in response to muscle contraction. In addition, osteoblasts secrete IL-6 to stimulate osteoclast formation.

IL-6 is one of the most important mediators of fever and of the acute phase response. In muscle and fatty tissue, IL-6 stimulates energy mobilisation, which leads to increased body temperature. IL-6 can be secreted by macrophages in response to specific microbial molecules, known as 'pathogen-associated molecular patterns' (PAMPs). These PAMPs bind to highly important detection molecules of the innate immune system called 'Toll-like receptors' (TLRs) that are present on the cell surface (or in intracellular compartments), which induces intracellular signalling cascades that give rise to inflammatory cytokine production. Inhibitors of IL-6 (including oestrogen) are used to treat postmenopausal osteoporosis.

## 2.45

*Answer: D*   Interleukin-10

Interleukin-10 (IL-10), also known as 'human cytokine synthesis inhibitory factor' (CSIF), is an anti-inflammatory cytokine. It is capable of inhibiting the synthesis of pro-inflammatory cytokines such as interferon-gamma, IL-2, IL-3, TNF-$\alpha$ and granulocyte macrophage colony-stimulating factor made by cells such as macrophages and the type 1 T-helper cells. IL-10 also displays a potent ability to suppress the antigen presentation capacity of antigen-presenting cells. However, it is also stimulatory towards certain T cells, mast cells and B cells. It is mainly expressed in monocytes and type 2 T-helper cells and mast cells and also in a particular subset of activated T cells and B cells. It is released by cytotoxic T cells to inhibit the actions of natural killer cells during the immune response to viral infection.

## 2.46

*Answer: C*   Interleukin-5

Interleukin-5 (IL-5) is a 115-amino-acid-long interleukin produced by T-helper-2 (TH2) cells and mast cells. It stimulates B-cell growth and increases immunoglobulin secretion. It is also a key mediator in eosinophil activation. It is a TH2 cytokine which is part of the haematopoietic family. Unlike other members of this cytokine family (IL-3 and granulocyte macrophage colony-stimulating factor [GM-CSF]), in its active form this glycoprotein is a homodimer. The IL-5 gene is located on chromosome 5 in humans, in close proximity to the genes encoding IL-3, IL-4 and GM-CSF, which are often co-expressed in TH2 cells. IL-5 is also expressed by eosinophils and has been observed in the mast cells of asthmatic airways after immunohistochemical staining. IL-5 expression is regulated by several transcription factors, including GATA-3.

IL-5 has long been associated with a number of allergic diseases, including allergic rhinitis and asthma, where a large increase in the number of circulating, airway-tissue, and induced sputum eosinophil numbers has been observed. Given that eosinophils are the primary IL-5R$\alpha$-expressing cells, it is not surprising that this cell type responds to IL-5. In fact, IL-5 was originally discovered as an eosinophil colony-stimulating factor, is a major regulator of eosinophil accumulation in tissues, and can modulate eosinophil behaviour at every stage from maturation to survival.

## 2.47

*Answer: D*   Prostaglandins

Arachidonic acid is a polyunsaturated fatty acid that is present in the phospholipids of cell membranes (especially phosphatidylethanolamine, phosphatidylcholine and phosphatidylinositides), and is abundant in the brain. Chemically, arachidonic acid is a carboxylic acid with a 20-carbon chain and four cis double bonds; the first double bond is located at the sixth carbon from the omega end. It is involved in cellular signalling as a second messenger. Arachidonic acid is freed from phospholipid

inflammation

molecules by the enzyme phospholipase A2, which cleaves off the fatty acid precursor (usually linoleic acid). Arachidonic acid is a precursor in the production of eicosanoids:

- The enzymes cyclo-oxygenase and peroxidase lead to prostaglandin H2 synthesis, which in turn is used to produce the prostaglandins, prostacyclin, and thromboxanes.

- The enzyme 5-lipoxygenase leads to 5-hydroperoxyeicosatetraenoic acid, which in turn is used to produce the leukotrienes.

- Arachidonic acid is also used in the biosynthesis of anandamide.

The production of these derivatives and their action in the body are collectively known as the 'arachidonic acid cascade'.

### 2.48

*Answer: B*    5-lipoxygenase

Leukotrienes are naturally produced eicosanoid lipid mediators, and they are thought to be responsible for a number of the effects of asthma and allergies. Leukotrienes use both autocrine signalling and paracrine signalling to regulate the body's response. Examples of leukotrienes are $LTA_4$, $LTB_4$, $LTC_4$, $LTD_4$, $LTE_4$ and $LTF_4$. $LTC_4$, $LTD_4$ and $LTE_4$ are often called 'cysteinyl leukotrienes' due to the presence of the amino acid cysteine in their structure. Collectively, the cysteinyl leukotrienes make up the slow-reacting substance of anaphylaxis (SRS-A). Another substance, $LTG_4$, has been postulated to exist, a metabolite of $LTE_4$, in which the cysteinyl moiety has been oxidised to an alpha-keto-acid (ie the cysteine has been replaced by a pyruvate). Very little is known about this putative leukotriene.

Leukotrienes are synthesised in the cell from arachidonic acid by 5-lipoxygenase. The catalytic mechanism involves the insertion of an oxygen moiety at a specific position in the arachidonic acid backbone. The lipoxygenase pathway is active in leukocytes, including mast cells, eosinophils, neutrophils, monocytes and basophils. When such cells are activated, arachidonic acid is liberated from cell membrane phospholipids by phospholipase A2 and donated by

inflammation

the 5-lipoxygenase-activating protein to 5-lipoxygenase, which converts it in two steps to leukotriene A$_4$, an unstable epoxide.

In cells equipped with LTA$_4$ hydrolase, such as neutrophils and monocytes, LTA$_4$ is converted to the dihydroxy acid leukotriene LTB$_4$, which is a powerful chemoattractant for neutrophils, acting at BLT$_1$ and BLT$_2$ receptors on the plasma membrane of these cells. In cells that express LTC$_4$ synthase, such as mast cells and eosinophils, LTA$_4$ is conjugated with the tripeptide glutathione to form the first of the cysteinyl-leukotrienes, LTC$_4$. Outside the cell, LTC$_4$ can be converted by ubiquitous enzymes to form, successively, LTD$_4$ and LTE$_4$, which retain biological activity.

The cysteinyl-leukotrienes act at their cell-surface receptors, CysLT1 and CystLT2, on target cells to contract bronchial and vascular smooth muscle to increase permeability of small blood vessels, to enhance the secretion of mucus in the airway and gut, and to recruit leukocytes to sites of inflammation. Both LTB$_4$ and the cysteinyl-leukotrienes (LTC$_4$, LTD$_4$, LTE$_4$) are partly degraded in local tissues, and ultimately become inactive metabolites in the liver.

## 2.49

*Answer: B*    Recycling of old red blood cells

Kupffer cells (or Browicz–Kupffer cells) are specialised macrophages located in the liver that form part of the reticuloendothelial system (mononuclear phagocyte system). The primary function of Kupffer cells is to recycle old red blood cells that are no longer functional. The red blood cell is broken down by phagocytic action and the haemoglobin molecule is split. The globin chains are reutilised, while the iron-containing portion or haem is further broken down into iron (which is reutilised) and bilirubin, which is conjugated with glucuronic acid within hepatocytes and secreted into the bile.

The cells were first observed by Karl Wilhelm von Kupffer in 1876. The scientist called them 'sternzellen' (star cells or stellate cells) but thought falsely that they were an integral part of the endothelium of the liver blood vessels and that they originated from it. In 1898, after several years of research, Tadeusz Browicz identified them correctly as macrophages.

Their development begins in the bone marrow with the genesis of promonocytes and monoblasts into monocytes and then on to peripheral blood monocytes, completing their differentiation into Kupffer cells.

## 2.50

*Answer: E*    Natural killer cell

Perforin is a cytolytic protein found in the granules of CD8 T cells and natural killer (NK) cells. On degranulation, perforin inserts itself into the target cell's plasma membrane, forming a pore. Although purified perforin is sufficient to lyse cells at high doses, the biology of perforin itself does not explain the ability of CD8 T cells and NK cells to induce apoptosis in target cells. This induction of apoptosis might require at least one other granule protein, granzyme B.

# SECTION 3: NEOPLASIA — ANSWERS

## 3.1

*Answer: B*   No metastases are found in the sampled lymph nodes

The lack of metastases suggests a lower stage and a better prognosis. Many breast cancers are oestrogen receptor-positive, which suggests that hormonal therapy will be helpful. Both aneuploidy and a high S-phase are characteristic of malignancy and suggest a worse prognosis. A history of breast cancer suggests a greater risk for breast cancer, but does not predict prognosis. A higher grade suggests a worse prognosis.

## 3.2

*Answer: B*   A K-*ras* mutation in the neoplastic cells

Many human carcinomas are associated with K-*ras* mutations that contribute to oncogenesis. Vimentin is a more typical marker for soft-tissue malignancies (sarcomas). Carcinomas are positive for cytokeratin by immunoperoxidase. Bacterial infections such as *Shigella flexneri* do not tend to increase the risk of adenocarcinoma. Adenocarcinomas are not generally seen significantly more frequently in people with immunodeficiency diseases. Adenocarcinomas are also generally not seen with significantly increased frequency in people with collagen vascular diseases and therefore a finding of a high titre of DNA topoisomerase I is less likely in this patient.

**3.3**

*Answer: E*   Uncontrolled (autonomous) growth

A neoplasm is new, uncontrolled growth of cells. Neoplasms and granulomas can both recur. Some neoplasms can increase in size quickly, but so can granulomas associated with certain infections. Response to therapy is not always a reliable indicator that the presumed disease was actually present. Any mass lesion can undergo necrosis, particularly if it is large and outgrows the blood supply.

**3.4**

*Answer: D*   A 15-year-old boy with a mass in the left femur and lung metastases

The pathological description of spindle-shaped, vimentin-positive cells is suggestive of an osteosarcoma with haematogenous metastases to the lung. The 35-year-old woman with a left breast mass and enlarged axillary lymph nodes will have cells that may be positive for oestrogen or progesterone. The 55-year-old woman with massive ascites and multiple peritoneal metastases probably has an ovarian carcinoma with peritoneal seeding. The 25-year-old man with an enlarged left testis probably has a germ cell tumour. The 55-year old man with a right renal mass has a renal cell carcinoma.

**3.5**

*Answer: E*   T4 N1 M1

This woman has a large invasive primary tumour mass with axillary node and lung metastases, making this stage T4 N1 M1. Looking at the other stems, T1 N1 M0 signifies a small primary cancer with nodal metastases but no distant metastases; T1 N0 M1 signifies a small primary cancer with no lymph node metastases but with distant metastases; T2 N1 M0 signifies a larger primary cancer with nodal metastases but no distant metastases; and T3 N0 M0 indicates a larger primary cancer with no metastases to either lymph nodes or to distant sites.

*neoplasia*

## 3.6

*Answer: C*   Invasion

Metastasis would be an even better indicator, but invasion suggests malignancy more than the other items listed here. While pleomorphism is more prominent in malignant neoplasms, it can be present in benign neoplasms too. Atypia can be part of benign or dysplastic processes that are not malignant. A high nuclear/cytoplasmic ratio is one feature of malignancy, but is not the best indicator. Necrosis can occur for many reasons, and even a benign tumour can cause pressure necrosis or outgrow its blood supply.

## 3.7

*Answer: D*   It is well differentiated and localised

A well-differentiated and localised neoplasm usually has both a low grade and a low stage. Criteria for malignancy must be satisfied first, then grading and staging follow. Grading and staging are most useful for epithelial malignancies, but are not reserved specifically for them. It can indeed spread to nodes, particularly if it is a carcinoma, but is less likely to do so if it is a low-grade tumour and it has not already done so. It may have an in-situ component, but the behaviour of most neoplasms is judged by the worst part of it.

## 3.8

*Answer: D*   Local recurrence

The description in this scenario is of a pleomorphic adenoma of the parotid gland. It is a benign tumour of the salivary glands. It is the most common type of salivary gland tumour and the most common tumour of the parotid gland. It derives its name from the architectural pleomorphism (ie variable appearance) seen by light microscopy. It is also known as 'mixed tumour', due to its pleomorphic appearance as opposed to its dual origin from epithelial and myoepithelial elements. The tumour is usually solitary and presents as a slow-growing, painless, firm, single nodular mass. Isolated nodules are generally outgrowths of the main nodule rather than a multinodular presentation. It is usually mobile unless found

neoplasia

in the palate and can cause atrophy of the mandibular ramus when located in the parotid gland. When found in the parotid tail, it can present as an eversion of the ear lobe. Though it is a benign tumour, pleomorphic adenomas have the capacity to grow quite large.

Histologically, it is highly variable in appearance, even within individual tumours. It is characterised by an admixture of epithelial and myoepithelial elements in a variable background stroma that can be mucoid, myxoid, cartilaginous or hyaline. Epithelial elements may be arranged in duct-like structures, sheets, clumps and/or interlacing strands and consist of polygonal, spindle-shaped or stellate-shaped cells. Areas of squamous metaplasia and epithelial pearls might be seen. The tumour is usually enveloped by a fibrous capsule of varying thickness, which is often incomplete. The tumour often extends through these discontinuities but this is not a sign of malignant transformation as it does not invade surrounding tissues. Recurrences are rare unless the tumour is treated too conservatively (enucleation can lead to spillage and seeding of tumour cells).

### 3.9

*Answer: E* PSA (prostate-specific antigen)

Prostate-specific antigen (PSA) is a protein produced by the cells of the prostate gland. PSA is present in small quantities in the serum of normal men and is often elevated in the presence of prostate cancer and in other prostate disorders. A blood test to measure PSA is the most effective test currently available for the early detection of prostate cancer. Higher than normal levels of PSA are associated with both localised and metastatic prostate cancer.

PSA (also known as 'kallikrein III', 'seminin', 'semenogelase', $\gamma$-seminoprotein' or 'P-30 antigen') is a glycoprotein produced almost exclusively by the prostate gland. PSA liquifies the semen and allows sperms to swim freely. It is also believed to be instrumental in dissolving the cervical mucus cap, allowing the entry of sperm. Biochemically, it is a serine protease enzyme, the gene of which is located on chromosome 19 (19q13).

*neoplasia*

Normal PSA levels lie in the range 0–4.0 ng/ml. Increased levels of PSA can suggest the presence of prostate cancer. However, prostate cancer can also be present in the complete absence of an elevated PSA level, in which case the test result would be a false negative. PSA levels can also be elevated due to prostate infection, irritation, benign prostatic hypertrophy or hyperplasia, or recent ejaculation, in which case it may give a false-positive result. It is a myth, however, that digital rectal examination raises the PSA level.

## 3.10

*Answer: E*    Seminoma

Seminoma is a very radiosensitive tumour. Standard treatment for seminoma after unilateral orchidectomy is radiation therapy, usually 20–40 Gy to the para-aortic regions up to the diaphragm (a higher dose is used for patients with a nodal mass); the ipsilateral ilioinguinal region is not treated routinely. Occasionally, the mediastinum and left supraclavicular regions are also irradiated, depending on the clinical stage.

## 3.11

*Answer: A*    Arrhenoblastoma

Arrhenoblastoma, also known as 'Sertoli–Leydig tumour', is a rare ovarian stromal neoplasm that secretes testosterone. Although it can occur at any age, it is mostly seen in women in the reproductive years. It is typically unilateral. The key clinical features of this tumour are related to its endocrine activity. The excessive production of testosterone leads to progressive masculinisation in a woman who typically had been normal beforehand: she might experience not only anovulation and amenorrhoea, but usually also acne and hirsutism, voice deepening, clitoromegaly, temporal hair recession, and an increase in musculature. On ultrasonography, a unilateral solid lesion can be seen in the ovary. The serum testosterone level is high. The treatment consists of surgical removal and the prognosis is generally good as the lesion tends to grow slowly and rarely metastasises.

neoplasia

## 3.12

*Answer: B*    Arsenic

The rare hepatic angiosarcomas are associated with distinct carcinogens, including arsenic (exposure to arsenical pesticides), Thorotrast (a radioactive contrast medium at one time widely used in radiology), and polyvinyl chloride (PVC, a widely used plastic). The increased frequency of angiosarcomas among workers in the PVC industry is one of the well-documented instances of chemical carcinogenesis in humans. With all three agents, there is a very long latent period of many years between exposure and the development of tumours.

## 3.13

*Answer: D*    *BRCA1* and *BRCA2* gene analysis

*BRCA1* is a human gene that belongs to a class of genes known as 'tumour suppressor genes'. Like many other tumour suppressor genes, *BRCA1* regulates the cycle of cell division by keeping cells from growing and dividing too rapidly or in an uncontrolled way. In particular, it inhibits the growth of cells that line the milk ducts in the breast. The protein made by *BRCA1* is directly involved in the repair of damaged DNA. In the nucleus of many types of normal cells, the BRCA1 protein interacts with the protein produced by the *RAD51* gene to mend breaks in DNA. These breaks can be caused by natural radiation or other exposures, but also occur when chromosomes exchange genetic material in preparation for cell division. The BRCA2 protein, which has a function similar to that of the BRCA1 protein, also interacts with the RAD51 protein. By repairing DNA, these three proteins play a role in maintaining the stability of the human genome.

Research suggests that both the BRCA1 and BRCA2 proteins regulate the activity of other genes and play a critical role in embryo development. The BRCA1 protein probably interacts with many other proteins, including tumour suppressors and regulators of the cell division cycle. *BRCA1* is located on the long (q) arm of chromosome 17 at position 21.

Certain variations of *BRCA1* lead to an increased risk for breast cancer. Researchers have identified more than 600 mutations in *BRCA1*, many of which are associated with an increased risk of cancer. These mutations can be changes in one or a small number of DNA base pairs. In some cases, large segments of DNA are rearranged. A mutated *BRCA1* gene usually makes a protein that does not function properly because it is abnormally short. Researchers believe that the defective BRCA1 protein is unable to help fix mutations that occur in other genes. These defects accumulate and may allow cells to grow and divide uncontrollably to form a tumour.

In addition to breast cancer, mutations in the *BRCA1* gene also increase the risk of ovarian, Fallopian tube, prostate and colon cancers. Moreover, precancerous lesions (dysplasia) within the Fallopian tube have been linked to *BRCA1* gene mutations.

*BRCA2* is another tumour suppressor , and although the structures of the *BRCA1* and *BRCA2* genes are very different, their functions appear to be similar. Like *BRCA1*, *BRCA2* probably regulates the activity of other genes and plays a critical role in embryo development. The *BRCA2* gene is located on the long (q) arm of chromosome 13 at position 12.3.

## 3.14

*Answer: D*    Increased level of PTH-related protein

Hypercalcaemia is probably the most common paraneoplastic syndrome. Overtly symptomatic hypercalcaemia is most often related to some form of cancer rather than to hyperparathyroidism. Two general processes are involved in cancer-associated hypercalcaemia: (1) osteolysis induced by cancer, whether primary in bone, such as multiple myeloma, or metastatic to bone from any primary lesion; and (2) the production of calcaemic humoral substances by extraosseous neoplasms. Note that hypercalcaemia due to skeletal metastases is not a paraneoplastic syndrome.

Several humoral factors have been associated with paraneoplastic hypercalcaemia of malignancy. Perhaps the most important is a molecule related to, but distinct from, parathyroid hormone (PTH). Parathyroid hormone-related protein (PTHRP) resembles the native hormone only in its amino terminus. It has some biological actions similar to those of PTH, and both hormones share a G-protein-coupled receptor known as PTH/PTHRP receptor (often referred to as PTH-R or PTHrP-R). In contrast to PTH, PTHrP is produced by many normal tissues, including keratinocytes, muscles, bone and ovary. The amounts produced by normal cells, however, are small. It is thought that PTHrP regulates calcium transport in the lactating breast and across the placenta. Tumours most often associated with paraneoplastic hypercalcaemia are carcinomas of the breast, lung, kidney and ovary. In breast cancers, PTHrP production is associated with osteolytic bone disease, bone metastasis and humoral hypercalcaemia. The most common lung neoplasm associated with hypercalcaemia is the squamous cell bronchogenic carcinoma (in contrast to the small-cell cancer of the lung, which is more often associated with endocrinopathies). In addition to PTHrP, several other factors, including interleukin-1, tumour growth factor-alpha, tumour necrosis factor and dihydroxyvitamin D, have also been implicated in causing the hypercalcaemia of malignancy.

## 3.15

*Answer: E*     Warthin's tumour

Warthin's tumour is a benign tumour of the salivary glands. It is also known as 'benign papillary cystadenoma lymphomatosum'. Its aetiology is unknown, but there is a strong association with cigarette smoking. Smokers are at an eight-fold greater risk of developing Warthin's tumour than non-smokers. The gland most likely to be affected is the parotid gland. Though much less common than pleomorphic adenoma, Warthin's tumour is the second most common benign parotid tumour.

Warthin's tumour is more likely to occur in older adults aged between 60 years and 70 years. There is only a slight male predilection according to recent studies, but historically it has been associated with a strong male predilection. This change is possibly due to the tumour's association with cigarette smoking and the growing use of cigarettes in women. The tumour is slow-growing, painless, and usually appears in the tail of the parotid gland, near the angle of the mandible. In 5%–14% of cases, Warthin's tumour is bilateral, but the two masses usually arise at different times.

neoplasia

The appearance of this tumour under the microscope is unique. There are cystic spaces surrounded by two uniform rows of cells with centrally placed, pyknotic nuclei. The cystic spaces have epithelium referred to as 'papillary infoldings' that protude into them. In addition, the epithelium has a lymphoid stroma with germinal centre formation.

## 3.16

*Answer: B*  Local invasion

The stage of a cancer is a descriptor (usually numbered I to IV) of how much the cancer has spread. The stage often takes into account the size of a tumour, how deep it has penetrated, whether it has invaded adjacent organs, if and how many lymph nodes it has metastasised to, and whether it has spread to distant organs. Staging of cancer is important because the stage at diagnosis is the most powerful predictor of survival, and treatments are often changed based on the stage.

Cancer staging can be divided into a clinical stage and a pathological stage. In the TNM (tumour-node-metastasis) system, clinical stage and pathological stage are denoted by a small 'c' or 'p' before the stage, for example cT3 N1 M0 or pT2 N0 M0:

- **Clinical stage** is based on all of the available information obtained before surgery to remove the tumour. This might include information about the tumour obtained by physical examination, radiological examination, and endoscopy.

- **Pathological stage** adds additional information gained by examination of the tumour microscopically.

Because they use different information, the clinical stage and pathological stage are often different. Pathological staging is usually considered the 'better' or 'truer' stage because it is based on direct examination of the tumour and its spread, in contrast to clinical staging, which is limited by the fact that the information is obtained by making indirect observations of a tumour which is still in the body. However, clinical staging and pathological staging should complement each other. Not every tumour is treated surgically, so

*neoplasia*

sometimes pathological staging is not available. Also, sometimes surgery is preceded by other treatments such as chemotherapy and radiotherapy which shrink the tumour, so the pathological stage might be an underestimate of the true stage.

Correct staging is critical because treatment is directly related to disease stage. Incorrect staging could lead to improper treatment, and reduced patient survival. Correct staging, however, can be difficult to achieve. Pathological staging, where a pathologist examines sections of tissue, can be particularly problematic for two reasons: visual discretion and random sampling of tissue. 'Visual discretion' means being able to identify single cancerous cells intermixed with healthy cells on a slide. Oversight of just one cell can lead to mis-staging and serious, unexpected spread of cancer. 'Random sampling' refers to the fact that lymph nodes are cherry-picked from patients and random samples of these are examined. If cancerous cells present in the lymph node happen not to be present in the slices of tissue viewed, incorrect staging and improper treatment can result.

Staging systems are specific for each type of cancer (eg systems for breast cancer and lung cancer). Some cancers, however, do not have a staging system. There are often competing staging systems for the same type of cancer. However, the universally accepted staging system is that of the Union Internationale Contre le Cancer (UICC), which has the same definitions of individual categories as the American Joint Committee on Cancer (AJCC).

## 3.17

*Answer: D   IIIA*

The staging of breast cancer based on the TNM classification is as follows.

### Primary tumour (T):

TX: primary tumour cannot be assessed
T0: no evidence of primary tumour
Tis: pure carcinoma in situ; intraductal carcinoma, lobular carcinoma in situ, or Paget disease of the nipple with no associated tumour mass

T1: tumour 2 cm or less in its greatest dimension

T2: tumour more than 2 cm in size, but not more than 5 cm in its greatest dimension

T3: tumour more than 5 cm in its greatest dimension

T4: tumour of any size growing into the chest wall or skin

## Regional lymph nodes (N) (pathological staging, based on microscopic examination):

NX: regional lymph nodes cannot be assessed

N0: cancer has not spread to regional lymph nodes

N1: cancer has spread to one to three axillary lymph node(s)

N2: cancer has spread to four to nine axillary lymph nodes

N3: cancer has spread to ten or more axillary lymph nodes or also involves lymph nodes in other areas around the breast

## Metastasis (M):

MX: presence of distant spread (metastasis) cannot be assessed

M0: no distant spread

M1: spread to distant organs is present

**Stage 0 breast cancer is Tis N0 M0 disease.** Ductal carcinoma in situ (DCIS) is the earliest form of breast cancer. In DCIS, cancer cells are located within a duct and have not invaded the surrounding fatty breast tissue. Lobular carcinoma in situ (LCIS) is sometimes classified as stage 0 breast cancer, but most oncologists believe it is not a true breast cancer. In LCIS, abnormal cells grow within the lobules or milk-producing glands, but they do not penetrate through the wall of these lobules. Paget's disease of the nipple is stage 0. In all cases the cancer has not spread to lymph nodes or distant sites.

**Stage I breast cancer is T1 N0 M0 disease.** The tumour is 2 cm or less in diameter and has not spread to lymph nodes or distant sites.

**Stage IIA breast cancer is T0 N1 M0, T1 N1 M0, or T2 N0 M0 disease.** No tumour is found in the breast but it is found in one to three axillary lymph nodes; or the tumour is less than 2 cm in size and has spread to one to three axillary lymph nodes; or the cancer is found by sentinel node biopsy as microscopic disease in internal mammary nodes, but not on imaging studies or by clinical examination; or the tumour is larger than 2 cm but less than 5 cm

*neoplasia*

in diameter, but has not spread to axillary nodes. In all cases the cancer has not spread to distant sites.

**Stage IIB breast cancer is T2 N1 M0 or T3 N0 M0 disease.** The tumour is larger than 2 cm but less than 5 cm in diameter and has spread to one to three axillary lymph nodes; or cancer is found by sentinel node biopsy as microscopic disease in internal mammary nodes; or the tumour is larger than 5 cm but does not grow into the chest wall and has not spread to lymph nodes. In all cases, the cancer has not spread to distant sites.

**Stage IIIA breast cancer is T0–2 N2 M0 or T3 N1-2 M0 disease.** The tumour is smaller than 5 cm in diameter and has spread to 4 to 9 axillary lymph nodes; or it is found through imaging studies or clinical exam to have spread to internal mammary nodes; or the tumour is larger than 5 cm and has spread to 1 to 9 axillary nodes, or to internal mammary nodes. In all cases, the cancer hasn't spread to distant sites.

**Stage IIIB breast cancer is T4 N0-2 M0 disease.** The tumour has grown into the chest wall or skin and may have spread to no lymph nodes or to as many as nine axillary nodes. It might or might not have spread to internal mammary nodes. The cancer has not spread to distant sites.

**Stage IIIC breast cancer is T0-4 N3 M0 disease.** The tumour can be of any size, has spread to ten or more nodes in the axilla; or to one or more lymph nodes under the clavicle (infraclavicular) or above the clavicle (supraclavicular); or to internal mammary lymph nodes, which are enlarged because of the cancer. All of these are on the same side as the breast cancer. The cancer has not spread to distant sites.

Inflammatory breast cancer is classified as stage III, unless it has spread to distant organs or lymph nodes that are not near the breast, in which case it would be stage IV.

**Stage IV breast cancer is T0-4 N0-3 M1 disease.** The cancer, regardless of its size, has spread to distant organs such as bone, liver or lung, or to lymph nodes far from the breast.

According to this staging system, therefore, the woman in this scenario has stage IIIA disease (see also *Answer* to **3.5**).

## 3.18

*Answer: D*     Solar keratosis

A premalignant condition is a disease, syndrome or finding that, if left untreated, can lead to cancer. Examples of premalignant conditions include solar (actinic) keratosis, Barrett's oesophagus and cervical dysplasia. Solar keratosis (also called 'actinic keratosis', 'senile keratosis', or 'AK') is a premalignant condition of thick, scaly, or crusty patches of skin. It is most common in fair-skinned people who are frequently exposed to the sun, because their skin pigment is not very protective. It is usually accompanied by solar damage. Because some of these pre-cancers progress to squamous cell carcinoma, they should be treated.

When skin is exposed to the sun constantly, thick, scaly, or crusty bumps appear. The scaly or crusty part of the bump is dry and rough. The growths start out as flat scaly areas, and later grow into a tough, wart-like area. A solar keratosis site commonly ranges in size between 2 mm and 6 mm, and can be dark or light, tan, pink, red, a combination of all these, or the same colour as the rest of the skin. It can appear on any sun-exposed area, such as the face, ears, neck, scalp, chest, the back of hands, forearms or lips. Solar keratosis can appear as early as 30 years of age in susceptible people who spend a lot of time outdoors. People with skin phototypes I and II are more likely to be affected, as are albinos and immunosuppressed patients. Up to 100% of elderly white people get AK, but it is rare in darker-skinned people. About 10% of people with AK eventually develop squamous cell carcinoma of the skin.

## 3.19

*Answer: B*     Liposarcoma

Liposarcoma is a malignant tumour that arises in fat cells in deep soft tissue, such as that inside the thigh or in the retroperitoneum. They are typically large bulky tumours which tend to have multiple smaller satellites extending beyond the main confines of the tumour. Patients usually notice a deep-seated mass in their soft tissue. Only when the tumour is very large do symptoms of pain or functional disturbances occur.

neoplasia

Retroperitoneal tumours can present with signs of weight loss and emaciation and abdominal pain. These tumours can also compress the kidney or ureter, leading to kidney failure. Most frequent in middle-aged and older adults (over the age of 40 years), liposarcomas are the most common of all soft-tissue sarcomas. The annual incidence is 2.5 per million. The prognosis varies, depending on the site of origin, the type of cancer cell, the tumour size, the depth, and the proximity to lymph nodes. Metastases are common. They are very radioresistant and the 5-year survival rate for a high-grade liposarcoma is less than 50%.

## 3.20

*Answer: C* IIB

In this case the tumour is larger than 2 cm and less than 5 cm in diameter and has spread to three axillary lymph nodes. According to the TNM staging system, this is stage IIB (see also *Answer* to **3.5** and **3.17**).

## 3.21

*Answer: D* Pap smear

The Papanicolaou test (also called 'Pap smear', 'Pap test', 'cervical smear', or 'smear test') is a medical screening method primarily designed to detect premalignant and malignant processes in the ectocervix. It may also detect infections and abnormalities in the endocervix and endometrium. The endocervix can be partially sampled with the device used to obtain the ectocervical sample but consistent and reliable sampling cannot be guaranteed because of the anatomy of this area, and abnormal endocervical cells might be sampled. The endometrium is not directly sampled with the device used to sample the ectocervix. Cells can exfoliate onto the cervix and be collected from there, so as with endocervical cells, abnormal cells can be recognised if present but the Pap test should not be used as a screening tool for endometrial malignancy.

The precancerous changes (dysplasias or cervical or endocervical intraepithelial neoplasia) are usually caused by sexually transmitted human papilloma viruses (HPVs). The test aims to detect and prevent the progression of HPV-induced cervical cancer and other abnormalities in the female genital tract by sampling cells from the outer opening of the cervix of the uterus and the endocervix. The sampling technique has changed very little since its invention by Georgios Papincolaou (1883–1962) to detect cyclic hormonal changes in vaginal cells in the early 20th century, until the development of liquid-based thin-layer technology. The test remains a highly effective, widely used method for early detection of cervical cancer and pre-cancer.

It is generally recommended that sexually active females undergo Pap smear testing annually, although guidelines vary from country to country. If results are abnormal, and depending on the nature of the abnormality, the test might need to be repeated in 3–12 months. If the abnormality requires closer scrutiny, the patient might be referred for detailed inspection of the cervix by colposcopy. The patient might also be referred for HPV DNA testing, which can serve as an adjunct (or even as an alternative) to Pap testing.

About 5%–7% of Pap smears produce abnormal results, such as dysplasia, possibly indicating a precancerous condition. Although many low-grade cervical dysplasias spontaneously regress without ever leading to cervical cancer, dysplasia can serve as an indication that increased vigilance is needed. Endocervical and endometrial abnormalities can also be detected, as can a number of infectious processes, including yeast and *Trichomonas vaginalis* infections. A small proportion of abnormalities are reported as being of 'uncertain significance'.

## 3.22

*Answer: D*   Nephroblastoma

Wilms' tumour is a neoplasm of the kidneys that typically occurs in children. It is named after Dr Max Wilms, a German surgeon (1867–1918) who first identified this form of cancer. It is also known as a 'nephroblastoma'. The majority (75%) occur in otherwise normal children; a minority (25%) are associated with other developmental abnormalities. It is highly responsive to treatment, with about 90% of patients surviving at least 5 years. Wilms' tumour can affect

neoplasia

any child, regardless of race, sex, country of origin or parental occupation. The disease is usually noticed around the age of 3 years, but has been recorded in people at the age of 32 years. Most people initially experience the following symptoms:

- Abdominal mass

- Haematuria

- Fever

- Anorexia, vomiting and malaise (less frequently).

It can be associated with a WAGR complex. This complex includes **W**ilms' tumour, **a**niridia, **g**enitourinary malformation, and mental/motor **r**etardation. It can also be associated with Beckwith–Wiedmann syndrome (hemihypertrophy, macroglossia, omphalocele).

### 3.23

*Answer: B*    Breast

Both *BRCA1* and *BRCA2* are tumour suppressor genes. Certain variations of the *BRCA1* and *BRCA2* genes lead to an increased risk for breast cancer. Researchers have found numerous mutations in these genes, many of which are associated with an increased risk of cancer. These mutations can be changes in one or a small number of DNA base pairs. In some cases, large segments of DNA are rearranged. A mutated *BRCA1* or *BRCA2* gene usually makes a protein that does not function properly because it is abnormally short. Researchers believe that the defective BRCA1 or BRCA2 protein is unable to help fix mutations that occur in other genes. These defects accumulate and may allow cells to grow and divide uncontrollably to form a tumour (see also *Answer* to **3.13**).

### 3.24

*Answer: B*    Carcinoembryonic antigen (CEA)

Carcinoembryonic antigen (CEA) is a glycoprotein involved in cell adhesion. It is normally produced during fetal development, but the production of CEA stops before birth. It is therefore not usually present in the blood of healthy adults, although levels are raised in heavy smokers. CEA was first identified in 1965 by Phil Gold and Samuel Freedman in human colon cancer tissue extracts. It was found that serum from individuals with colorectal, gastric, pancreatic, lung and breast carcinomas had higher levels of CEA than those found in healthy individuals. CEA measurement is mainly used to identify recurrences after surgical resection. Elevated CEA levels should return to normal after surgical resection, and elevation of CEA during follow-up is an indicator of recurrence of tumour. CEA levels can also be raised in some non-neoplastic conditions such as ulcerative colitis, pancreatitis and cirrhosis. CEA and related genes make up the CEA family and belong to the immunoglobulin superfamily. In humans, the carcinoembryonic antigen family consists of 29 genes, 18 of which are normally expressed.

## 3.25

*Answer: A* CA-125

CA-125 (or CA125) is an abbreviation for cancer antigen-125. CA-125 is a tumour marker or biomarker that can be elevated in the blood of some people with specific types of cancers. CA-125 is a mucinous glycoprotein and is the product of the *MUC16* gene. It is best known as a marker for ovarian cancer, but it can also be elevated in other malignant cancers, including those originating in the endometrium, Fallopian tubes, lungs, breast and gastrointestinal tract. CA-125 can also be elevated in a number of relatively benign conditions, such as endometriosis, several diseases of the ovary, and in pregnancy. It also tends to be elevated in the presence of any inflammatory condition in the abdominal area, whether cancerous and benign. CA-125 is therefore not completely specific for cancer nor is it 100% sensitive since not every patient with cancer will have elevated levels of CA-125 in the blood. For example, 79% of all ovarian cancers are positive for CA-125, whereas the remainder do not express this antigen at all.

CA-125 is clinically approved for following the response to treatment and predicting prognosis after treatment. It is especially useful for detecting the recurrence of ovarian cancer. Its potential role for the early detection of ovarian cancer is controversial and it has not yet been adopted for widespread screening programmes in

neoplasia

asymptomatic women. The key problems in using the CA-125 test as a screening tool are its lack of specificity and its inability to detect early-stage cancers.

### 3.26

*Answer: A*   Asbestos

Mesothelioma is the most common malignant tumour of the pleura. It is a highly invasive lesion and has been linked to inhalation of asbestos fibres, especially by workers in the shipbuilding and insulation industries. A history of smoking dramatically increases the risk of developing a mesothelioma. Histologically, the tumour can be either sarcomatous (composed of mesenchymal stromal cells), carcinomatous (resembling tubular or papillary structures), or a combination of these two types. These tumours are highly malignant and most patients die within 1 year of diagnosis.

### 3.27

*Answer: D*   Osteosarcoma

Paget's disease of bone can lead to osteosarcoma. It should not be confused with Paget's disease of the breast, which is closely associated with an underlying duct carcinoma.

### 3.28

*Answer: E*   Papillary carcinoma

Papillary carcinoma is by far the most common primary malignant tumour of the thyroid.

### 3.29

*Answer: B*   Is predisposed to by erythroplasia

Carcinoma of the oral cavity accounts for approximately 54% of all human malignancies. More than 90% are squamous cell type and precursor lesions include dysplastic leukoplakia and erythroplasia, with transformation rates of approximately 15% and 50% respectively. It is more common in men. Smoking, tobacco chewing, chronic irritation, heat exposure and irradiation are all thought to contribute to carcinogenesis. The lower lip is the most common site, followed by the floor of the mouth, anterior tongue, palate and posterior tongue. The prognosis varies according to site but is best for lesions of the lip and worst for lesions in the floor of the mouth.

## 3.30

*Answer: B*    Osteochondroma

Osteochondroma is also referred to as 'exostosis'. It is benign new bone growth that often protrudes from the outer contour of bones and is capped by growing cartilage. The multifocal and clearly hereditary form of this lesion is known as 'hereditary multiple cartilaginous exostosis'. Whether multiple or isolated, nearly 80% of these lesions are noted prior to the age of 21 years.

## 3.31

*Answer: A*    Cerebellar vermis

A highly malignant and uniformly malignant neoplasm, medulloblastoma (neuroblastoma, granuloblastoma) represents 84% of all neuroglial neoplasms. It occurs predominantly in children; the greatest incidence is in children aged between 5 years and 9 years. Most of the tumours originate at the region of the cerebellar vermis, possibly from microscopic remnants of the cerebellar external granular layer.

## 3.32

*Answer: C*    Dermoid cyst

Benign cystic teratoma, also known as 'dermoid cyst', is the most common ovarian tumour found in premenopausal women. A dermoid cyst originates from the germ-cell component of the ovary. The tumour can therefore contain tissues that are characteristic of all

neoplasia

three germ cell layers: endoderm, mesoderm and ectoderm. The dermoid tumour is benign; the malignant counterpart is known as an 'immature teratoma'.

## 3.33

*Answer: E*   Osteosarcoma

When an osteogenic sarcoma (osteosarcoma) penetrates the bone cortex, it elevates the periosteum. This periosteal elevation usually produces an acute angle with the underlying remaining cortical bone, which is known as 'Codman's triangle'. A significant radiographic sign, Codman's triangle aids in the diagnosis of osteogenic sarcoma.

## 3.34

*Answer: B*   Burkitt's lymphoma – *c-myc* oncogene

Burkitt's lymphoma is associated with the c-*myc* oncogene, which is involved in the synthesis of nuclear regulatory proteins necessary for the growth process of B lymphocytes. Some breast cancers (eg comedocarcinomas) are associated with overexpression of the *erb*-B3 oncogene. The presence of this oncogene implies a poor prognosis for the patient. Chronic myelogenous leukaemia is associated with the c-*abl* oncogene, which is normally involved in non-receptor tyrosine kinase activity for the generation of second messengers. Colon cancer is associated with the *ras* oncogene, which is normally involved in guanosine-5-triphosphate (GTP) binding and the generation of second messengers. Neuroblastomas have an abnormality in the N-*myc* oncogene, which normally involved in the generation of nuclear regulatory proteins.

## 3.35

*Answer: E*   Thymoma – pure red blood cell aplasia

Thymomas are often associated with pure red blood cell aplasia, this sign sometimes leading to the discovery of the underlying thymoma. Paraneoplastic syndromes often indicate the presence

neoplasia

of an underlying neoplasm before it has progressed to an advanced stage. Unfortunately, they only occur in 10% to 15% of cases. To qualify as a paraneoplastic sydrome, the syndrome must not be caused by the direct effects of tumour invasion or metastasis. For example, hypercalcaemia caused by lysis of bone by metastatic tumour does not qualify, but secretion of a parathormone-like peptide producing the hypercalcemia does qualify.

Small-cell carcinoma of the lung is associated with an increase in antidiuretic hormone or adrenocorticotrophic hormone. Pancreatic carcinoma is associated with Trousseau's superficial migratory thrombophlebitis. Gastric carcinoma is associated with acanthosis nigricans. Breast carcinoma is associated with dermatomyositis.

### 3.36

*Answer: A*     Neuroblastoma – chromosome 1

Neuroblastoma is associated with a deletion on chromosome 1 and inactivation of a suppressor gene. Neurofibromas are associated with an abnormality on chromosome 17, in which there is a neurofibromatosis-1 gene that down-regulates the function of the *ras* oncogene in producing second messengers. Osteogenic sarcoma is associated with an abnormality on chromosome 17, particularly a point mutation with inactivation of the *TP53* suppressor gene. Retinoblastoma (Rb) is associated with an abnormality on chromosome 13, with inactivation of a Rb-suppressor gene that normally inhibits the growth of retinal cells. Wilms' tumours of the kidney are associated with an abnormality on chromosome 11, with loss of a suppressor gene.

### 3.37

*Answer: D*     Lung

The lungs are a more common primary site for a tumour in adults than in children. Other tumour sites that are more common in adults than in children are the skin (eg basal-cell carcinoma, malignant melanoma), the breast (eg infiltrating ductal carcinoma), the prostate and the colon. The most important risk factor for breast,

neoplasia

prostate and colon cancer is increasing age. Exposure of the skin to ultraviolet light increases the risk of skin cancer.

## 3.38

*Answer: E*    Skin cancer

Carcinomas of the skin are the most common cancers in organ transplant recipients. There is 4- to 21-fold higher incidence than that of the general population. The skin cancers differ from the carcinomas in the general population because they have increased aggressiveness, are of squamous cell origin, and occur more frequently in relatively young patients. Other common cancers in transplant recipients are: anogenital cancer (eg carcinoma of the cervix, vulva, perineum, penis and anus, possibly associated with the human papilloma viruses); non-Hodgkin's lymphoma, particulary large-cell and immunoblastic types (most non-Hodgkin's lymphomas are of B-cell origin and are commonly associated with central nervous system involvement); and Kaposi's sarcoma, which has a 400 times to 500 times higher incidence in these patients compared with the incidence in the general population. Kaposi's sarcoma has an endothelial-cell origin and is highly aggressive.

## 3.39

*Answer: D*    Renal adenocarcinoma

The distinction between a benign renal adenoma and renal adenocarcinoma is commonly made on the basis of size, tumours less than 2 cm in size rarely being malignant and those greater than 3 cm in size behaving in a malignant fashion. This distinction is also made for carcinoid tumours, which most commonly occur in the appendix. These tumours rarely metastasise because they are less than 2 cm. Carcinoids in the small intestine, however, commonly metastasise because they are often larger than 2 cm. Although size is an important criterion in staging breast, prostate, colon and lung cancers, the relationship between tumour size and malignant potential is much more marked for renal adenocarcinoma and carcinoid tumours.

## 3.40

*Answer: D*    Sacrococcygeal area

Tumours derived from all three cell layers are called 'teratomas'. In a newborn infant, the most common location is the sacrococcygeal area. Overall, however, a haemangioma is the most common tumour in infancy, and the majority of these regress over time.

## 3.41

*Answer: D*    T3

The staging of all non-small-cell lung cancer follows the TNM system. The current TNM staging system came into effect in 1997 after revisions for stage groupings for stages I, II and III. According to TNM staging for primary lung cancer, the tumour (T) stages are as follows:

TX: positive malignant cytology results, no lesion seen

T1: diameter smaller than or equal to 3 cm

T2: diameter larger than 3 cm

T3: extension to pleura, chest wall, diaphragm, pericardium, within 2 cm of carina or total atelectasis

T4: invasion of mediastinal organs (eg oesophagus, trachea, great vessels, heart), malignant pleural effusion, or satellite nodules within the primary lobe

In this scenario, therefore, the patient has a T3 tumour.

## 3.42

*Answer: C*    N2

The most important prognostic indicator in lung cancer is the extent of disease. The American Joint Committee for Cancer (AJCC) developed the TNM staging system, which takes into account the degree of spread of primary tumour, the extent of regional lymph-node involvement, and the presence or absence of distant metastases. The TNM system is used for all lung carcinomas except small-cell lung carcinomas. According to the TNM staging system,

neoplasia

regional lymph-node involvement (N) is as follows:

N0: no lymph nodes involved

N1: ipsilateral bronchopulmonary or hilar nodes involved

N2: ipsilateral mediastinal or subcarinal nodes

N3: contralateral mediastinal or hilar, or any supraclavicular nodes involved

In this scenario, therefore, the patient has N2 disease.

### 3.43

*Answer: B*    Gastro-oesophageal reflux disease

Gastro-oesophageal reflux disease (GORD) is the most common predisposing factor for adenocarcinoma of the oesophagus. As a consequence of the irritation caused by the reflux of acid and bile, 10%–15% of patients who undergo endoscopy for evaluation of GORD symptoms are found to have Barrett's epithelium. Adenocarcinoma can develop in these patients, representing the last event of a sequence that starts with the development of GORD and progresses to Barrett's metaplasia, low-grade dysplasia, high-grade dysplasia and adenocarcinoma. With the premalignant nature of Barrett's oesophagus well established, many investigators have searched for markers of oesophageal carcinoma that could facilitate earlier diagnosis and follow-up of tumour recurrence. The risk of adenocarcinoma among patients with Barrett's metaplasia has been estimated to be 30–60 times that of the general population. The oncosuppressor gene, *TP53* and various oncogenes, particularly *erb-b2*, have been studied as potential markers. Casson and colleagues have identified mutations in the *TP53* gene in patients with Barrett's epithelium that are associated with adenocarcinoma.

### 3.44

*Answer: C*    30%–60%

An excellent correlation exists between stage and 5-year survival rate in patients with colon cancer. For stage I or Dukes' stage A disease, the 5-year survival rate after surgical resection exceeds

90%. For stage II or Dukes' stage B disease, the 5-year survival rate is 70%–85% after resection, with or without adjuvant therapy. For stage III or Dukes' stage C disease, the 5-year survival rate is 30%–60% after resection and adjuvant chemotherapy. For stage IV or Dukes' stage D disease, the 5-year survival rate is poor (approximately 5%).

## 3.45

*Answer: D*   Small-cell carcinoma

Small-cell lung cancer (SCLC) is considered to be distinct from the other lung cancers (the so-called 'non-small-cell lung cancers' or NSCLCs), because of its clinical and biological characteristics. SCLC exhibits aggressive behaviour, with rapid growth, early spread to distant sites, exquisite sensitivity to chemotherapy and radiation and frequent association with distinct paraneoplastic syndromes. Surgery usually plays no role in its management, except in rare situations where it presents at a very early stage as a solitary pulmonary nodule (<5% of patients). Even then, adjuvant chemotherapy after surgical resection is recommended because SCLC should always be considered to be a systemic disease. Approximately 65%–70% of patients with SCLC have disseminated disease at presentation. Late-stage SCLCs are incurable, and patients with extensive disease have a median survival of less than 1 year. Even patients presenting with localised disease have a median survival of less than 2 years. The overall 5-year survival rate for SCLC is less than 20%.

## 3.46

*Answer: B*   Lung cancer

Lambert–Eaton myasthenic syndrome is a rare disorder of the neuromuscular junction. In terms of both the aetiology and the clinical findings, it can resemble myasthenia gravis, but there are several substantial differences between the clinical presentations and pathogenetic features of the two disorders.

The disease is usually observed in middle-aged and older people but children and young people can also be affected. Because of its

neoplasia

rarity, the exact incidence is unknown. Lambert–Eaton myasthenic syndrome is usually a solitary diagnosis but it can also occur as a paraneoplastic syndrome associated with lung cancer (small-cell histology). It can also be associated with cancers such as lymphoma, non-Hodgkin's lymphoma, T-cell leukaemia, non-small-cell lung cancer, prostate cancer and thymoma. In both conditions, the disease is of autoimmune origin, caused by antibodies that are directed against the antigens of the neuromuscular junction. In 1989 the antibodies were demonstrated to be directed against presynaptic calcium channels, which are located in the neuromuscular junction and are responsible for the efficient release of acetylcholine. The antibodies prevent normal functioning of calcium channels and so prevent the release of acetylcholine that is essential for normal nerve–muscle interactions, which in turn maintain the normal muscle strength.

The major clinical finding is progressive weakness that does not usually involve the respiratory muscles and the muscles of the face. In patients with affected ocular and respiratory muscles, the involvement is not as severe as in myasthenia gravis. The proximal parts of the legs and arms are predominantly affected. Many patients have autonomic symptoms such as dry mouth or impotence. Reflexes are usually reduced or absent.

## 3.47

*Answer: D    T3*

The Union Internationale Contre le Cancer (UICC) and the American Joint Committee on Cancer (AJCC) developed the tumour-node-metastasis (TNM) staging system, which is used to stage bladder cancer. Ta and T1 tumours and carcinoma in situ (CIS) are considered to be superficial bladder tumours. T2, T3 and T4 tumours are invasive bladder tumours. Transitional cell carcinoma (TCC) is histologically graded as low-grade (formerly graded 1–2) or high-grade (formerly graded as 3). CIS is characterised by full-mucosal-thickness and high-grade dysplasia of the bladder epithelium and is associated with a poorer prognosis.

The following is the TNM staging system for bladder cancer:

CIS: carcinoma in situ, high-grade dysplasia, confined to the epithelium

Ta: papillary tumour confined to the epithelium

T1: tumour invasion into the lamina propria

T2: tumour invasion into the muscularis propria

T3: tumour involvement of the perivesical fat

T4: tumour involvement of adjacent organs such as prostate, rectum or side wall of the pelvis

N+: lymph-node metastasis

M+: metastasis

The patient in this scenario therefore has a T3 tumour.

## 3.48

*Answer: E*    Smoking

Exposure to environmental carcinogens of various types is responsible for the development of nearly 80% of bladder cancers. Smoking is the most commonly associated risk factor and accounts for approximately 50% of all bladder cancers. Nitrosamine, 2-naphthylamine and 4-aminobiphenyl are possible carcinogenic agents found in cigarette smoke. Bladder cancer is also associated with industrial exposure to aromatic amines in dyes, paints, solvents, leather dust, inks, combustion products, rubber and textiles. Higher-risk occupations associated with bladder cancer therefore include painting, driving trucks and working with metal.

Several medical risk factors are associated with bladder cancer. Patients with prior exposure to radiation treatment of the pelvis have an increased risk of bladder cancer. Chemotherapy with cyclophosphamide increases the risk of bladder cancer via exposure to acrolein, a urinary metabolite of cyclophosphamide. Patients with spinal cord injuries who have long-term indwelling catheters have a 16- to 20-fold increased risk of developing squamous cell carcinoma of the bladder.

Coffee consumption does not increase the risk of developing bladder cancer and there is no significant correlation between artificial sweeteners (eg saccharin, cyclamate) and bladder cancer.

neoplasia

Although no convincing evidence exists for a hereditary factor in the development of bladder cancer, familial clusters of bladder cancer have been reported. Several genetic mutations have been identified in bladder cancer. Mutations of the tumour suppressor gene for p53, found on chromosome 17, are associated with high-grade bladder cancer and CIS. Mutations of the tumour suppressor gene for p15 and p16, found on chromosome 9, are associated with low-grade and superficial tumours. Retinoblastoma (Rb) tumour suppressor gene mutations have also been noted. Bladder cancer is associated with increased expression of the epidermal growth factor gene and the *erb*-b2 oncogene, and mutations of the oncogenes *p21 ras*, c-*myc*, and c-*jun*.

## 3.49

*Answer: D*    Stage III

Renal cell carcinomas can be staged by using the American Joint Committee on Cancer (AJCC) TNM (tumour-node-metastasis) classification, as follows:

Stage I: tumours that are 7 cm or smaller and confined to the kidney

Stage II: tumours that are larger than 7 cm but still confined to the kidney

Stage III: tumours extending into the renal vein or vena cava, involving the ipsilateral adrenal gland and/or perinephric fat, or which have spread to one local lymph node

Stage IV: tumours extending beyond Gerota's fascia, to more than one local node, or with distant metastases

Recent literature has questioned whether the cut-off in size between stage I and stage II tumours should be 5 cm instead of 7 cm.

The patient in this scenario therefore has a stage III tumour.

## 3.50

*Answer: B*    T2

The TNM staging system used for head and neck cancers is a clinical staging system that allows physicians to compare results across patients, assess prognosis, and design appropriate treatment regimens: 'T' refers to tumour size at the primary site, 'N' refers to the status of the cervical chain of lymph nodes, and 'M' refers to the presence or absence of distant metastases. The same system is employed for laryngeal tumours. The basic premise of these systems is that smaller cancers with no nodal disease have a better prognosis than a larger lesion with positive neck nodes.

## Primary tumour (T):

Tis: pre-invasive cancer (carcinoma in situ)

T0: no evidence of primary tumour

T1: tumour 2 cm or less in its greatest dimension

T2: tumour more than 2 cm but not more than 4 cm

T3: tumour larger than 4 cm

T4: tumour with extension to bone, muscle, skin, antrum, neck, etc

TX: minimum requirements to assess primary tumour cannot be met

## Regional lymph nodes (N):

N0: no evidence of regional lymph node involvement

N1: evidence of involvement of movable homolateral regional lymph nodes

N2: evidence of involvement of movable contralateral or bilateral regional lymph nodes

N3: evidence of involvement of fixed regional lymph nodes

NX: Minimum requirements to assess the regional nodes cannot be met

## Distant metastases (M):

M0: no evidence of distant metastases

M1: evidence of distant metastases

MX: minimum requirements to assess the presence of distant metastases cannot be met

## Staging:

Stage I: T1 N0 M0

Stage II: T2 N0 M0

neoplasia

Stage III: $T_2NOMO$, $T_3N_1MO$

Stage IV: $T_4N_1M_0$, Any $TN_2M_0$, Any $TN_3M_0$, Any T Any $NM_1$

The depth of infiltration is predictive of the prognosis. With increasing depth of invasion of the primary tumour, the risk of nodal metastasis increases and survival decreases.

The patient in this scenario therefore has a T2 tumour.

# SECTION 4: MICROBIOLOGY — ANSWERS

## 4.1

*Answer: B*    Endotoxin

Endotoxins are potentially toxic natural compounds found inside pathogens such as bacteria. Classically, an 'endotoxin' is a toxin which, unlike an 'exotoxin', is not secreted in soluble form by live bacteria, but is a structural component in the bacterium itself and which is released mainly when bacteria are lysed. The prototypical examples of endotoxin are lipopolysaccharides (LPS) or lipo-oligo-saccharides found in the outer membrane of various Gram-negative bacteria. The term 'LPS' is often used interchangeably with 'endotoxin' because of the history of its discovery: in the early nineteenth century it became understood that bacteria could secrete toxins into their environment, which became broadly known as 'exotoxin'. The term 'endotoxin' resulted from the discovery that portions of Gram-negative bacteria can cause toxicity, hence the name 'endotoxin'. Studies of endotoxin over the next 50 years revealed that the effects of 'endotoxin' were in fact due to lipopolysaccharide.

There are, however, endotoxins other than LPS. For example, delta endotoxin of *Bacillus thuringiensis* makes crystal-like inclusion bodies next to the endospore inside the bacteria. It is toxic to larvae of insects feeding on plants, but is harmless to humans (as we do not possess the enzymes and receptors necessary for its processing followed by toxicity). The only Gram-positive bacteria that produces endotoxin is *Listeria monocytogenes*.

LPS consist of a polysaccharide (sugar) chain and a lipid moiety, known as lipid A, which is responsible for the toxic effects. The polysaccharide chain is highly variable between different bacteria. Endotoxins are approximately 10 kDa in size but can form large aggregates of up to 1000 kDa. Humans are able to produce antibodies to endotoxins after exposure but these are generally directed at the polysaccharide chain and do not protect against a wide variety of endotoxins. Injection of a small amount of endotoxin in human volunteers produced fever, a lowering of the blood pressure, and activation of inflammation and coagulation. Endotoxins are in large part responsible for the dramatic clinical manifestations of infections with pathogenic Gram-negative bacteria such as *Neisseria meningitidis* (also simply known as 'meningococcus'), the pathogen that causes fulminant meningitis. The clinical features in this scenario are also suggestive of meningitis.

## 4.2

*Answer:* C  *Escherichia coli*

*Escherichia coli* is one of the main species of bacteria living in the lower intestines of mammals, known as the 'gut flora'. When located in the large instestine, it actually assists with waste processing, vitamin K production and food absorption. Discovered in 1885 by Theodor Escherich, a German paediatrician and bacteriologist, *E. coli* are abundant: the number of individual *E. coli* bacteria in the faeces that a human defecates in 1 day averages between 100 billion and 10 trillion.

As with all Gram-negative organisms, *E. coli* are unable to sporulate. Treatments which kill all active bacteria, such as pasteurisation or simple boiling, are therefore effective for their eradication, without requiring the more rigorous sterilisation which also deactivates spores. As a result of their adaptation to mammalian intestines, *E. coli* grow best in vivo or at the higher temperatures characteristic of such an environment, rather than the cooler temperatures found in soil and other environments.

*E. coli* can generally cause several intestinal and extra-intestinal infections, including urinary tract infections, meningitis, peritonitis, mastitis, septicaemia and Gram-negative pneumonia. Although it is more common in females due to the shorter urinary tract, urinary tract infection is seen in both males and females. It is found in roughly equal proportions in elderly men and women. Because bacteria invariably enter the urinary tract through the urethra ('ascending infections'), poor toilet habits can predispose to infection, but other factors are also important (pregnancy in women, prostate enlargement in men) and in many cases the initiating event is unclear. While ascending infections are generally the rule for lower urinary tract infections and cystitis, the same may not necessarily hold for upper urinary tract infections such as pyelonephritis, which can be haematogenous in origin. Most cases of lower urinary tract infections in women are benign and do not need exhaustive laboratory investigations. However, young infants with urinary tract infections must undergo some form of imaging study, typically a retrograde urethrogram, to investigate for congenital urinary tract anomalies. Males with urinary tract infections also must be investigated further.

The clinical features and laboratory findings point to *E. coli* septicaemia in this patient.

## 4.3

*Answer: A*   Epstein–Barr virus

These are the findings of infectious mononucleosis, which is typically acquired through close personal contact. Infectious mononucleosis, also known as 'the kissing disease', 'Pfeiffer's disease', 'mono', or 'glandular fever', is a disease seen most commonly in adolescents and young adults, and is characterised by fever, sore throat, muscle soreness and fatigue. White patches on the tonsils or in the back of the throat can also be seen. Mononucleosis is usually caused by the Epstein–Barr virus (EBV), which infects B lymphocytes, producing a reactive lymphocytosis and atypical T lymphocytes known as 'Downey bodies'.

The virus is typically transmitted from asymptomatic individuals through blood or saliva, or by sharing a drink or eating utensils, though the disease is far less contagious than is commonly thought. In rare cases a person may have a high resistance to infection. The mononuclear leukocyte count is significantly raised. There are two main types of mononuclear leukocytes, monocytes and lymphocytes. They normally account for about 35% of all white blood cells. In infectious mononucleosis, this can rise to 50%–70%. In addition, the overall white blood cell count is almost invariably raised, and can increase to $10$–$20 \times 10^9/l$.

microbiology

Mononucleosis leads to the production of heterophile antibodies, which cause agglutination of non-human red blood cells: the Monospot test is a non-specific test that screens for mononucleosis by looking for these antibodies. Confirmation of the exact cause of the infection can be obtained through tests to detect specific antibodies to the causative viruses. The Monospot test might be negative in the first week, so negative tests are often repeated at a later date. Because the Monospot test is usually negative in children under the age of 6–8 years, EBV serology should be requested if mononucleosis is suspected. An older test for heterophile antibodies is the Paul–Bunnell test, in which the patient's serum is mixed with sheep red blood cells and checked for agglutination of these cells.

## 4.4

*Answer: C     Lactobacillus* species

*Lactobacillus* is a genus of Gram-positive facultative anaerobic bacteria. They are a major part of the lactic acid bacteria group, named as such because most of its members convert lactose and other sugars to lactic acid. They are common and usually benign. In humans they are present in the vagina and the gastrointestinal tract, where they are symbiotic and make up a small portion of the gut flora. Many species are prominent in decaying plant material. The production of lactic acid makes its environment acidic, which inhibits the growth of some harmful bacteria. Several members of the genus have had their genome sequenced.

## 4.5

*Answer: E     Outer membrane

Gram-negative bacteria do not retain crystal violet dye in the Gram staining protocol. Gram-positive bacteria will retain the dark-blue dye after an alcohol wash. In a Gram stain test, a counterstain (commonly Safranin) is added after the crystal violet, which colours all Gram-negative bacteria a red or pink colour. The test itself is useful in classifying two distinctly different types of bacteria on the basis of structural differences in their cell walls.

microbiology

Many species of Gram-negative bacteria are pathogenic, meaning they can cause disease in a host organism. This pathogenic capability is usually associated with certain components of Gram-negative cell walls, in particular the lipopolysaccharide (LPS) or endotoxin layer. The LPS is the trigger which the body's innate immune response receptors sense to begin a cytokine reaction. It is toxic to the host. It is this response which begins the inflammation cycle in tissues and blood vessels.

The following characteristics are displayed by Gram-negative bacteria:

- The cell walls only contain a few layers of peptidoglycan (which is present in much higher levels in Gram-positive bacteria).

- The cells are surrounded by an outer membrane containing lipopolysaccharide (which consists of lipid A, core polysaccharide and O-polysaccharide) outside the peptidoglycan layer.

- Porins exist in the outer membrane, which act like pores for particular molecules.

- There is a space between the layers of peptidoglycan and the secondary cell membrane called the 'periplasmic space'.

- The S-layer is directly attached to the outer membrane, rather than to the peptidoglycan.

- If present, flagella have four supporting rings instead of two.

- No teichoic acids or lipoteichoic acids are present.

- Lipoproteins are attached to the polysaccharide backbone, in contrast to Gram-positive bacteria, in which no lipoproteins are present.

- Most do not sporulate (*Coxiella burnetii* forms spore-like structures).

microbiology

**4.6**

*Answer: E*    Rifampicin + isoniazid + pyrazinamide + ethambutol

Tuberculosis is treated in two phases, an initial phase using four drugs and a continuation phase using two drugs in fully sensitive cases. Treatment requires specialised knowledge, particularly where the disease involves resistant organisms or non-respiratory organs.

The regimens given below are recommended for the treatment of tuberculosis in the UK; variations occur in other countries. Either the unsupervised regimen or the supervised regimen described below should be used; the two regimens should not be used concurrently.

**Initial phase.** The concurrent use of four drugs during the initial phase is designed to reduce the bacterial population as rapidly as possible and to prevent the emergence of drug-resistant bacteria. The drugs are best given as combination preparations unless one of the components cannot be given because of resistance or intolerance. The treatment of choice for the initial phase is the daily use of isoniazid, rifampicin, pyrazinamide and ethambutol. Streptomycin is rarely used in the UK but it can be used in the initial phase of treatment if resistance to isoniazid has been established before therapy is commenced. Treatment should be started without waiting for culture results if clinical features or histology results are consistent with tuberculosis; treatment should be continued even if initial culture results are negative. The initial phase drugs should be continued for 2 months. Where a positive culture for *Mycobacterium tuberculosis* has been obtained, but susceptibility results are not available after 2 months, treatment with rifampicin, isoniazid, pyrazinamide and ethambutol should be continued until full susceptibility is confirmed, even if this is for longer than 2 months.

**Continuation phase.** After the initial phase, treatment is continued for a further 4 months with isoniazid and rifampicin (preferably given as a combination preparation). Longer treatment is necessary for meningitis, direct spinal cord involvement, and for resistant organisms (which might also require modification of the regimen).

## 4.7

*Answer: A     Bacteroides fragilis*

*Bacteroides* is a genus of Gram-negative, rod-shaped bacteria. *Bacteroides* species are non-endospore-forming anaerobes, and can either be motile or non-motile, depending on the species. The DNA base composition is 40%–48% GC. Unusual in bacterial organisms, *Bacteroides* organisms' membranes contain sphingolipids. They also contain meso-diaminopimelic acid in their peptidoglycan layer. *Bacteroides* are normally commensal, making up the most substantial portion of the mammalian gastrointestinal flora, where they play a fundamental role in the processing of complex molecules to simpler ones in the host intestine. As many as $10^{10}$–$10^{11}$ cells per gram of human faeces has been reported. They can use simple sugars when available, but their main source of energy is polysaccharide from plant sources.

*Bacteroides fragilis* is an obligate anaerobe of the gut. It is involved in 90% of anaerobic peritoneal infections. *B. fragilis* is generally susceptible to metronidazole, carbapenems, and beta-lactam/beta-lactamase inhibitor combinations, but it has inherent high-level resistance to penicillin. Clindamycin is no longer recommended as the first-line agent for *B. fragilis* due to emerging high-level resistance (>30% in some reports).

## 4.8

*Answer: B     Cholera toxin*

Cholera toxin is a protein complex secreted by the bacterium *Vibrio cholerae*. Cholera toxin is responsible for the harmful effects of cholera infection. The cholera toxin is an oligomeric complex made up of six protein subunits: a single copy of the A subunit and five copies of the B subunit. The five B subunits, each weighing 12 kDa, form a five-membered ring. The A subunit has two important segments: the A1 portion of the chain (CTA1) is a globular enzyme payload, while the A2 chain (CTA2) forms an extended alpha helix which sits snugly in the central pore of the B subunit ring. This structure is similar in shape, mechanism and sequence to the heat-labile enterotoxin secreted by some strains of the *Escherichia coli* bacterium.

microbiology

Once secreted, the B subunit ring of cholera toxin will bind to GM1 gangliosides on the surface of the host's cells. After binding takes place, the entire cholera toxin complex is internalised by the cell and the CTA1 chain is released by the reduction of a disulphide bridge. CTA1 is then free to bind with a human partner protein called 'ADP-ribosylation factor 6' (Arf6); binding to Arf6 drives a change in the conformation of CTA1, which exposes its active site and enables its catalytic activity. The CTA1 fragment catalyses ADP ribosylation from NAD to the regulatory component of adenylate cyclase, thereby activating it. Increased adenylate cyclase activity increases cyclic AMP synthesis, causing massive fluid and electrolyte efflux, resulting in diarrhoea.

## 4.9

*Answer: B      Clostridium botulinum*

Botulism (from the Latin *botulus*, sausage) is a rare but serious paralytic illness caused by a nerve toxin, botulin, that is produced by the bacterium *Clostridium botulinum*. Botulinum toxin is one of the most powerful known, with a lethal dose of a microgram. It acts by blocking nerve function and leads to respiratory and musculoskeletal paralysis.

There are three main kinds of botulism:

- **Food-borne botulism** is a form of food-borne illness and is caused by eating foods that contain the botulinum toxin.

- **Infant botulism** is caused by consuming the spores of the botulinum bacteria, which then grow in the intestines and release toxin.

- **Wound botulism** is caused by toxin produced from a wound infected with *C. botulinum*. This is the rarest type of botulism.

All forms of botulism can be fatal and are considered medical emergencies. Food-borne botulism can be especially dangerous as a public health problem because many people can be poisoned from a single contaminated food source.

## 4.10

*Answer: E*    *Staphylococcus aureus*

Folliculitis is inflammation of one or more hair follicles. The condition can occur anywhere on the skin. Most carbuncles and furuncles and other cases of folliculitis develop as a result of *Staphylococcus aureus* infection. This organism is a bit different from the regular staphylococcus found on the skin, mostly within the nostrils. *S. aureus* is an important pathogen as most of the important skin infections are caused by it. Folliculitis starts when hair follicles are damaged by friction from clothing, blockage of the follicle or shaving. In most cases of folliculitis, the damaged follicles are then infected with *S. aureus*.

## 4.11

*Answer: D*    Sputum culture

Sputum culture is used to detect and identify bacteria or fungi that are infecting the lungs or breathing passages. Sputum is a thick fluid produced in the lungs and in the airways leading to the lungs. A sample of sputum is placed in a container with substances that promote the growth of bacteria or fungi. If no bacteria or fungi grow, the culture is negative. If pathogenic organisms do grow, the culture is positive. The type of bacterium or fungus is identified by microscopy or using chemical tests. If bacteria or fungi that can cause infection grow in the culture, other tests can be performed in order to determine which antibiotic will be most effective in treating the infection, ie susceptibility or sensitivity testing. The test is done on a sample of sputum that is usually collected by coughing. For people who cannot cough deeply enough to produce a sample, a suction tube or needle may be inserted into the airway to collect the sputum.

microbiology

## 4.12

*Answer: C*    Ciprofloxacin

Treatment for anthrax infection includes large doses of intravenous and oral antibiotics, such as ciprofloxacin, doxycycline, erythromycin and vancomycin. For inhalation infections, antibiotic treatment is not very effective unless initiated within 1 day of exposure, before any symptoms appear. Antibiotic treatment is crucial in cases of pulmonary anthrax to prevent death. Antibiotic-resistant strains of *Bacillus anthracis* are known.

## 4.13

*Answer: E*    *Salmonella typhi*

The Widal test is a serological test for *Salmonella typhi*. It is a demonstration of salmonella antibodies against antigens O-somatic and H-flagellar in the blood. It is used to ascertain the presence of typhoid fever. However, it is not a very accurate method because patients are often exposed to other bacteria in this species that induce cross-reactivity (eg *S. enteritidis*, *S. typhimurium*). Many people have antibodies against these enteric pathogens, which also react with the antigens in the Widal test, leading to a false-positive result. Typhidot is the other test used to diagnose typhoid fever. As with all serological tests, the rise in antibody levels needed to make the diagnosis takes 7–14 days, which limits their usefulness. Other means of diagnosing *S. typhi* (and paratyphus infections) include cultures of blood, urine and faeces. The organism also produces hydrogen sulphide from thiosulphate.

## 4.14

*Answer: D*    Respiratory tract

Blastomycosis is a pulmonary and occasionally haematogenous fungal infection caused by the organism *Blastomyces dermatitidis*. Endemic in parts of North America, blastomycosis causes clinical symptoms similar to histoplasmosis. Infection occurs by inhalation of the spores of the fungus from its natural soil habitat. Once inhaled into the lungs, the fungus multiplies and can disseminate through the blood and lymphatics to other organs, including the skin, bone, genitourinary tract and brain. The incubation period is 30–100 days, although infection can be asymptomatic.

## 4.15

*Answer: D*   Exotoxin

*Pseudomonas aeruginosa* is a Gram-negative, aerobic, rod-shaped bacterium with unipolar motility. *P. aeruginosa* is an opportunistic human pathogen. Like other *Pseudomonas* organisms, *P. aeruginosa* secretes a variety of pigments, including pyocyanin (blue-green), fluorescein (yellow-green and fluorescent, now also known as 'pyoverdin'), and pyorubin (red-brown).

An opportunistic pathogen in immunocompromised individuals, *P. aeruginosa* typically infects the pulmonary tract, urinary tract, burns and wounds, and also causes other blood infections. *Pseudomonas* can occasionally cause community-acquired pneumonias, as well as ventilator-associated pneumonias (being one of the most common agents isolated in these infections in several studies). One in ten hospital-acquired infections are caused by *Pseudomonas*. Patients with cystic fibrosis are also predisposed to *P. aeruginosa* infection of the lungs. *P. aeruginosa* is also the typical cause of 'hot-tub rash' (dermatitis), which is caused by lack of proper, periodic attention to water quality. The most common cause of burn infections is *P. aeruginosa*.

*P. aeruginosa* uses the virulence factor exotoxin A to ADP-ribosylate eukaryotic elongation factor 2 in the host cell, much as the diphtheria toxin does. Without elongation factor 2, eukaryotic cells cannot synthesise proteins and necrose. The release of intracellular contents induces an immunological response in immunocompetent patients.

microbiology

## 4.16

*Answer: D*    *Staphylococus aureus*

*Staphylococus aureus* is commonly found on the skin and can attack either healthy or deformed valves. This organism is responsible for 10% to 20% of cases of infective endocarditis. *S. aureus* is the main offender in intravenous drug abusers.

## 4.17

*Answer: A*    Caseation necrosis

The tuberculous granuloma (caseating tubercle) has central caseous necrosis bordered by giant multinucleated cells (Langerhans cells), and surrounded by epithelioid cell aggregates, lymphocytes and fibroblasts. Granulomatous tubercles tend to become confluent. Multinucleated giant cells (mature, Langerhans-type) are 50–100 μm in diameter, with numerous small nuclei (over 20) lying peripherally in the cell (in a crown or horseshoe distribution). They have abundant eosinophilic cytoplasm. They are formed when activated macrophages merge. Epithelioid cells are activated macrophages that resemble epithelial cells. They are elongated, with finely granular, pale eosinophilic (pink) cytoplasm and a central, ovoid nucleus. They have indistinct shape and contour and form aggregates. At the periphery of the tubercle are the lymphocytes (T cells) and rare plasma cells and fibroblasts. Caseous necrosis is a central area, amorphous, finely granular, and eosinophilic. If recent, it can contain nuclear fragments. The caseous material is the result of the accumulated destruction of giant cells and epithelioid cells.

## 4.18

*Answer: A*    Toxin and enzyme production

'Virulence' refers to the degree of pathogenicity of a microbe, in other words, the relative ability of a microbe to cause disease. The virulence factors of bacteria are typically proteins or other molecules that are synthesised by protein enzymes. These proteins are coded for by genes in chromosomal DNA, bacteriophage DNA or plasmids. Factors which affect pathogens' ability to cause disease include adhesion, colonisation, invasion, immune response inhibition and toxins:

- **Adhesion**. Many bacteria must first bind to host cell surfaces. Many bacterial and host molecules that are involved in the adhesion of bacteria to host cells have been identified. Often, the host cell receptors for bacteria are essential proteins for other functions.

- **Colonisation**. Some virulent bacteria produce special proteins that allow them to colonise parts of the host body. *Helicobacter pylori* is able to survive in the acidic environment of the human stomach by producing the enzyme urease, for example. Colonisation of the stomach lining by this bacterium can lead to gastric ulcer and cancer. The virulence of various strains of *H. pylori* tends to correlate with the level of production of urease.

- **Invasion**. Some virulent bacteria produce proteins that either disrupt host cell membranes or stimulate endocytosis into host cells. These virulence factors allow the bacteria to enter host cells and facilitate entry into the body across epithelial tissue layers at the body surface.

- **Immune response inhibitors**. Many bacteria produce virulence factors that inhibit the host's immune system defences. For example, a common bacterial strategy is to produce proteins that bind host antibodies. The polysaccharide capsule of *Streptococcus pneumoniae* inhibits phagocytosis of the bacterium by host immune cells, for example.

- **Toxins**. Many virulence factors are proteins made by bacteria that poison host cells and cause tissue damage. For example, there are many food-poisoning toxins produced by bacteria that can contaminate human foods. Some of these can remain in 'spoiled' food even after cooking and cause illness when the contaminated food is consumed. Some bacterial toxins are chemically altered and inactivated by the heat of cooking.

microbiology

## 4.19

*Answer: E*    Unpasteurised milk

Brucellosis, also called 'undulant fever' or 'Malta fever', is a zoonosis (an infectious disease transmitted from animals to humans) caused by bacteria of the genus *Brucella*. It is primarily a disease of domestic animals (goats, pigs, cattle, dogs, etc) and humans and has a worldwide distribution, mainly now in developing countries.

The disease is transmitted either through contaminated or untreated milk (and its derivatives) or through direct contact with infected animals, which can include dogs, pigs, camels and ruminants, but primarily includes sheep, goats and cattle. This also includes contact with their carcasses. Parturition rests are extremely rich in highly virulent *Brucella* organisms. Along with *Leptospira*, *Brucella* organisms have the unique property of being able to penetrate through intact human skin, so infection by mere hand contact with infectious material is likely to occur.

The disease is now usually associated with the consumption of unpasteurised milk and soft cheeses made from the milk of infected animals and with occupational exposure of veterinarians and slaughterhouse workers. Some vaccines used in livestock management, most notably derived from the *B. abortus* strain 19, can also cause disease in humans if accidentally injected. The incubation period of brucellosis is usually 1–3 weeks, but the disease can occasionally take several months to surface.

## 4.20

*Answer: A*    Actinomycosis

Actinomycosis is usually caused by *Actinomyces israelii* and is frequently misdiagnosed as a neoplasm. In health, *A. israelii* colonises the vagina, colon and mouth. Infection is established first by a breach of the mucosal barrier through various procedures (eg dental, gastrointestinal), aspiration, or pathological conditions such as diverticulitis. The chronic phase of this disease is also known as the 'classic phase' because the acute early phase is often missed. This is characterised by slow contiguous growth that ignores tissue planes and forms a sinus tract that can spontaneously heal

microbiology

and recur, leading to a densely fibrotic lesion. This lesion is often described as 'wooden'. Sulphur granules form in a central purulence surrounded by neutrophils. This conglomeration of organisms is virtually diagnostic of *A. israelii*.

Oral-cervicofacial disease is the most common form of actinomycosis. It is characterised by a painless 'lumpy jaw'. Lymphadenopathy is uncommon in this form of the disease. Another form of actinomycosis is thoracic disease, which is often misdiagnosed as a neoplasm, as it forms a mass that extends to the chest wall. It arises through aspiration of organisms from the oropharynx. Symptoms include chest pain, fever and weight loss. Abdominal disease is another manifestation of actinomycosis. This can lead to a sinus tract that drains to the abdominal wall or the perianal area. Pelvic actinomycosis is often caused by intrauterine devices. Symptoms include fever, abdominal pain and weight loss.

## 4.21

*Answer: B    Pseudomonas aeruginosa*

The colour of the pus gives a clue to the likely causative pathogen here. Definitive clinical identification of *Pseudomonas aeruginosa* often includes identifying the production of both pyocyanin (blue-green) and fluorescein (yellow-green and fluorescent), which are responsible for the greenish colour of the pus.

## 4.22

*Answer: A    Cryptosporidium parvum*

*Cryptosporidium parvum* is one of several species that cause cryptosporidiosis. *C. parvum* infection is a protozoal infection that causes an acute diarrhoea in immunocompromised patients. In HIV infection, it can cause a watery diarrhoea which can be associated with anorexia, nausea, vomiting and abdominal pain. There is no effective treatment (other than supportive treatment) for this infection apart from an antibiotic called paromomycin. This drug can have a limited effect on the diarrhoea.

microbiology

**4.23**

*Answer: D*   *Streptococcus viridans*

Endocarditis of native but previously damaged or otherwise abnormal valves is caused most commonly (in 50%–60% of cases) by *Streptococcus viridans*. It is, however, important to remember that *S. viridans* is not the organism responsible for rheumatic disease.

**4.24**

*Answer: E*   Iron deficiency anaemia

Worldwide, the most common cause of iron deficiency anemia is parasitic infestation (hookworm, amoebiasis, schistosomiasis and whipworm).

**4.25**

*Answer: B*   Epstein–Barr virus

Epstein–Barr virus (EBV), also called human herpesvirus 4 (HHV-4), is a virus of the herpes family (which includes herpes simplex virus and cytomegalovirus). Its host is humans and most people become infected with EBV. Infection with EBV is often asymptomatic but it commonly causes infectious mononucleosis. EBV is also statistically associated with and likely has a causal role in Burkitt's lymphoma, certain B-cell tumours in immunocompromised patients, and nasopharyngeal carcinoma. It is named after Michael Epstein and Yvonne Barr, who together with Bert Achong discovered the virus in 1964 (see also *Answer* to **4.3**).

**4.26**

*Answer: C*   Inhibition of bacterial wall synthesis

Meropenem is an ultra-broad-spectrum, beta-lactam, injectable antibiotic used to treat a wide variety of infections, including meningitis and pneumonia. It belongs to the subgroup of carbapenem and is similar to imipenem and ertapenem. It penetrates well into many tissues and body fluids, including the cerebrospinal fluid, bile, heart valves, lung and peritoneal fluid. Meropenem is bactericidal except against *Listeria monocytogenes* (where it is bacteriostatic). It inhibits bacterial wall synthesis like other beta-lactam antibiotics. In contrast to other beta-lactams, however, it is highly resistant to degradation by beta-lactamases or cephalosporinases. Resistance generally arises due to mutations in penicillin-binding proteins, production of metallo-beta-lactamases, or resistance to diffusion across the bacterial outer membrane. Unlike imipenem, it is stable to dehydropeptidase-1 and can therefore be given without cilastatin.

## 4.27

*Answer: E*    Prevents the amino-acyl t-RNA from binding to the A site of the ribosome

Doxycycline is a member of the tetracycline antibiotic group. As well as the general indications for all members of the tetracycline antibiotic group, doxycycline is frequently used to treat chronic prostatitis, sinusitis, syphilis, chlamydia infections, pelvic inflammatory disease, acne and rosacea. In addition, it is used in the treatment and prophylaxis of anthrax and malaria. Its mechanism of action against malaria is to specifically impair in the progeny the apicoplast genes resulting in their abnormal cell division.

It is also effective against *Yersinia pestis* (the infectious agent of bubonic plague) and is prescribed for the treatment of Lyme disease and Rocky Mountain spotted fever. Doxycycline, like other antibiotics, will not work for colds, flu or other viral infections.

Elephantiasis is a disease caused by a nematode *Wuchereria bancrofti*. It causes swollen limbs and genitals (filariasis) and affects over 120 million people in the world. Previous anti-nematode treatments have been limited by poor levels of effectiveness, drug side-effects and high costs. In 2003 doxycycyline was shown to kill the symbiotic *Wolbachia* bacteria which the nematodes depend on. Field trials in 2005 showed that doxycycline almost completely eliminates blood-borne filaria when given as an 8-week course.

microbiology

Doxycycline like other tetracyclines inhibits cell growth by inhibiting translation. It binds to the 16S part of the 30S ribosomal subunit and prevents the amino-acyl t-RNA from binding to the A site of the ribosome. The binding is reversible in nature.

## 4.28

*Answer: D*   Sulphonamides

Stevens–Johnson syndrome (SJS) is a severe and life-threatening condition. It is thought to be a hypersensitivity complex affecting the skin and the mucous membranes. SJS has been classified as a severe expression of erythema multiforme, and is sometimes referred to as 'erythema multiforme major'. This terminology is not consistent; medical texts often distinguish between causes of SJS, referring to the drug-induced syndrome as SJS and applying the term 'erythema multiforme' to cases with a viral aetiology. SJS is a rare condition, with a reported incidence of around one case per million people per year.

SJS is characterised by a flu-like prodromal period of fever, sore throat and headache, followed by the sudden development of circular mucocutaneous lesions that can cover the majority of the skin. These lesions begin as macules and can develop into papules, vesicles, blisters or urticarial weals.

Stevens–Johnson syndrome is the term usually used to describe those cases where less than 10% of body surface is involved. When more than 30% of the body surface area is involved the condition is called toxic epidermal necrolysis syndrome (TENS) or Lyell's syndrome. Intermediate cases (10%–30% body surface involved) are classified as 'SJS/TENS' overlap.

SJS can be caused by infections (usually viral infections such as herpes simplex, influenza, mumps, cat-scratch fever, histoplasmosis, Epstein–Barr virus infection), allergic reactions to drugs, (valdecoxib, penicillins, barbiturates, sulphonamides, phenytoin, lamotrigine, nevirapine, ibuprofen, ethosuximide, carbamazepine), malignancy (carcinomas and lymphomas), or idiopathic factors (up to 50% of cases). SJS has also been consistently reported as an uncommon side-effect of herbal supplements containing ginseng. SJS can also be caused by cocaine usage.

## 4.29

*Answer: B*    Blockage of bacterial DNA replication

Ciprofloxacin, belonging to a group called 'fluoroquinolones', is a broad-spectrum antibiotic that is active against both Gram-positive and Gram-negative bacteria. Ciprofloxacin is bactericidal. Its mode of action depends on blocking bacterial DNA replication by binding itself to the enzyme DNA gyrase (topoisomerase), thereby causing double-stranded breaks in the bacterial choromosome.

## 4.30

*Answer: D*    Inhibition of protein synthesis by binding to the 30S subunit of the bacterial ribosome

Amikacin is an aminoglycoside antibiotic used to treat different types of bacterial infections. Amikacin works by binding to the bacterial 30S ribosomal subunit, causing misreading of mRNA and leaving the bacterium unable to synthesise proteins vital to its growth. Amikacin can be administered once or twice a day but must be given by the intravenous or intramuscular routes and tends to be painful. There is no oral form available. The dosage must be adjusted in people with kidney failure. Amikacin is most often used for treating severe, hospital-acquired infections with multidrug-resistant Gram-negative bacteria such as *Pseudomonas aeruginosa*, *Acinetobacter*, and enterobacteria. Amikacin can be combined with a beta-lactam antibiotic for empirical therapy for people with neutropenia and fever.

Side-effects of amikacin are similar to those of other aminoglycosides. Kidney damage and hearing loss are the most important effects. Because of this potential, blood levels of the drug and markers of kidney function (creatinine) should be monitored.

microbiology

## 4.31

*Answer: B*   *Escherichia coli* with pili

Piliated strains of *Escherichia coli* ascend the urethra to infect the bladder and kidney. Infections of the kidney cause pyelonephritis. The vast majority of cases of bacterial pyelonephritis, cystitis, and other urinary tract infections are caused by *E. coli*. Introduction of catheters into the urethra has been associated with the occurrence of urinary tract infections. *Clostridium difficile* is the cause of pseudomembranous colitis. *Staphylococcus aureus* is usually the cause of boils, skin sepsis, postoperative wound infections, scalded skin syndrome, food-borne infection, septicaemia, endocarditis, toxic shock syndrome, osteomyelitis and pneumonia. *Pseudomonas aeruginosa* is usually the cause of infections of skin and burns. It is also the major pathogen in cystic fibrosis, and can cause urinary infections, but not as commonly as *E. coli*. *Streptococcus pneumoniae* is the most common micro-organism that causes pneumonia.

## 4.32

*Answer: C*   Identification of the organism that is causing the pneumonia

The patient described in the question probably has acquired immunodeficiency syndrome (AIDS). Such individuals will be lymphopenic and have greatly reduced immunity. People with AIDS commonly develop *Pneumocystis carinii* pneumonia. The most important evaluative procedure for the patient described here is determination of the cause of the pneumonia so the problem can be corrected. Identifying the infecting organism might assist in the overall diagnosis. About 30% of patients with HIV infection have *P. carinii* pneumonia as the initial AIDS-defining diagnosis, and over 80% of AIDS patients have this infection at some time if prophylaxis is not given. Patients with HIV infection become vulnerable to *P. jiroveci* pneumonia when the CD4+ helper cell count is less than 200/$\mu$l.

Choices B to E involve innate immunity, either complement activity or phagocytic cell functions, and would not be of much diagnostic assistance.

## 4.33

*Answer:* C    Methicillin

The boy in this scenario appears to be suffering from meningitis due to *S. aureus,* which should always be assumed to be a betaβ-lactamase-producing organism until the laboratory reports its antibiotic sensitivity. Methicillin is a betaβ-lactamase-resistant penicillin that would be the drug of choice among those listed. It is also bactericidal and is not associated with toxicity, which is a feature of streptomycin and chloramphenicol. Other antibiotics that might be used include the cephalosporins, gentamicin, or vancomycin, which can be injected intrathecally.

## 4.34

*Answer:* E    Start rabies vaccine and give antirabies serum

If exposure to rabies virus appears definite, as in this case, treatment with human diploid-cell live-derived vaccine and hyperimmune antirabies gamma globulin should be started immediately. Serum antibodies provide an immediate barrier to the growth of virus; meanwhile, antibodies are elicited by the vaccine. If the level of exposure is minimal (ie there is no skin puncture) and the animal probably is not rabid, vaccine is not recommended. Ordering a search for the attacking dog for autopsy to determine if it has rabies is like searching for a needle in a haystack, and therefore not the best approach to address a possible rabies infection, which requires immediate action. Initiation of rabies vaccine will lead to production of antibodies against the rabies virus, but it will require approximately two weeks to develop protective antibodies. By that time, severe damage could have already occurred. Post-exposure immunisation and human rabies immunoglobulin is the best approach. Observation of the patient or reporting of the incident to the local police do not address the real needs of an individual running the risk of rabies.

microbiology

## 4.35

*Answer: E*    Receive prophylactic isoniazid

Exposure to the tuberculosis (TB) bacillus does not assure disease, but a positive skin test makes the diagnosis more likely. Chemoprophylaxis with isoniazid would be the treatment of choice for contacts of actively infected people. Ethambutol is very effective against most mycobacteria, but would be used in the therapy of TB, not in prophylaxis. The skin test is the most sensitive index of infection, and for individuals who have already shown a positive response, chest X-ray would not add much information. Sequential X-rays taken months apart might indicate if a lesion was increasing in size, but that is certainly not a high-priority procedure for the people described in the question. Immunisation with the live attenuated TB strain bacillus Calmette–Guérin (BCG) would be pointless because the contacts have already experienced an infection with *Mycobacterium tuberculosis*. Immunisation with purified protein derivative does not give protection against tuberculosis. It is used to determine exposure to *M. tuberculosis*.

## 4.36

*Answer: B*    Causes the formation of pyrimidine dimers

The mode of action of ultraviolet light on micro-organisms is related to its absorption by the DNA. This absorption leads to the formation of covalent bonds between adjacent pyrimidine bases. These pyrimidine dimers alter the form of the DNA and thus interfere with normal base pairing during the synthesis of DNA. Disruption of the bacterial cell membrane, removal of free sulphhydryl groups, protein denaturation, and addition of alkyl groups to cellular components are caused by detergents, heavy metals, heat or alcoholic compounds, and ethylene oxide or formaldehyde, respectively.

## 4.37

*Answer: E*    T-cell deficiency

An undesirable side-effect of chemotherapy used to treat malignancies is the destruction of T cells, which play a key role in the development of immunity against viral infections. This is especially true for viral diseases in which the causative agent remains dormant in the body. Varicella-zoster is an excellent example of such a virus and flare-ups of varicella-zoster infections are well-known occurrences in cancer patients who receive chemotherapy. The varicella-zoster virus is a single entity. It is a medium-sized (100–200 nm), double-stranded DNA virus of the herpesvirus group, with only one serological type. Primary infection with the varicella-zoster virus causes chickenpox. Immunity develops, but the virus remains in the body. Immunosuppression by chemotherapy reactivates the varicella-zoster virus and causes shingles. Deficiency in the third component of complement is associated with enhanced susceptibility to pyogenic extracellular bacteria, but not to viruses. Hypogammaglobulinaemia has not been shown to cause disseminated varicella-zoster infection.

## 4.38

*Answer: D*    Production of an exotoxin by the causative agent

Diphtheria is typically a toxaemic disease. The causative agent, *Corynebacterium diphtheriae* remains localised in the nose and throat, where it produces diphtheria exotoxin, which has a selective action on certain organs, such as the heart, kidneys, adrenals and diaphragm. The exotoxin inhibits protein synthesis by ADP ribosylation of elongation factor 2. Tumour necrosis factor is an inflammatory substance produced by macrophages, and might therefore contribute to the pathogenesis of diphtheria but does not explain the toxigenicity of *C. diphtheriae*. *C. diphtheriae* has not been shown to possess a capsule that plays a major role in the pathogenesis of diphtheria. *C. diphtheriae* has not been shown to have any envelope enzymes that kill natural killer T lymphocytes. Immune complex formation has been shown to be involved in the pathogenicity of acute glomerulonephritis, type III hypersensitivity and various autoimmune diseases, but not diphtheria.

microbiology

**4.39**

*Answer: A*　Coagulase

In a laboratory test used to identify *Staphylococcus aureus*, coagulase reacts with a prothrombin-like compound in plasma to produce an active enzyme (a complex of thrombin and coagulase) that converts fibrinogen to fibrin. This activity of *S. aureus* has a very high correlation with the organism's virulence, although coagulase-negative organisms can cause less severe disease. Coagulase reactive factor is a plasma protein with which coagulase reacts. This protein is presumably a modified derivative of prothrombin. Prothrombin is the substrate from which coagulase splits a number of amino acids to convert it to thrombin. Thrombin is the proteolytic enzyme that converts fibrinogen to fibrin, forming the clot. Plasmin is a plasma protein associated with the destruction of such a clot.

**4.40**

*Answer: D*　Ketoconazole

Ketoconazole inhibits the biosynthesis of ergosterol by blocking demethylation at the C14 site of the ergosterol precursor lanosterol. This results in the accumulation of lanosterol-like sterols in the cell, which alters the properties of the cell membrane, and permits the leakage of potassium ions. Amphotericin B and nystatin impair the permeability of the cell membrane by directly complexing with the membrane sterol. The target of griseofulvin is the microtubules. Flucytosine is incorporated into RNA after being deaminated and then phosphorylated. It also interferes with DNA synthesis because it is a non-competitive inhibitor of thymidylate synthetase.

microbiology

# SECTION 5: DISORDERS OF FLUIDS AND ELECTROLYTES — ANSWERS

## 5.1

*Answer: E*    pH 7.50, $p(CO_2)$ 47 mmHg, $HCO_3^-$ 35 mmol/l

Metabolic alkalosis results in decreased hydrogen ion concentration (increased pH) with accompanying increased bicarbonate and carbon dioxide concentrations. The organ systems involved are mainly the kidneys and gastrointestinal tract. The pathogenesis of metabolic alkalosis involves two processes, the generation of metabolic alkalosis and the maintenance of metabolic alkalosis, events that usually overlap.

The generation of metabolic alkalosis occurs with the loss of acid, the gain of alkali, or the contraction of the extracellular fluid compartment, with a consequent change in bicarbonate concentration. The kidneys usually have an enormous capacity to excrete excess bicarbonate generated and to restore normal acid–base balance by the following mechanisms: (1) less reabsorption of bicarbonate because infused sodium bicarbonate leads to volume expansion, which reduces reabsorption of sodium ions and bicarbonate in the proximal tubule, and (2) bicarbonate secretion by B-type intercalated cells in the collecting duct that exchange bicarbonate for chloride via the apical chloride/bicarbonate countertransporter. Therefore, to sustain metabolic alkalosis, the kidneys must participate to maintain the alkalosis by overriding these mechanisms.

## 5.2

*Answer: A*    Decreased colloid osmotic pressure

Nephrotic syndrome is a disorder where the kidneys have been damaged, causing them to leak protein from the blood into the urine. It is a fairly benign disease when it occurs in childhood, but it

fluids

can lead to chronic renal failure, especially in adults, or be a sign of an underlying serious disease such as systemic lupus erythematosus or a malignancy. Nephrotic syndrome is characterised by proteinuria and low plasma albumin levels. As a compensation, the liver begins to make more of all its proteins, and levels of large proteins (such as alpha-2-macroglobulin) increase. Oedema usually occurs due to salt and water retention by the diseased kidneys as well as due to the reduced colloid osmotic pressure (because of reduced albumin in the plasma). Oedema might also be caused by congestive heart failure.

## 5.3

*Answer: D*    Isotonic saline

Fluid replacement or fluid resuscitation is the practice of replenishing bodily fluid lost through sweating, bleeding, fluid shifts or other pathological processes. Fluids can be replaced via oral administration (drinking), intravenous administration, or hypodermoclysis, the direct injection of fluid into the subcutaneous tissue. Fluids administered by the oral and hypodermic routes are absorbed more slowly than those given intravenously. In severe dehydration, intravenous fluid replacement is preferred, and may be life-saving. Physiological normal saline, or 0.9% sodium chloride solution, is often used because it is isotonic, and therefore will not cause potentially dangerous fluid shifts. If given intravenously, normal saline remains in the circulation, boosting blood pressure and preventing the complications of inadequate circulation.

## 5.4

*Answer: D*    Increased serum ADH (vasopressin) concentration

Dehydration is a state of negative fluid balance that can be caused by a number of disease entities, though diarrhoeal illnesses are the most common cause. The negative fluid balance causing dehydration results from decreased intake, increased output (renal, gastrointestinal or insensible losses) or fluid shift (ascites, effusions, and capillary leak states such as burns and sepsis). The decrease in total body water causes reductions in both the intracellular and

fluids

extracellular fluid volumes. Clinical manifestations of dehydration are most closely related to intravascular volume depletion. As dehydration progresses, hypovolaemic shock eventually develops, resulting in end-organ failure and death.

Dehydration is often categorised according to serum sodium concentration as isonatraemic (130–150 mmol/l), hyponatraemic (<135 mmol/l), or hypernatraemic (>150 mmol/l). Isonatraemic dehydration is the most common (80%). Hypernatraemic and hyponatraemic dehydration each comprise 5%–10% of cases. Variations in serum sodium reflect the composition of the fluids lost and have different pathophysiological effects. Isonatraemic (isotonic) dehydration occurs when the lost fluid is similar in sodium concentration to the blood. Sodium and water losses are of the same relative magnitude in both the intravascular and extravascular fluid compartments. Hyponatraemic (hypotonic) dehydration occurs when the lost fluid contains more sodium than the blood (loss of hypertonic fluid). Relatively more sodium than water is lost. Because the serum sodium is low, intravascular water shifts to the extravascular space, exaggerating intravascular volume depletion for a given amount of total body water loss. Hypernatraemic (hypertonic) dehydration occurs when the lost fluid contains less sodium than the blood (loss of hypotonic fluid). Relatively less sodium than water is lost. Because the serum sodium is high, extravascular water shifts to the intravascular space, minimising intravascular volume depletion for a given amount of total body water loss. Compensatory reponses to dehydration will include increased release of antidiuretic hormone (ADH) in an attempt to conserve body water.

### 5.5

*Answer: E*   Wide anion gap metabolic acidosis

To distinguish between the main types of metabolic acidosis, a clinical tool called the 'anion gap' is considered very useful. It is calculated by subtracting the chloride and bicarbonate levels from the sodium plus potassium levels:

$$\text{Anion gap} = ([Na^+] + [K^+]) - ([Cl^-] + [HCO_3^-])$$

fluids

As sodium is the main extracellular cation and chloride and bicarbonate are the main anions, the result should reflect the remaining anions. Normally, this concentration is about 8–16 mmol/l (12 ± 4). An elevated anion gap (ie >16 mmol/l) can indicate particular types of metabolic acidosis, particularly acidosis due to certain poisons, lactate acidosis and ketoacidosis.

**5.6**

*Answer: B*   Hypovolaemia

Oliguria and anuria are the decreased or absent production of urine, respectively. The decreased production of urine may be a sign of dehydration/hypovolaemia, renal failure or urinary obstruction/urinary retention. Patients usually have a decrease in urine output after a major operation that may be a normal physiological response to:

- Fluid/blood loss — decreased glomerular filtration rate secondary to hypovolaemia and/or hypotension

- Response of adrenal cortex to stress — increase in aldosterone (sodium and water retention) and antidiuretic hormone release.

**5.7**

*Answer: C*   Multiple blood transfusions

Hyperkalaemia is an elevated blood level of potassium (>5.0 mmol/l). Extreme degrees of hyperkalaemia are considered a medical emergency due to the risk of potentially fatal arrhythmias. Causes of hyperkalaemia include ineffective elimination of potassium from the body, excessive release of potassium from cells, and excessive potassium intake.

Ineffective elimination of potassium from the body can be due to:

- Renal insufficiency

- Medication that interferes with urinary excretion:

  o angiotensin-converting enzyme (ACE) inhibitors and angiotensin-receptor blockers

fluids

- o potassium-sparing diuretics (eg amiloride and spironolactone)
- o non-steroidal anti-inflammatory drugs (NSAIDs), such as ibuprofen, naproxen or celecoxib
- o the calcineurin-inhibitor immunosuppressants, ciclosporin and tacrolimus
- o trimethoprim
- o pentamidine

- Mineralocorticoid deficiency or resistance:

  - o Addison's disease
  - o some forms of congenital adrenal hyperplasia
  - o type IV renal tubular acidosis (resistance of renal tubules to aldosterone)
- Gordon syndrome (familial hypertension with hyperkalaemia), a rare genetic disorder caused by defective modulators of salt transporters, including the thiazide-sensitive sodium chloride cotransporter.

Excessive release of potassium from cells can occur as a result of:

- Rhabdomyolysis, burns or any cause of rapid tissue necrosis, including tumour lysis syndrome

- Massive blood transfusion or massive haemolysis

- Shifts/transport out of cells caused by acidosis, low insulin levels, beta-blocker therapy, digoxin overdose, or the paralysing anaesthetic, succinylcholine.

Excessive intake of potassium can be caused by:

- Intoxication with salt-substitute, potassium-containing dietary supplements, or potassium chloride infusion. Note that for a person with normal kidney function and nothing interfering with normal elimination (see above), hyperkalaemia due to potassium intoxication would only be seen with large infusions of potassium chloride or massive doses of oral potassium chloride supplements.

fluids

## 5.8

*Answer: B*   Metabolic alkalosis

Metabolic alkalosis is a primary increase in serum bicarbonate ($HCO_3^-$) concentration. This occurs as a consequence of a loss of $H^+$ from the body or a gain in $HCO_3^-$. In its pure form, it manifests as alkalemia (pH >7.40). As a compensatory mechanism, metabolic alkalosis leads to alveolar hypoventilation with a rise in arterial carbon dioxide tension $p(CO_2)$, which diminishes the change in pH that would otherwise occur.

Normally, arterial $p(CO_2)$ increases by 0.5–0.7 mmHg for every 1 mmol/l increase in plasma bicarbonate concentration, a compensatory response that occurs very rapidly. If the change in $p(CO_2)$ is not within this range, then a mixed acid–base disturbance occurs. For example, if the increase in $p(CO_2)$ is more than 0.7 times the increase in bicarbonate, then metabolic alkalosis coexists with primary respiratory acidosis. Likewise, if the increase in $p(CO_2)$ is less than the expected change, then a primary respiratory alkalosis is also present.

The first clue to metabolic alkalosis is often an elevated bicarbonate concentration that is observed when serum electrolytes are obtained. Remember that an elevated serum bicarbonate concentration can also be observed as a compensatory response to primary respiratory acidosis. However, a bicarbonate concentration greater than 35 mmol/l is almost always caused by metabolic alkalosis (as is the case in this clinical scenario).

Calculation of the serum anion gap can also help to differentiate between primary metabolic alkalosis and the metabolic compensation for respiratory acidosis. The anion gap is frequently elevated to a modest degree in metabolic alkalosis because of the increase in the negative charge of albumin and the enhanced production of lactate. However, the only definitive way to diagnose metabolic alkalosis is by performing a simultaneous blood gases analysis, which reveals elevation of both pH and arterial $p(CO_2)$ and increased calculated bicarbonate.

There are two ways to determine the serum bicarbonate concentration. The first method is calculating serum bicarbonate concentration from a blood gas sample using the Henderson–

Hasselbalch equation, as follows:

$$pH = 6.10 + \log[HCO_3^-] \div 0.03 \times p(CO_2)$$

Alternatively:

$$[HCO_3^-] = 24 \times p(CO_2) \div [H^+]$$

Because pH and $p(CO_2)$ are measured directly, bicarbonate can be calculated.

The second method is by measuring the total carbon dioxide content in serum, which is routinely measured with serum electrolytes obtained from venous blood. In this method, a strong acid is added to serum, which interacts with bicarbonate in the serum sample, forming carbonic acid. Carbonic acid dissociates to form carbon dioxide and water and then the carbon dioxide is measured. Note that the carbon dioxide measured includes bicarbonate and dissolved carbon dioxide. The contribution of dissolved carbon dioxide is quite small ($0.03 \times p(CO_2)$) and is usually ignored, although it accounts for a difference of 1–3 mmol/l between the measured total carbon dioxide content in venous blood and the calculated bicarbonate in arterial blood. Thus, at a $p(CO_2)$ of 40 mmHg, a total carbon dioxide content of 25 means a true bicarbonate concentration of 23.8 mmol/l (ie, $25 - 0.03 \times 40$) (see also *Answer* to **5.1**).

## 5.9

*Answer: D*   Tented T waves

Electrocardiography (ECG) is generally done early on in order to identify any influences on the heart, as hyperkalaemia can cause fatal arrhythmias. With moderate hyperkalaemia, there is reduction of the size of the P wave and development of tent-shaped T waves. Further hyperkalaemia will lead to widening of the QRS complex, which ultimately can become sinusoidal in shape. There appears to be a direct effect of elevated potassium on some of the potassium channels which increases their activity and speeds membrane repolarisation. Also, hyperkalaemia causes an overall membrane depolarisation that inactivates many sodium channels. The faster repolarisation of the cardiac action potential causes the tenting of the T waves, and the inactivation of sodium channels causes a

fluids

sluggish conduction of the electrical wave around the heart, which leads to smaller P waves and widening of the QRS complex.

## 5.10

*Answer: D*    Na+

The electrolyte disturbance hyponatraemia is defined as a plasma sodium concentration below 135 mmol/l and reflects an excess of total body water content relative to total body sodium content. At lower levels, water intoxication can result, a very dangerous condition. Hyponatraemia is an abnormality that can occur in isolation or, most commonly, as a complication of other medical illnesses. An abnormally low plasma sodium level is best considered in conjunction with the person's plasma osmolarity and extracellular fluid volume status.

Most cases of hyponatraemia are associated with reduced plasma osmolarity. In fact, the vast majority of adult cases are due to increased antidiuretic hormone (ADH). ADH is a hormone that causes retention of water, but not salt. It is the physician's task to identify the cause of the increased ADH activity in each case. In patients who are volume-depleted, that is their blood volume is too low, ADH secretion is increased, because volume depletion is a potent stimulus for ADH secretion. As a result, the kidneys of such patients hold on to water and produce a very concentrated urine. Treatment is simple (if not without risk) — simply restore the patient's blood volume, thereby turning off the stimulus for ongoing ADH release and water retention.

Some patients with hyponatraemia have normal blood volume. In these patients the increased ADH activity and subsequent water retention might be due to 'physiological' causes of ADH release, such as pain or nausea. Alternatively, they might have the syndrome of inappropriate ADH secretion (SIADH). In SIADH there is sustained, non-physiological release of ADH and this most often occurs as a side-effect of certain medicines, lung problems such as pneumonia or abscess, brain disease, or certain cancers (most often small-cell lung carcinoma).

A third group of patients with hyponatraemia are often said to be hypervolaemic. They are identified by the presence of peripheral

fluids

oedema. In fact, the term 'hypervolaemic' is misleading because their blood volume is actually low. The oedema underscores the fact that fluid has left the circulation, meaning that the oedema represents fluid that has exited the circulation and settled in dependent areas. Because such patients do, in fact, have reduced blood volume, and because reduced blood volume is a potent stimulus for ADH release, it is easy to see why they have retained water and become hyponatraemic. Treatment of these patients involves treating the underlying disease that caused the fluid to leak out of the circulation in the first place. In many cases, this is easier said than done because the responsible underlying conditions are diseases such as liver cirrhosis or heart failure, conditions that are notoriously difficult to manage, let alone cure.

Hyponatraemia can result from dysfunction of the mineralocorticoid aldosterone (ie hypoaldosteronism) due to adrenal insufficiency, congenital adrenal hyperplasia or some drugs. Hyponatraemia also occurs in the setting of diuretic use. Patients taking diuretic medications such as furosemide, hydrochlorothiazide and chlorthalidone become volume-depleted. That is to say that their diuretic medicine, by design, has caused their kidneys to produce more urine than they would otherwise make. This extra urine represents blood volume that is no longer there, that has been lost from the body. As a result, their blood volume is reduced. As mentioned above, lack of adequate blood volume is a potent stimulus for ADH secretion and therefore for water retention.

## 5.11

*Answer: D*    Hypokalaemia

Cardiac effects of hypokalaemia are usually minimal until plasma potassium levels are less than 3 mmol/l. Hypokalaemia leads to sagging of the ST segment, depression of the T wave and elevation of the U wave. With marked hypokalaemia, the T wave becomes progressively smaller and the U wave becomes increasingly larger. Sometimes, a flat or positive T wave merges with a positive U wave, which can be confused with QT prolongation. Hypokalemia can also cause premature ventricular and atrial contractions, ventricular and atrial tachyarrhythmias, and second- or third-degree atrioventricular block. Such arrhythmias become more severe with increasingly

fluids

severe hypokalaemia; eventually, ventricular fibrillation can occur. Patients with significant pre-existing heart disease and/or those receiving digoxin are at risk of cardiac conduction abnormalities, even with mild hypokalaemia.

## 5.12

*Answer: B*    Liddle syndrome

Hypokalaemia can be caused by decreased intake of potassium but is usually caused by excessive losses of potassium in the urine or from the gastrointestinal tract. Liddle syndrome is a rare autosomal dominant disorder characterised by severe hypertension and hypokalaemia. Liddle syndrome is caused by unrestrained sodium reabsorption in the distal nephron due to one of several mutations found in genes encoding for epithelial sodium channel subunits. Inappropriately high reabsorption of sodium results in both hypertension and renal potassium wasting.

## 5.13

*Answer: E*    Spironolactone

Hyperkalaemia resulting from total body potassium excess is particularly common in oliguric states (especially acute renal failure) and with rhabdomyolysis, burns, bleeding into soft tissue or the gastrointestinal tract and in adrenal insufficiency. In chronic renal failure hyperkalaemia is uncommon until the glomerular filtration rate (GFR) falls to less than 10–15 ml/minute unless dietary potassium intake is excessive or another source of excess potassium load is present, such as oral or parenteral potassium therapy, gastrointestinal bleeding, tissue injury or haemolysis. Other potential causes of hyperkalaemia in chronic renal failure are hyporeninaemic hypoaldosteronism (type 4 renal tubular acidosis), angiotensin-converting enzyme (ACE) inhibitors, potassium-sparing diuretics such as spironolactone, fasting (suppression of insulin secretion), beta-blockers, and non-steroidal anti-inflammatory drugs (NSAIDs). If sufficient potassium chloride is ingested or given parenterally, severe hyperkalaemia can result, even with normal renal function. Causes are usually iatrogenic, such as giving potassium

fluids

supplements to patients taking ACE inhibitors. Other drugs that can limit renal potassium output, thereby leading to hyperkalaemia, include ciclosporin, lithium, heparin and trimethoprim.

## 5.14

*Answer:* C   Respiratory depression

Hypermagnesaemia defined as a plasma magnesium concentration over 1.05 mmol/l. At plasma magnesium concentrations of 2.5–5 mmol/l the electrocardiogram shows prolongation of the PR interval, widening of the QRS complex and increased T-wave amplitude. Deep tendon reflexes disappear as the plasma magnesium level approaches 5.0 mmol/l; hypotension, respiratory depression, and narcosis develop with increasing hypermagnesemia. Cardiac arrest can occur when blood magnesium levels exceed 6.0–7.5 mmol/l).

## 5.15

*Answer:* D   Renal insufficiency

Hyperphosphataemia is defined as a serum phosphate concentration greater than 1.46 mmol/l. Hyperphosphataemia generally results from a decrease in renal excretion of phosphate. Advanced renal insufficiency, with a glomerular filtration rate of less than 20 ml/minute, reduces excretion sufficiently to increase plasma phosphate. Defects in renal excretion of phosphate in the absence of renal failure also occur in pseudohypoparathyroidism and hypoparathyroidism. Hyperphosphataemia can also occur with excessive oral phosphate administration and occasionally with overzealous use of phosphate-containing enemas.

Hyperphosphataemia occasionally results from a transcellular shift of phosphate into the extracellular space that is so large that the renal excretory capacity is overwhelmed. This occurs most frequently in diabetic ketoacidosis (despite total body phosphate depletion), crush injuries and non-traumatic rhabdomyolysis, as well as in overwhelming systemic infections and tumour lysis syndrome. Hyperphosphataemia also plays a critical role in the development

fluids

of secondary hyperparathyroidism and renal osteodystrophy in patients on dialysis. Lastly, hyperphosphataemia can be spurious in cases of hyperproteinaemia (in multiple myeloma or Waldenström's macroglobulinaemia, for example), hyperlipidaemia, haemolysis or hyperbilirubinaemia.

## 5.16

*Answer: D* Psychosis

In euvolemic hyponatraemia the total body sodium and so the extracellular fluid volume are normal; however, total body water is increased. Primary polydipsia can cause hyponatraemia only when water intake overwhelms the kidneys' ability to excrete water. Because normal kidneys can excrete up to 25 litres of urine a day, hyponatraemia due solely to polydipsia results only from the ingestion of large amounts of water or from defects in renal diluting ability. Patients affected include those with psychosis or more modest degrees of polydipsia plus renal insufficiency. Dilutional hyponatraemia can also result from excessive water intake without sodium retention in the presence of Addison's disease, myxoedema or non-osmotic antidiuretic hormone (ADH) secretion (due to: stress; postoperative states; or the use of drugs such as chlorpropamide or tolbutamide, opioids, barbiturates, vincristine, clofibrate or carbamazepine). Postoperative hyponatraemia occurs because of a combination of non-osmotic ADH release and excessive administration of hypotonic fluids after surgery. Certain drugs (eg cyclophosphamide, non-steroidal anti-inflammatory drugs, chlorpropamide) potentiate the renal effect of endogenous ADH, whereas others (eg oxytocin) have a direct ADH-like effect on the kidney. A deficiency in water excretion is common in all these conditions.

## 5.17

*Answer: A* Cirrhosis

Hypervolaemic hyponatraemia is characterised by an increase in both total body sodium (and thus extracellular fluid volume) and total body water, with a relatively greater increase in total body water.

Various oedematous disorders, including heart failure and cirrhosis, cause hypervolaemic hyponatraemia. Rarely, hyponatraemia occurs in nephrotic syndrome, although pseudohyponatraemia can be due to interference with sodium measurement by elevated lipids. In each of these disorders, a decrease in effective circulating volume results in the release of antidiuretic hormone (ADH) and angiotensin II. Hyponatraemia results from the antidiuretic effect of ADH on the kidney as well as the direct impairment of renal water excretion by angiotensin II. Decreased glomerular filtration rate and stimulation of thirst by angiotensin II also potentiate the development of hyponatraemia. Urine sodium excretion is usually <10 mmo//l and urine osmolality is high relative to plasma osmolality.

## 5.18

*Answer: C*   Nephrotic syndrome

An increase in total body sodium is the key pathophysiological event in extracellular fluid volume expansion. It increases osmolality, which triggers compensatory mechanisms that produce water retention. Movement of fluid between interstitial and intravascular spaces depends on Starling's forces at the capillaries: increased capillary hydrostatic pressure (as in heart failure), decreased plasma oncotic pressure (as in nephrotic syndrome) or a combination of these factors (as in severe cirrhosis) shift fluid into the interstitial space, producing oedema. In these conditions, subsequent intravascular volume depletion increases renal sodium retention, which maintains fluid overload.

## 5.19

*Answer: A*   Hypoparathyroidism

Hypoparathyroidism is characterised by hypocalcaemia and hyperphosphataemia and often causes chronic tetany. Hypoparathyroidism results from deficient parathyroid hormone, and this often occurs as a result of accidental removal of or damage to parathyroid glands during thyroidectomy. Transient hypoparathyroidism is common after subtotal thyroidectomy. Permanent hypoparathyroidism occurs after fewer than 3% of

fluids

thyroidectomies performed by experienced surgeons. Manifestations of hypocalcaemia usually begin about 24–48 hours postoperatively but can occur after months or years. Parathyroid hormone deficiency is more common after radical thyroidectomy for cancer or as the result of surgery on the parathyroid itself (subtotal or total parathyroidectomy). Risk factors for severe hypocalcaemia after subtotal parathyroidectomy include severe preoperative hypercalcaemia, removal of a large adenoma, and elevated alkaline phosphatase.

Idiopathic hypoparathyroidism is an uncommon sporadic or inherited condition in which the parathyroid glands are absent or atrophied. It manifests in childhood. The parathyroid glands are occasionally absent with thymic aplasia and abnormalities of the arteries arising from the branchial arches (DiGeorge syndrome). Other inherited forms include the X-linked genetic syndrome of hypoparathyroidism, Addison's disease and mucocutaneous candidiasis.

## 5.20

*Answer: A    1%*

Despite its important intracellular roles, roughly 99% of body calcium is in bone, mainly as hydroxyapatite crystals. Roughly 1% of bone calcium is freely exchangeable with the extracellular fluid and therefore is available for buffering changes in calcium ion balance. The normal total plasma calcium range is 2.20–2.60 mmol/l. About 40% of the total blood calcium is bound to plasma proteins, primarily albumin. The remaining 60% includes ionized calcium plus calcium complexed with phosphate and citrate. Total calcium (ie protein-bound plus complexed plus ionised calcium) is usually what is determined by clinical laboratory measurement. Ideally, the ionised or free calcium should be determined, because this is the physiologically active form of calcium in plasma; this determination, because of its technical difficulty, is usually restricted to patients in whom significant alteration of protein binding of plasma calcium is suspected, however. Ionised calcium is generally assumed to be roughly 50% of the total plasma calcium.

fluids

## 5.21

*Answer: A*  Hypoalbuminaemia

Decreased anion gap is unrelated to metabolic acidosis but is caused by hypoalbuminaemia (decreased anions); hypercalcaemia, hypermagnesaemia, lithium intoxication, and hypergammaglobulinaemia (increased cations); or by hyperviscosity or halide (bromide or iodide) intoxication. The effect of low albumin can be accounted for by adjusting the anion gap 2.5 mmol/l upwards for every 10 g/l fall in albumin.

## 5.22

*Answer: E*  Lactic acidosis

An increased anion gap is most commonly caused by metabolic acidosis in which negatively charged acids (mostly ketones, lactate, sulphates or metabolites of methanol, ethylene glycol and salicylate) consume (are buffered by) bicarbonate ion. Other causes of increased anion gap include hyperalbuminaemia and uraemia (increased anions) and hypocalcaemia or hypomagnesaemia (decreased cations).

## 5.23

*Answer: B*  Hypokalaemia

Metabolic alkalosis may be generated by one of the following mechanisms:

- **Loss of hydrogen ions**. Whenever a hydrogen ion is excreted, a bicarbonate ion is gained into the extracellular space. Hydrogen ions can be lost through the kidneys or the gastrointestinal tract. Vomiting or nasogastric suction generates metabolic alkalosis by the loss of gastric secretions, which are rich in hydrochloric acid. Renal losses of hydrogen ions occur whenever the distal delivery of sodium increases in the presence of excess aldosterone, which stimulates the electrogenic epithelial sodium channel in the

fluids

collecting duct. As this channel reabsorbs sodium ions, the tubular lumen becomes more negative, leading to the secretion of hydrogen ions and potassium ions into the lumen.

- **Shift of hydrogen ions into the intracellular space**. This mainly develops with hypokaalemia. As the extracellular potassium concentration decreases, potassium ions move out of the cells. To maintain neutrality, hydrogen ions move into the intracellular space.

- **Alkali administration.** Administration of sodium bicarbonate in amounts that exceed the capacity of the kidneys to excrete this excess bicarbonate can cause metabolic alkalosis. This capacity is reduced when a reduction in filtered bicarbonate occurs, as observed in renal failure, or when enhanced tubular reabsorption of bicarbonate occurs, as observed in volume depletion.

- **Contraction alkalosis**. Loss of bicarbonate-poor, chloride-rich extracellular fluid, as observed with thiazide diuretics or loop diuretic therapy or chloride diarrhoea, leads to contraction of the extracellular fluid volume. Because the original bicarbonate mass is now dissolved in a smaller volume of fluid, an increase in bicarbonate concentration occurs. This increase in bicarbonate causes, at most, a 2–4-mmol/l rise in bicarbonate concentration.

## 5.24

*Answer: B*    Cerebral perfusion is decreased

Severe metabolic alkalosis (blood pH >7.55) is a serious medical problem. Mortality rates have been reported as 45% in patients with an arterial blood pH of 7.55 and 80% when the pH was greater than 7.65. Severe alkalosis causes diffuse arteriolar constriction, with reduction in tissue perfusion. By decreasing cerebral blood flow, alkalosis can lead to tetany, seizures and decreased mental status. Metabolic alkalosis also decreases coronary blood flow and predisposes to refractory arrhythmias. Metabolic alkalosis causes hypoventilation, which can cause hypoxaemia, especially in patients with poor respiratory reserve, and it can impair weaning from mechanical ventilation. Alkalosis decreases the serum concentration of ionised calcium by increasing calcium-ion binding to albumin. In addition, metabolic alkalosis is almost always associated with hypokalaemia, which can cause neuromuscular weakness and arrhythmias and, by increasing ammonia production, can precipitate hepatic encephalopathy in susceptible individuals.

## 5.25

*Answer: B*    0.8–1.45 mmol/l

Phosphorus is one of the most abundant elements in the human body. Most phosphorus in the body is complexed with oxygen as phosphate ($PO_4^{3-}$). About 85% of the roughly 500–700 g of phosphate in the body is contained in bone, where it is an important constituent of hydroxyapatite. In soft tissues, phosphate is mainly found in the intracellular compartment as an integral component of several organic compounds, including nucleic acids and cell membrane phospholipids. Phosphate is also involved in aerobic and anaerobic energy metabolism. Red blood cell 2,3-diphosphoglycerate (2,3-DPG) plays a crucial role in the delivery of oxygen to tissues. Adenosine diphosphate (ADP) and adenosine triphosphate (ATP) contain phosphate and use chemical bonds between $PO_4^{3-}$ groups to store energy. Inorganic phosphate is a major intracellular anion but is also present in plasma. The normal plasma inorganic phosphate concentration in adults ranges from 0.8 mmol/l to 1.45 mmol/l. Phosphate levels are up to 50% higher in infants and 30% higher in children, possibly because additional phosphate is required for growth.

## 5.26

*Answer: D*    Seizures

The primary clinical findings in hypomagnesaemia are neuromuscular irritability, central nervous system (CNS) hyperexcitability and cardiac arrhythmias. The severity of symptoms is not related

fluids

directly to the magnesium level. The reference range for serum magnesium level is 0.75–1.05 mmol/l, and patients usually become symptomatic at levels of around 0.75 mmol/l, although the typical physical findings might not be present in all cases. The clinical manifestations are as follows:

- Neuromuscular irritability:
  - hyperactive deep tendon reflexes
  - muscle cramps
  - muscle fibrillation
  - Trousseau's and Chvostek's signs
  - dysarthria and dysphagia due to oesophageal dysmotility.

- CNS hyperexcitability:
  - irritability and combativeness
  - disorientation
  - psychosis
  - ataxia, vertigo, nystagmus and seizures (at levels <0.5 mmol/l).

- Cardiac arrhythmias, which can be caused by hypomagnesaemia alone or concomitant hypokalaemia, result from decreased activity of ATPase:
  - paroxysmal atrial and ventricular dysrhythmias
  - repolarisation alternans.

### 5.27

*Answer: C*    Metastatic calcification

Hyperphosphataemia causes hypocalcaemia by precipitating calcium, decreasing vitamin D production, and interfering with parathyroid hormone-mediated bone resorption. Severe life-threatening hypocalcaemia can result. Signs and symptoms of acute hyperphosphataemia are due to the effects of hypocalcaemia. Prolonged hyperphosphataemia promotes metastatic calcification, an abnormal deposition of calcium phosphate in previously healthy connective tissues such as cardiac valves and in solid organs such as muscles. The calcium-phosphate product predicts the risk of metastatic calcification.

Excess free serum phosphorus is taken up into vascular smooth muscle via a sodium–phosphate cotransporter. The increased cellular phosphate activates a gene (*cbfa-1*) that promotes calcium deposition in the vascular cell, making smooth muscle cells engage in osteogenesis. Vascular walls become calcified and arteriosclerotic, leading to increased systolic blood pressure, widened pulse pressure and, eventually, left ventricular hypertrophy.

Hyperphosphataemia is an independent risk factor contributing to the increased incidence of aortic and mitral stenosis and other cardiovascular disease among dialysis-dependent patients. A peripheral form known as 'calcific uraemic arteriolopathy' (or 'calciphylaxis') can induce necrotic ulceration and gangrene in affected extremities. Hyperphosphataemia-induced resistance to parathyroid hormone contributes to secondary hyperparathyroidism and renal osteodystrophy.

## 5.28

*Answer: D*   Hypokalaemia

Ammonia ($NH_3$) buffering occurs via the following reaction:

$$NH_3 + H^+ \leftrightarrow NH_4^+$$

$NH_3$ is produced in the proximal tubule from the amino acid glutamine, and this reaction is enhanced by an acid load and by hypokalaemia. Ammonia is converted to ammonium ion ($NH_4^+$) by intracellular $H^+$ and is secreted into the proximal tubular lumen by the apical $Na^+/H^+(NH_4^+)$ antiporter. The apical $Na^+/K^+(NH_4^+)/2Cl^-$ cotransporter in the thick ascending limb of the loop of Henle then transports $NH_4^+$ into the medullary interstitium, where it dissociates back into $NH_3$ and $H^+$. The $NH_3$ diffuses into the lumen of the collecting duct, where it is available to buffer $H^+$ ions and becomes $NH_4^+$. $NH_4^+$ is trapped in the lumen and excreted as the chloride salt, and every $H^+$ ion buffered is an $HCO_3^-$ gained to the systemic circulation.

The increased secretion of $H^+$ in the collecting duct shifts the

*fluids*

equation to the right and decreases the $NH_3$ concentration, facilitating continued diffusion of $NH_3$ from the interstitium down its concentration gradient and allowing more $H^+$ to be buffered. The kidneys can adjust the amount of $NH_3$ synthesised to meet demand, making this a powerful system to buffer secreted $H^+$ in the urine.

Renal production of $NH_3$ is increased in hypokalaemia, resulting in an increase in renal acid excretion. The increase in $NH_3$ production by the kidneys can be significant enough to precipitate hepatic encephalopathy in patients who have advanced liver disease. Correcting the hypokalaemia can reverse this process.

**5.29**

*Answer: A*   Type A

Lactic acidosis was described and classified by Cohen and Woods into two categories: type A lactic acidosis occurs with decreased tissue ATP in the setting of poor tissue perfusion or oxygenation; and type B lactic acidosis occurs when evidence of poor tissue perfusion or oxygenation is absent. However, in many cases of type B lactic acidosis, occult tissue hypoperfusion is now recognised as an accompanying factor. Type B lactic acidosis is further divided into three subtypes on the basis of the underlying aetiology:

- Type B1 lactic acidosis occurs in association with systemic disease such as renal and hepatic failure, diabetes and/or malignancy.

- Type B2 lactic acidosis is caused by several classes of drugs and toxins, including biguanides, alcohols, iron, isoniazid and salicylates.

- Type B3 lactic acidosis is due to inborn errors of metabolism.

fluids

## 5.30

*Answer: D*   Hyperalimentation

Hypernatraemia in rare cases is associated with volume overload. In this case, hypernatraemia results from a grossly elevated sodium intake associated with limited access to water. One example is excessive administration of hypertonic sodium bicarbonate given during cardiopulmonary rescuscitation or during the treatment of lactic acidosis. Hypernatraemia can also be caused by the administration of hypertonic saline or hyperalimentation.

fluids

# SECTION 6:
# BLEEDING AND HAEMOSTASIS
# — ANSWERS

## 6.1

*Answer: B*    Disseminated intravascular coagulopathy

Disseminated intravascular coagulation (DIC), also called 'consumptive coagulopathy', is a pathological process that involves excessive, abnormal generation of thrombin and fibrin in the circulating blood. During the process, platelet aggregation and coagulation factors' consumption occur. This depletes the body of its platelets and coagulation factors, and there is a paradoxically increased risk of haemorrhage. It occurs in critically ill patients, especially in those with Gram-negative sepsis and in acute promyelocytic leukaemia.

There are a variety of causes of DIC, all usually causing the release of chemicals into the blood that instigates the coagulation:

- Sepsis, particularly with Gram-negative bacteria.

- Obstetric complications (most common cause), with chemicals from the uterus being released into the blood, or from amniotic fluid embolism, and eclampsia can be causes. Another obstetric condition which can cause DIC is abruptio placentae.

- Tissue trauma, such as burns, accidents, surgery or shock.

- Liver disease.

- Incompatible blood transfusion reactions or massive blood transfusion (more than the total circulatory volume).

- Malignant cancers or hypersensitivity reactions can produce the chemicals leading to DIC.

bleeding

- Acute promyelocytic leukaemia.

- Viral haemorrhagic fevers bring about their frank effects, paradoxically, by causing DIC.

- Envenomation by some species of venomous snakes, such as those belonging to the genus *Echis* (saw-scaled vipers).

Under homeostatic conditions, the body is maintained in a finely tuned balance of coagulation and fibrinolysis. The activation of the coagulation cascade yields thrombin that converts fibrinogen to fibrin; the stable fibrin clot being the final product of haemostasis. The fibrinolytic system then functions to break down fibrinogen and fibrin. Activation of the fibrinolytic system generates plasmin (in the presence of thrombin), which is responsible for the lysis of fibrin clots. The breakdown of fibrinogen and fibrin results in polypeptides called 'fibrin degradation products' (FDPs) or 'fibrin split products' (FSPs). In a state of homeostasis, the presence of thrombin is critical because it is the central proteolytic enzyme of coagulation and is also necessary for the breakdown of clots, or fibrinolysis.

In DIC, the processes of coagulation and fibrinolysis lose control, and the result is widespread clotting with resultant bleeding. Regardless of the triggering event of DIC, once initiated, the pathophysiology of DIC is similar in all conditions. One critical mediator of DIC is the release of a transmembrane glycoprotein called 'tissue factor' (TF). TF is present on the surface of many cell types (including endothelial cells, macrophages and monocytes) and is not normally in contact with the general circulation, but is exposed to the circulation after vascular damage. For example, TF is released in response to exposure to cytokines (particularly interleukin), tumour necrosis factor and endotoxin. This plays a major role in the development of DIC in septic conditions. TF is also abundant in tissues of the lungs, brain and placenta. This helps to explain why DIC develops so readily in patients with extensive trauma. Once activated, TF binds with coagulation factors that then trigger both the intrinsic and the extrinsic pathways of coagulation.

Excess circulating thrombin results from the excess activation of the coagulation cascade. The excess thrombin cleaves fibrinogen, which ultimately leaves behind multiple fibrin clots in the circulation.

bleeding

These excess clots trap platelets to become larger clots, which leads to microvascular and macrovascular thrombosis. This lodging of clots in the microcirculation, in the large vessels and in the organs is what leads to the ischaemia, impaired organ perfusion and end-organ damage that occurs with DIC.

Coagulation inhibitors are also consumed in this process. Decreased inhibitor levels will permit more clotting so that a feedback system develops in which increased clotting leads to more clotting. At the same time, thrombocytopenia occurs because of the entrapment of platelets. Clotting factors are consumed in the development of multiple clots, which contributes to the bleeding seen with DIC.

Simultaneously, excess circulating thrombin assists in the conversion of plasminogen to plasmin, resulting in fibrinolysis. The breakdown of clots results in excess amounts of FDPs, which have powerful anticoagulant properties, contributing to haemorrhage. The excess plasmin also activates the complement and kinin systems. Activation of these systems leads to many of the clinical symptoms that patients experiencing DIC exhibit, such as shock, hypotension and increased vascular permeability. The acute form of DIC is considered to be an extreme expression of the intravascular coagulation process, with a complete breakdown of the normal homeostatic boundaries. DIC is associated with a poor prognosis and a high mortality.

Although numerous blood tests are often performed on patients prone to develop DIC, the important measures are: full blood count (especially the platelet count), FDPs or D-dimer tests (markers of fibrinolysis), bleeding time and fibrinogen levels. Decreased platelets, elevated FDPs or D-dimers, prolonged bleeding time and decreased fibrinogen are markers of DIC.

## 6.2

*Answer: A*   Epistaxis

Platelets (thrombocytes) are the cell fragments circulating in the blood that are involved in the cellular mechanisms of primary haemostasis that lead to the formation of blood clots. Dysfunction or low levels of platelets predisposes to bleeding. Epistaxis, petechiae and purpura are likely findings with platelet abnormalities. A normal platelet count in a healthy person is $150–400 \times 10^9/l$: 95% of healthy

bleeding

people will have platelet counts in this range. Some will have statistically abnormal platelet counts while having no abnormality, although the likelihood increases if the platelet count is either very low or very high.

Generally, low platelet counts increase the risk of bleeding (although there are exceptions, such as immune heparin-induced thrombocytopenia). Low platelet counts are generally not corrected by transfusion unless the patient is bleeding or the count has fallen below $5 \times 10^9/l$; it is contraindicated in thrombotic thrombocytopenic purpura (TTP) as it fuels the coagulopathy. In patients having surgery, a level below $50 \times 10^9/l$) is associated with abnormal surgical bleeding, and regional anaesthetic procedures such as epidurals are avoided if levels are below $80–100 \times 10^9/l$.

Normal platelet counts are not a guarantee of adequate function. In some states the platelets, while being adequate in number, are dysfunctional. For instance, aspirin irreversibly disrupts platelet function by inhibiting cyclo-oxygenase-1 (COX1), and therefore also disrupts normal haemostasis; normal platelet function might not return until the aspirin has been stopped and all the affected platelets have been replaced by new ones, which can take over a week. Similarly, uraemia (resulting from renal failure) leads to platelet dysfunction that can be ameliorated by the administration of desmopressin.

## 6.3

*Answer:* C    Scurvy

Scurvy is a deficiency disease that results from lack of vitamin C, which is required for normal collagen synthesis in humans. Vitamin C is essential for wound healing and facilitates recovery from burns. The scientific name of vitamin C, ascorbic acid, is derived from the Latin name of scurvy, *scorbutus*. Scurvy leads to the formation of petechiae on the skin, spongy gums, and bleeding from all mucous membranes. The spots are most abundant on the thighs and legs, and a person with the ailment looks pale, feels depressed, and is partially immobilised. In advanced scurvy there are open, suppurating wounds and loss of teeth. Scurvy was at one time common among sailors who spent longer periods at sea than perishable fruits and vegetables could be stored for and by soldiers who were similarly separated from these foods for extended periods. It was described by Hippocrates (c. 460 BC to c. 380 BC). Its cause and cure has been known in many native cultures since prehistory.

The bleeding is due to capillary fragility and not to some defect of coagulation. Normal collagen synthesis depends on the hydroxylation of proline and lysine residues in the endoplasmic reticulum, to form hydroxyproline and hydroxylysine respectively. Prolyl and lysyl hydroxylase, the enzymes that catalyse the hydroxylation, require ascorbic acid to function correctly. With no ascorbic acid, the enzymes cannot hydroxylate proline and lysine, and so normal collagen synthesis cannot be performed.

## 6.4

*Answer: E*    Transfusion of factor VIII concentrate is helpful

Haemophilia A is a clotting disorder caused by a mutation of the factor VIII gene, leading to a deficiency in factor VIII. It is the most common haemophilia. Inheritance is X-linked recessive, and so males are affected while females are carriers or (very rarely) display a mild phenotype; 1 in 10,000 males are affected. Haemophilia leads to a severely increased risk of bleeding from common injuries. The sites of bleeding are joints, muscles, digestive tract and brain. The muscle and joint haemorrhages are quite typical of haemophilia.

Coagulation testing reveals a prolonged partial thromboplastin time in the context of a normal prothrombin time and normal bleeding time. The diagnosis is made in the presence of very low levels of factor VIII (<10 IU). A family history is frequently present, although not essential. Nowadays, genetic testing might also be performed.

The most important differential diagnosis is that of haemophilia B (also known as 'Christmas disease') or von Willebrand's disease: the former is usually considered if factor VIII levels are normal in a person with a haemophilia phenotype; the latter is excluded on routine testing for that condition. A very small minority of patients have antibodies against factor VIII that impair its functioning.

Most people with haemophilia require regular supplementation with intravenous recombinant factor VIII. This is highly individually

bleeding

determined. Apart from 'routine' supplementation, extra factor concentrate is given around surgical procedures and after trauma. Some patients are managed on desmopressin if the clotting factor is still partially active.

## 6.5

*Answer: A*   A myeloproliferative disorder

All cell lines can be increased with myeloproliferative disorders. Thrombocytosis is one manifestation. The myeloproliferative diseases are a group of diseases of the bone marrow in which excess cells are produced. They are related to, and can evolve into, myelodysplastic syndrome and acute myeloid leukaemia, although the myeloproliferative diseases on the whole have a much better prognosis than these conditions.

## 6.6

*Answer: C*   Antithrombin III

Antithrombin III is a member of a larger family of antithrombins (numbered I–VI). They are all are serpins. Only antithromin III (and possibly antithrombin I) is medically significant and this is often referred to simply as 'antithrombin'. Antithrombin III deficiency is a rare hereditary disorder that generally only comes to light when a patient suffers recurrent venous thrombosis and pulmonary embolism. The patients are treated with anticoagulants or, more rarely, with antithrombin concentrate. In renal failure, and especially in nephrotic syndrome, antithrombin is lost in the urine, leading to a higher activity of factor II and factor X and an increased tendency to thrombosis.

## 6.7

*Answer: A*   It may result from endothelial cell injury

This patient has disseminated intravascular coagulation (DIC). One way for this to happen is through the release of endotoxins from Gram-negative bacteria with sepsis. The result is widespread activation of the coagulation system leading to DIC (see also *Answer* to **6.1**).

## 6.8

*Answer: D*   Haemarthrosis

Haemarthrosis is more of a complication with haemophilia. von Willebrand's disease (vWD) is the most common hereditary coagulation abnormality described in humans, although it can also be acquired as a result of other medical conditions. It arises from a qualitative or quantitative deficiency of von Willebrand factor (vWF), a multimeric protein that is required for platelet adhesion. There are three types of hereditary vWD, but other factors such as ABO blood group may also play a part in the cause of the condition.

When suspected, blood plasma of a patient needs to be investigated for quantitative and qualitative deficiencies of vWF, by measuring the amount of vWF in a vWF antigen assay and the functionallity of vWF with a glycoprotein (GP)Ib binding assay, a collagen binding assay, or a ristocetin cofactor activity (RiCof) or ristocetin-induced platelet agglutination (RIPA) assay. Factor VIII levels are also measured because factor VIII is bound to vWF, which protects the factor VIII from rapid breakdown within the blood. Deficiency of vWF can therefore lead to a reduction in factor VIII levels. Normal levels do not exclude all forms of vWD, particularly type II vWD, which might only be revealed by investigating platelet interaction with subendothelium under flow, a highly specialised coagulation study not routinely performed in most medical laboratories. A platelet aggregation assay will show an abnormal response to ristocetin with normal responses to the other agonists used. A platelet function assay will give an abnormal collagen/adrenaline closure time but a normal collagen/ADP time.

bleeding

## 6.9

*Answer: B*    Factor XII

Factor XII (Hageman factor) deficiency is a rare hereditary disorder with a prevalance of about one in a million, although it is a little more common among Asians. Deficiency does not cause excessive haemorrhage as the other coagulation factors compensate for it. It can increase the risk of thrombosis, due to inadequate activation of the fibrinolytic pathway. The deficiency leads to activated partial thromboplastin times (PTT) greater than 200 seconds.

## 6.10

*Answer: A*    d-Dimer test

D-Dimer is a blood test performed in the medical laboratory to diagnose thrombosis. Since its introduction in the 1990s, it has become an important test performed in patients suspected of thrombotic disorders. While a negative result practically rules out thrombosis, a positive result can indicate thrombosis but does not rule out other potential underlying conditions. Its main use, therefore, is to exclude thromboembolic disease where the probability is low.

D-Dimer testing is of clinical use when there is a suspicion of deep venous thrombosis or pulmonary embolism. In patients suspected of disseminated intravascular coagulation, D-dimers can aid in the diagnosis. Most sampling kits have a normal range of 0–300 ng/ml; values exceeding 250 ng/ml, 300 ng/ml or 500 ng/ml (different for various kits) are considered positive.

## 6.11

*Answer: D*    Thrombotic thrombocytopenic purpura

Thrombotic thrombocytopenic purpura (TTP) or 'Moschcowitz disease' is a rare disorder of the blood coagulation system. Most cases of TTP arise from deficiency or inhibition of the enzyme ADAMTS 13, which is responsible for cleaving large multimers of von Willebrand factor. This leads to haemolysis and end-organ damage, and can require plasmapheresis therapy.

bleeding

Classically, the following five symptoms are indicative of TTP:

- Fluctuating neurological symptoms, such as bizarre behaviour, altered mental status, stroke or headaches (65%)

- Kidney failure (46%)

- Fever (33%)

- Thrombocytopenia (low platelet count), leading to bruising or frank purpura

- Microangiopathic haemolytic anaemia.

A patient might notice dark urine, a result of the haemolytic anemia. Because of the many small areas of ischaemia produced by hyaline thrombi in the microvasculature, symptoms can be diffuse and fluctuating, including the classical bruising, confusion and headache. Nausea and vomiting (resulting from ischaemia in the gastrointestinal tract or from central nervous system involvement), chest pain (resulting from cardiac ischaemia), seizures and muscle and joint pain can also occur.

## 6.12

*Answer: B*   Factor VIII deficiency

Joint haemorrhages (haemarthroses) are typical of haemophilia. The diagnosis might be suspected as coagulation testing reveals an increased partial thromboplastin time in the context of a normal prothrombin time and a normal bleeding time. The diagnosis is made in the presence of very low levels of factor VIII (<10 IU). A family history is frequently present, although not essential (see also *Answer* to 6.4).

## 6.13

*Answer: A*   Factor IX deficiency

Mutations of the factor IX gene leads to an increased propensity for haemorrhage. This occurs in response to mild trauma or can even occur spontaneously, for example into joints (haemarthrosis)

bleeding

or muscles. Deficiency of factor IX causes Christmas disease (haemophilia B). Over 100 mutations of factor IX have been described: some cause no symptoms, but many lead to a significant bleeding disorder.

## 6.14

*Answer: B* von Willebrand's disease

von Willebrand's disease (vWD) is a bleeding disorder caused by a defect or deficiency of a blood clotting protein called von Willebrand factor (vWF). The disease is estimated to occur in 1% to 2% of the population. The disease was first described by Erik von Willebrand, a Finnish physician who reported a new type of bleeding disorder among island people in Sweden and Finland. vWF is a protein critical to the initial stages of blood clotting. This protein, produced by the endothelial cells, interacts with platelets to form a plug which prevents the blood from flowing at the site of injury. People with vWD are unable to make this plug because they do not have enough von Willebrand factor or their factor is abnormal.

Researchers have identified many variations of the disease, but most fall into the following classifications:

- **Type I vWD.** This is the most common and mildest form of von Willebrand's disease. Levels of vWF are lower than normal, and levels of factor VIII can also be reduced.

- **Type II vWD.** In these people, the vWF factor itself has an abnormality. Depending on the abnormality, they may be classified as having type IIa or type IIb vWD. In type IIa vWD, the level of vWF is reduced, as is the ability of platelets to clump together. In type IIb vWD, although the factor itself is defective, the ability of platelets to clump together is actually increased.

- **Type III vWD.** This is severe von Willebrand's disease. These people can have a total absence of vWF, and factor VIII levels are often less than 10% normal.

- **Pseudo- (or platelet-type) vWD.** This disorder resembles type IIb vWD, but the defects appear to be in the platelets, rather than in vWF.

bleeding

vWD is a genetic disease that can be inherited from either parent. It affects males and females equally. A man or woman with vWD has a 50% chance of passing the gene on to his or her child. There are no racial or ethnic associations with the disorder. A family history of a bleeding disorder is the primary risk factor (see also *Answer* to **6.8**).

## 6.15

*Answer: B*   Acetylsalicylic acid

Aspirin, or acetylsalicylic acid, is a drug in the family of salicylates, often used as an analgesic and antipyretic, and as an anti-inflammatory agent. It also has an antiplatelet effect and is used chronically in low doses to prevent myocardial infarction and thrombus formation in hypercoaguable states. Low-dose, long-term aspirin use irreversibly blocks the formation of thromboxane $A_2$ in platelets, producing an inhibitory effect on platelet aggregation.

## 6.16

*Answer: E*   Tissue factor

Tissue factor (TF), also called 'thromboplastin' or 'factor III', is a protein present in subendothelial tissue, platelets and leukocytes that is necessary for the initiation of thrombin formation from the zymogen prothrombin. Thrombin formation ultimately leads to the coagulation of blood. TF is the cell surface receptor for the serine protease factor VIIa. The best-known function of TF is its role in blood coagulation. The complex of TF with factor VIIa catalyses the conversion of the inactive protease factor X into the active protease factor Xa.

Together with factor VII, TF forms the tissue factor or extrinsic pathway of coagulation. The intrinsic (amplification) pathway involves both activated factor IX and factor VIII. Both pathways lead to the activation of factor X (the common pathway), which combines with activated factor V in the presence of calcium and phospholipid to produce thrombin (thromboplastin activity).

bleeding

TF is expressed by cells which are normally not exposed to flowing blood, such as subendothelial cells (eg smooth muscle cells) and cells surrounding blood vessels (eg fibroblasts). This can change when the blood vessel is damaged, for example by physical injury or rupture of atherosclerotic plaques. Exposure of TF-expressing cells during injury allows the complex formation of TF with factor VIIa, accelerating activity of factor VIIa about a thousand-fold.

The inner surface of the blood vessel consists of endothelial cells. Endothelial cells do not express TF except when they are exposed to inflammatory molecules such as tumour necrosis factor-alpha (TNF-$\alpha$). Another cell type that expresses TF on the cell surface in inflammatory conditions is the monocyte, a white blood cell.

## 6.17

*Answer: A*   D-Dimer

A schistocyte is a red blood cell undergoing fragmentation, or a fragmented part of a red blood cell. Schistocytes can be seen in disseminated intravascular coagulation (DIC) and the clinical scenario in this scenario fits with DIC. Measurements of D-dimer are ordered, along with other tests, to help diagnose DIC. DIC is a complex acute condition that can arise from a variety of situations, including some surgical procedures, septic shock, poisonous snake bites and liver disease, and can occur postpartum. With DIC, clotting factors are activated and then used up throughout the body. This creates numerous minute blood clots and at the same time leaves the patient vulnerable to excessive bleeding. Steps are taken to support the patient while the underlying condition resolves. D-Dimer levels can be used to monitor the effectiveness of DIC treatment (see also *Answer* to **6.10**).

## 6.18

*Answer: C*   Factor VII deficiency

The main role of factor VII (FVII) is to initiate the process of coagulation in conjunction with tissue factor (TF). Tissue factor is found on the outside of blood vessels and is not normally exposed to the bloodstream. When a vessel is injured, tissue factor is exposed to the blood and circulating factor VII. Once bound to TF, FVII is activated to form FVIIa by different proteases, among which are thrombin (factor IIa), activated factor X and the FVIIa-TF complex itself. The most important substrates for FVIIa-TF are factor IX and factor X. Factor VII is vitamin K-dependent; it is produced in the liver and its production can be affected by liver disease. Warfarin and similar anticoagulants also impair its function.

## 6.19

*Answer: A*   A fibrinolytic agent

Aspirin inhibits platelet function, but has no effect on a clot that is already formed. Once the clot has formed, neither warfarin nor heparin are suitable as initial therapy for the condition. Fibrinolytic drugs are given once a clot is formed. Fibrinolytic drugs are used, for example, to reperfuse the myocardium by dissolving the thrombus blocking the cornary arteries and in massive pulmonary embolism. This process is called 'thrombolysis'. Thrombolysis requires the use of thrombolytic or fibrinolytic drugs, which are either derived from *Streptomyces* species or (more recently) by recombinant technology, where human activators of plasminogen (eg tissue plasminogen activator, tPA) are manufactured by bacteria.

Some commonly used thrombolytics are:

- Streptokinase

- Urokinase

- Alteplase (recombinant tissue plasminogen activator or rtPA)

- Reteplase

- Tenecteplase.

All thrombolytic agents work by activating the enzyme plasminogen, which clears the cross-linked fibrin mesh (the backbone of a clot). This makes the clot soluble and subject to further proteolysis by other enzymes, and restores blood flow in occluded blood vessels.

bleeding

## 6.20

*Answer: B*   If he also takes aspirin, the dosage of warfarin must be decreased

Warfarin is an anticoagulant medication that is administered orally or, very rarely, by injection. It is used for the prophylaxis of thrombosis and embolism in many disorders. Its activity has to be monitored by frequent blood testing for the international normalised ratio (INR). Warfarin is a synthetic derivative of coumarin, a chemical found naturally in many plants, notably woodruff, and at lower levels in liquorice, lavender and various other species. Warfarin decreases blood coagulation by interfering with vitamin K metabolism and for this reason it is referred to as a vitamin K antagonist.

Warfarin inhibits the synthesis of biologically active forms of the vitamin K-dependent clotting factors II, VII, IX and X, as well as the regulatory factors, protein C, protein S and protein Z. Other proteins not involved in blood clotting, such as osteocalcin, or matrix Gla protein, can also be affected.

The precursors of these factors require carboxylation of their glutamic acid residues to allow the coagulation factors to bind to phospholipid surfaces inside blood vessels, on the vascular endothelium. The enzyme that carries out the carboxylation of glutamic acid is gamma-glutamyl carboxylase. The carboxylation reaction will only proceed if the carboxylase enzyme is able to convert a reduced form of vitamin K (vitamin K hydroquinone) to vitamin K epoxide at the same time. The vitamin K epoxide is in turn recycled back to vitamin K and vitamin K hydroquinone by another enzyme, the vitamin K epoxide reductase. Warfarin inhibits epoxide reductase, thereby diminishing available vitamin K and vitamin K hydroquinone in the tissues, which inhibits the carboxylation activity of the glutamyl carboxylase. When this occurs, the coagulation factors are no longer carboxylated at certain glutamic acid residues, and are incapable of binding to the endothelial surface of blood vessels, and are thus biologically inactive. As the body stores of previously produced active factors degrade (over several days) and are replaced by inactive factors, the anticoagulation effect becomes apparent. The coagulation factors are produced, but have decreased functionality due to undercarboxylation; they are collectively referred to as PIVKAs (proteins induced [by] vitamin K absence/antagonism). The effect of warfarin, therefore, is to diminish blood clotting in the patient.

Concomitant intake of aspirin can displace warfarin from plasma protein, leading to a warfarin overdose. If aspirin is prescribed, then dose of warfarin must be decreased.

## 6.21

*Answer:* C    Normal PT, increased PTT, low factor VIII AHF, normal vWFAg

The partial thromboplastin time will be increased with classic haemophilia and factor VIII antihaemophilic factor (also called 'factor VIIIc') is decreased, but von Willebrand factor antigen is usually normal or increased (see also *Answer* to **6.4**).

## 6.22

*Answer:* C    Disseminated intravascular coagulation

The patient in this scenario has disseminated intravascular coagulation (DIC) due to Gram-negative sepsis. Bacterial infection, in particular septicaemia, is commonly associated with DIC. No difference exists in the incidence of DIC in patients with Gram-negative sepsis or Gram-positive sepsis. In addition, systemic infections with other micro-organisms, such as viruses and parasites, can also lead to DIC. Factors involved in the development of DIC in patients with infections can be specific cell membrane components of the micro-organism (lipopolysaccharide or endotoxin) or bacterial exotoxins (eg staphylococcal alpha toxin). These components cause a generalised inflammatory response, characterised by the systemic dissemination of pro-inflammatory cytokines (see also *Answer* to **6.1**).

## 6.23

*Answer:* A    Antiphospholipid syndrome

Antiphospholipid syndrome (APS) is a disorder of coagulation in which there is thrombosis in both arteries and veins, as well as

bleeding

pregnancy-related complications such as miscarriage, preterm delivery, or severe pre-eclampsia. The syndrome occurs as a result of autoimmune production of antiphospholipid (aPL) antibodies. The aPL antibodies include anticardiolipin antibodies and lupus anticoagulant. The name 'antiphospholipid syndrome' is a misnomer, in fact, because the target antigen of aPL is not phospholipids but the plasma proteins that bind to phospholipids. The term 'primary antiphospholipid syndrome' is used when APS occurs in the absence of any other autoimmune disease. APS is often seen in conjunction with other autoimmune diseases, such as systemic lupus erythematosus (SLE), when the term 'secondary antiphospholipid syndrome' is used.

Antiphosphilipid syndrome can cause arterial or venous blood clots in any organ system or can lead to pregnancy-related complications (especially miscarriage in the second or third trimester). The most common venous event is deep venous thrombosis of the lower extremities and the most common arterial event is stroke. Other common findings, although not part of the APS classification criteria, are thrombocytopenia, heart valve disease and the skin condition, livedo reticularis. Some patients report headaches and migraines. Antiphospholipid syndrome can rarely mimic multiple sclerosis and it is estimated that 10% of patients are misdiagnosed. Very few patients with primary APS go on to develop SLE.

## 6.24

*Answer: E* Thrombocytopenia

The platelets are responsible for dealing with small leaks in vessels. Thrombocytopenia is marked by petechiae and purpura. Generally speaking, the normal range for the platelet count is $150-450 \times 10^9/l$. Decreased platelet counts can be due to decreased production or to increased destruction of platelets; medication-induced low counts can be caused by either.

### Causes of decreased production of platelets:

- Vitamin $B_{12}$ or folic acid deficiency
- Leukaemia or myelodysplastic syndrome

- Decreased production of thrombopoietin by the liver in liver failure

- Sepsis, systemic viral or bacterial infections

- Dengue fever, due to direct infection of bone marrow megakaryocytes as well as immunologically mediated shortened platelet survival

- Hereditary syndromes:

  o Congenital amegakaryocytic thrombocytopenia

  o Thrombocytopenia absent radius syndrome

  o Fanconi's anaemia

  o Bernard–Soulier syndrome (associated with large platelets)

  o May–Hegglin anomaly, the combination of thrombocytopenia, pale-blue leukocyte inclusions and giant platelets

  o Grey platelet syndrome

  o Alport syndrome.

## Causes of increased destruction of platelets:

- Idiopathic thrombocytopenic purpura (ITP)

- Thrombotic thrombocytopenic purpura (TTP)

- Haemolytic-uraemic syndrome (HUS)

- Disseminated intravascular coagulation (DIC)

- Paroxysmal nocturnal haemoglobinuria (PNH)

- Antiphospholipid syndrome

- Systemic lupus erythematosus (SLE)

- Post-transfusion purpura

- Neonatal alloimmune thrombocytopenia (NAITP)

- Splenic sequestration of platelets due to hypersplenism

- Dengue fever (see above).

bleeding

## Causes of medication-induced thrombocytopenia:

- Heparin
- Valproic acid
- Sulfonamides
- Clopidogrel
- Vancomycin.

If the cause of the low platelet count remains unclear, bone marrow biopsy is often undertaken in order to assess whether the low platelet count is due to decreased production or peripheral destruction.

### 6.25

*Answer: B*  Fresh frozen plasma

Fresh frozen plasma (FFP) is an effective treatment for coagulopathies resulting from disseminated intravascular coagulation, liver disease, and massive transfusion. FFP is defined as the fluid portion of one unit of human blood that has been centrifuged, separated, and frozen solid at −18 °C (or colder) within 6 hours of collection. FFP contains the labile as well as the stable components of the coagulation, fibrinolytic and complement systems; the proteins that maintain oncotic pressure and modulate immunity; and other proteins that have diverse activities. In addition, fats, carbohydrates and minerals are present in concentrations similar to those in the circulation. Although well-defined indications exist for the use of FFP in single or multiple coagulation deficiencies, indications for many of its other uses is often empirical.

FFP is efficacious for the treatment of deficiencies of factors II, V, VII, IX, X and XI when specific component therapy is either not available or not appropriate. Requirements for FFP vary with the specific factor being replaced. For example, haemostatic levels of factor IX in a patient with severe deficiency are difficult to achieve with FFP alone, whereas patients with severe factor X deficiency require factor levels of about 10% to achieve haemostasis and are easily treated with FFP.

bleeding

The risks of administering FFP include disease transmission, anaphylactoid reactions, alloimmunisation and excessive intravascular volume. The potential viral infectivity of FFP is probably similar to that of whole blood and of red blood cells. The rate of post-transfusion hepatitis depends on many factors, including donor selection. In rare instances, acquired immunodeficiency syndrome (AIDS) is transmitted by blood transfusions and possibly also by FFP. Allergic or anaphylactoid reactions can occur in response to FFP administration and can vary from hives to fatal non-cardiac pulmonary oedema. The potential for alloimmunisation is present, as demonstrated by the infrequent formation of Rh antibodies. As with any intravenously administered fluid, excessive amounts of FFP can result in hypervolaemia and cardiac failure.

In this scenario the patient has coagulopathy due to possible deficiency of coagulation factors, as suggested by prolonged partial thromboplastin time.

## 6.26

*Answer: E*    Liver damage

The prothrombin time (PT) and its derived measures of prothrombin ratio (PR) and international normalised ratio (INR) are measures of the extrinsic pathway of coagulation. The reference range for prothrombin time is usually around 12–15 seconds; the normal range for the INR is 0.8–1.2. PT measures factors II, V, VII, and X and fibrinogen. It is used in conjunction with the activated partial thromboplastin time (aPTT), which measures the intrinsic pathway. The speed of the extrinsic pathway is greatly affected by levels of factor VII in the body. Factor VII has a short half-life and its synthesis requires vitamin K. The prothrombin time can be prolonged as a result of deficiencies in vitamin K, which can be caused by warfarin, malabsorption, or a lack of intestinal colonisation by bacteria (eg in newborns). In addition, poor factor VII synthesis (due to liver disease) or increased consumption (in disseminated intravascular coagulation) can prolong the PT.

bleeding

**6.27**

*Answer: C*    Hypofibrinogenaemia

The thrombin clotting time (TCT), also known as the 'thrombin time' (TT), is a coagulation assay that is usually performed in order to assess for the therapeutic level of heparin. It is also sensitive in detecting the presence of fibrinogen abnormalities. The reference interval of the TCT is generally less than 21 seconds, depending on the method and the patient population. Results outside of the reference interval indicate heparin therapy, fibrinogen abnormality or the presence of lupus anticoagulant.

**6.28**

*Answer: C*    Factor VII

Factor VII (formerly known as 'proconvertin') is one of the central proteins in the coagulation cascade. It is an enzyme of the serine protease class. The main role of factor VII (FVII) is to initiate the process of coagulation in conjunction with tissue factor (TF). TF is found on the outside of blood vessels and so not normally exposed to the bloodstream. On vessel injury, TF is exposed to the blood and circulating factor VII. Once bound to TF, FVII is activated to FVIIa by different proteases, among which are thrombin (factor IIa), activated factor X and the FVIIa-TF complex itself. The most important substrates for FVIIa-TF are factor X and factor IX.

The action of factor VII is impeded by tissue factor pathway inhibitor (TFPI), which is released almost immediately after initiation of coagulation. Factor VII is vitamin K-dependent, and is produced in the liver. The use of warfarin or similar anticoagulants impairs its function.

**6.29**

*Answer: C*    Protein C

Warfarin necrosis is an acquired protein C deficiency due to treatment with the vitamin K-inhibitor anticoagulant, warfarin. It is a feared (but rare) complication of warfarin treatment. This rare reaction usually occurs between the third and tenth days of therapy

bleeding

with warfarin derivatives, usually in women. Lesions are sharply demarcated, erythematous, indurated and purpuric, and can either resolve or progress to form large, irregular, haemorrhagic bullae, with eventual necrosis and slow-healing eschar formation. Development of the syndrome is unrelated to drug dose or underlying condition. The most usual sites affected are breasts, thighs and buttocks. The course is not altered by discontinuation of the drug once the lesions have appeared. In initial stages of action, inhibition of protein C can be stronger than inhibition of the vitamin K-dependent coagulation factors (factors II, VII, IX and X), leading to paradoxical activation of coagulation and necrosis of skin areas. It occurs mainly in patients with a deficiency of protein C. Protein C is an innate anticoagulant, and as warfarin further decreases protein C levels by inhibiting vitamin K, this can lead to massive thrombosis, with necrosis and gangrene of the limbs.

## 6.30

*Answer:* C    It functions as a cofactor to protein C

Protein S is a vitamin K-dependent plasma glycoprotein that is synthesised in the liver. In the circulation, protein S exists in two forms: a free form and a complex form bound to complement protein C4b. The best characterised function of protein S is its role in the anticoagulation pathway, where it functions as a cofactor to protein C in the inactivation of factors Va and VIIIa. Only the free form has cofactor activity.

Protein S can bind to negatively charged phospholipids via the carboxylated GLA domain. This property allows protein S to function in the removal of cells which are undergoing apoptosis. Apoptosis is a form of cell death that is used by the body to remove unwanted or damaged cells from tissues. Cells which are apoptotic no longer actively manage the distribution of phospholipids in their outer membrane and so begin to display negatively charged phospholipids, such as phosphatidyl serine on the cell surface. In healthy cells, an adenosine triphosphate- (ATP-) dependent enzyme removes these from the outer leaflet of the cell membrane. These negatively charged phospholipids are recognised by phagocytes such as macrophages. Protein S can bind to the negatively charged phospholipids and function as a bridging molecule between the

bleeding

apoptotic cell and the phagocyte. The bridging property of protein S enhances the phagocytosis of the apoptotic cell, allowing it to be removed 'cleanly' without any symptoms of tissue damage (such as inflammation).

Protein S deficiency is a rare blood disorder which can lead to an increased risk of thrombosis.

## 6.31

*Answer: E*    Factor XIII

Factor XIII (FXIII), or 'fibrin stabilising factor' is an enzyme of the coagulation cascade that cross-links fibrin. When thrombin has converted fibrinogen to fibrin, the latter forms a proteinaceous network in which every E unit is cross-linked to only one D unit. Factor XIII is activated by thrombin into factor XIIIa; its activation into factor XIIIa requires calcium as a cofactor. FXIII is known also as 'Laki–Lorand' factor, after the scientists who first proposed its existence in 1948. Factor XIII deficiency is a rare deficiency, and can cause a severe bleeding tendency. The incidence is 1 in 1 million to 1 in 5 million people.

## 6.32

*Answer: B*    Factor V

The coagulation factors are generally serine proteases. There are some exceptions. For example, factor VIII and factor V are glycoproteins and factor XIII is a transglutaminase. Factor V is occasionally referred to as 'pro-accelerin' or 'labile factor'. In contrast to most other coagulation factors, it is not enzymatically active but functions as a cofactor. Deficiency leads to predisposition to haemorrhage, while some mutations (most notably factor V Leiden) predispose to thrombosis.

Factor V circulates in plasma as a single-chain molecule with a plasma half-life of about 12 hours, though this has been reported to be up to 36 hours. Factor V is able to bind to activated platelets and is activated by thrombin. On activation, factor V is spliced into two chains (a heavy and a light chain, with molecular masses of 110 kDa

bleeding

and 73 kDa respectively) which are non-convalently bound to each other by calcium. Factor V is active as a cofactor of the thrombinase complex. The activated factor X (FXa) enzyme requires calcium and activated factor V to convert prothrombin to thrombin on the cell surface membrane. This is considered to be part of the common pathway in the coagulation cascade.

Factor Va is degraded by activated protein C, one of the principal physiological inhibitors of coagulation. In the presence of thrombomodulin, thrombin acts to decrease clotting by activating protein C, so the concentration and action of protein C are important determinants in the negative feedback loop through which thrombin limits its own activation.

## 6.33

*Answer: E*    Thrombomodulin

Thrombomodulin is an integral membrane protein expressed on the surface of endothelial cells. The protein has a molecular mass of 74 kDa, and consists of a single chain with five distinct domains. It functions as a cofactor in the thrombin-induced activation of protein C in the anticoagulant pathway by forming a 1 : 1 stochiometric complex with thrombin. This raises the speed of protein C activation 1000-fold. Thrombomodulin-bound thrombin has no pro-coagulant effect. The thrombomodulin-thrombin complex also inhibits fibrinolysis by cleaving thrombin-activatable fibrinolysis inhibitor (TAFI) into its active form.

## 6.34

*Answer: D*    Mast cells

Heparin is a naturally occurring anticoagulant produced by basophils and mast cells. A highly sulphated glycosaminoglycan, heparin is widely used as an injectable anticoagulant and has the highest negative charge density of any known biological molecule. Pharmaceutical-grade heparin is commonly derived from mucosal tissues of slaughtered meat animals such as porcine intestine or bovine lung.

bleeding

## 6.35

*Answer: A*    Activation of antithrombin III

Heparin binds to the enzyme inhibitor, antithrombin III (AT-III), causing a conformational change that results in its active site being exposed. The activated AT-III then inactivates thrombin and other proteases involved in blood clotting, most notably factor Xa. The rate of inactivation of these proteases by AT-III increases 1000-fold due to the binding of heparin. AT-III binds to a specific pentasaccharide sulphation sequence contained within the heparin polymer (GlcNAc/NS(6S)-GlcA-GlcNS(3S,6S)-IdoA(2S)-GlcNS(6S)). The conformational change in AT-III on heparin binding mediates its inhibition of factor Xa. For thrombin inhibition, however, thrombin must also bind to the heparin polymer at a site proximal to the pentasaccharide. The highly negative charge density of heparin contributes to its very strong electrostatic interaction with thrombin. The formation of a ternary complex between AT-III, thrombin and heparin results in the inactivation of thrombin. For this reason heparin's activity against thrombin is size-dependent, the ternary complex requiring at least 18 saccharide units for efficient formation. In contrast, anti-factor Xa activity only requires the pentasaccharide binding site.

## 6.36

*Answer: B*    Inhibition of factor Xa

Low-molecular-weight heparins (LMWHs) consist of only short chains of polysaccharide. LMWHs are defined as heparin salts which have an average molecular weight of less than 8000 Da and in which at least 60% of all chains have a molecular weight less than 8000 Da. These salts are manufactured using various methods of fractionation or depolymerisation of polymeric heparin. They have a potency of greater than 70 units/mg of anti-factor Xa activity and a ratio of anti-factor Xa activity to antithrombin activity of more than 1 : 5. LMWHs target anti-factor Xa activity rather than antithrombin (IIa) activity, with the aim of facilitating a more subtle regulation of coagulation and an improved therapeutic index.

bleeding

## 6.37

*Answer: D*    Factor X

Factor X, also known by the eponymous 'Stuart–Prower factor' or as 'thrombokinase', is an enzyme of the coagulation cascade. It is a serine endopeptidase. Factor X is synthesised in the liver and requires vitamin K for its synthesis. Factor X is activated into factor Xa by both factor IX (with its cofactor, factor VIII in a complex known as 'intrinsic Xase') and factor VII with its cofactor, tissue factor (a complex known as 'extrinsic Xase'). It is therefore the first member of the final common pathway or thrombin pathway. It acts by cleaving prothrombin in two places (an arg-thr and then an arg-ile bond), which yields the active thrombin. This process requires factor V as a cofactor.

Factor Xa is inactivated by a protein Z-dependent protease inhibitor, a serine protease inhibitor (serpin). The affinity of this protein for factor Xa is increased 1000-fold by the presence of protein Z, while it does not require protein Z for inactivation of factor XI. Defects in protein Z lead to increased factor Xa activity and a propensity for thrombosis. The half-life of factor X is 40–45 hours.

Inborn deficiency of factor X is very uncommon (1 in 500,000) and can present with epistaxis, haemarthrosis and gastrointestinal blood loss. Apart from congenital deficiency, low factor X levels can occasionally occur in a number of disease states. Deficiency of vitamin K or antagonism by warfarin (or similar medications) leads to the production of an inactive factor X. (In warfarin therapy, this is desirable to prevent thrombosis.)

## 6.38

*Answer: D*    Factor XI

Deficiency of factor XI causes the rare haemophilia C. This mainly occurs in Ashkenazi Jews and is believed to affect approximately 8% of that population (both sexes). One per cent of cases occur in other population groups. It is an autosomal recessive disorder. There is little spontaneous bleeding, but surgical procedures can cause excessive blood loss, and prophylaxis is required.

bleeding

## 6.39

*Answer: D*  Factor XI

Factor XI (or plasma thromboplastin antecedent) is one of the enzymes of the coagulation cascade. Like many other coagulation factors, it is a serine protease. Factor XI (FXI) is produced by the liver and circulates as a homo-dimer in its inactive form. The plasma half-life of FXI is approximately 52 hours. The zymogen factor is activated into factor XIa by factor XIIa (FXIIa), thrombin, and it is also autocatalytic. FXI is a member of the 'contact pathway' due to activation by FXIIa (with includes high-molecular-weight kininogen, prekallikrein, factor XII, factor XI and factor IX). Factor XIa activates factor IX by selectively cleaving arg-ala and arg-val peptide bonds. Factor IXa, in turn, activates factor X.

## 6.40

*Answer: A*  Alpha granules

Grey platelet syndrome (GPS) is characterised by thrombocytopenia, abnormally large, agranular platelets in peripheral blood smears, and almost total absence of platelet alpha granules and their constituents. The defect in GPS is the failure of megakaryocytes to package secretory proteins into alpha granules. The alpha granules in platelets contain a number of growth factors (such as insulin-like growth factor, platelet-derived growth factor, transforming growth factor-beta), platetet factor 4 (which is a heparin-binding chemokine), and other clotting proteins (such as thrombospondin and fibronectin.) The alpha granules express the adhesion molecule P-selectin. Patients with GPS are affected by mild to moderate bleeding tendencies.

bleeding

# SECTION 7:
# CARDIOVASCULAR PATHOLOGY
# — ANSWERS

## 7.1

*Answer:* C   Hypovolaemic shock

Shock, or cardiovascular collapse, is the final common pathway for a number of potentially lethal clinical events, including severe haemorrhage, extensive trauma or burns, a large myocardial infarction, massive pulmonary embolism and microbial sepsis. Regardless of the underlying pathology, shock gives rise to systemic hypoperfusion caused by reduction either in cardiac output or in the effective circulating blood volume. The end results are hypotension, followed by impaired tissue perfusion and cellular hypoxia. Although the hypoxic and metabolic effects of hypoperfusion initially cause only reversible cellular injury, persistence of shock eventually causes irreversible tissue injury and can culminate in the death of the patient.

Shock may be grouped into three general categories:

- **Cardiogenic shock** results from myocardial pump failure. This can be caused by intrinsic myocardial damage (infarction), ventricular arrhythmias, extrinsic compression (cardiac tamponade) or outflow obstruction (eg due to pulmonary embolism).

- **Hypovolaemic shock** results from loss of blood or plasma volume. This can be caused by haemorrhage as in this case, fluid loss from severe burns or trauma.

- **Septic shock** is caused by systemic microbial infection. Most commonly, this occurs in the setting of Gram-negative infections (endotoxic shock), but it can also occur with Gram-positive and fungal infections.

The mechanisms underlying cardiogenic and hypovolaemic shock are fairly straightforward, essentially involving low cardiac output. Septic shock, in comparison, is substantially more complicated and results from a complex interplay of peripheral vasodilation and pooling of blood, endothelial activation/injury, leukocyte-induced damage, disseminated intravascular coagulation, and activation of cytokine cascades.

Less commonly, shock can occur in the setting of anaesthetic accident or spinal cord injury (neurogenic shock), owing to loss of vascular tone and peripheral pooling of blood. Anaphylactic shock, initiated by a generalised IgE-mediated hypersensitivity response, is associated with systemic vasodilation and increased vascular permeability. In these instances, widespread vasodilatation causes a sudden increase in the vascular bed capacitance, which is not adequately filled by the normal circulating blood volume. Hypotension, tissue hypoperfusion and cellular anoxia result.

## 7.2

*Answer: E    Streptococcus viridans*

Infective endocarditis, one of the most serious of all infections, is characterised by colonisation or invasion of the heart valves or the mural endocardium by a microbe, leading to the formation of bulky, friable vegetations composed of thrombotic debris and organisms, often associated with destruction of the underlying cardiac tissues. The aorta, aneurysmal sacs, other blood vessels and prosthetic devices can also become infected. Although fungi, rickettsiae (Q fever), and chlamydiae have at one time or another been responsible for these infections, most cases are bacterial. Prompt diagnosis and effective treatment of infective endocarditis can significantly alter the outlook for the patient.

Infective endocarditis can develop on previously normal valves, but a variety of cardiac and vascular abnormalities predispose to this form of infection. In years past, rheumatic heart disease was the major antecedent disorder, but more common now are myxomatous mitral valve, degenerative calcific valvular stenosis, bicuspid aortic valve (whether calcified or not) and artificial (prosthetic) valves. Host factors such as neutropenia, immunodeficiency, malignancy, therapeutic immunosuppression, diabetes mellitus, and alcohol or intravenous drug abuse are predisposing influences. Sterile platelet-fibrin deposits that accumulate at sites of impingement of jet-streams caused by pre-existing cardiac disease or indwelling vascular catheters can also be important in the development of endocarditis.

The causative organisms differ somewhat in the major high-risk groups. Endocarditis of native but previously damaged or otherwise abnormal valves is caused most commonly by *Streptococcus viridans* (50%–60% of cases). Note that this is not the organism responsible for rheumatic disease. In contrast, the more virulent *Staphylococcus aureus* organisms commonly found on the skin can attack either healthy or deformed valves and are responsible for 10%–20% of cases overall; *S. aureus* is the major offender in intravenous drug abusers. The roster of the remaining bacteria includes enterococci and the so-called HACEK group (*Haemophilus*, *Actinobacillus*, *Cardiobacterium*, *Eikenella*, and *Kingella*), all commensals in the oral cavity. Prosthetic valve endocarditis is caused most commonly by coagulase-negative staphylococci (eg *S. epidermidis*). Other agents causing endocarditis include Gram-negative bacilli and fungi. In about 10% of all cases of endocarditis, no organism can be isolated from the blood ('culture-negative' endocarditis) because of prior antibiotic therapy, difficulties in isolating the offending agent, or because deeply embedded organisms within the enlarging vegetation are not released into the blood.

## 7.3

*Answer: D*   Temporal arteritis

Giant-cell (temporal) arteritis, the most common form of systemic vasculitis in adults, is an acute or chronic, often granulomatous, inflammation of arteries of large to small size. It affects principally the arteries in the head, especially the temporal arteries, but also the vertebral and ophthalmic arteries and the aorta, where it can cause thoracic aortic aneurysm. Ophthalmic arterial involvement can lead to permanent blindness, and visual loss caused by giant-cell arteritis is a medical emergency that requires prompt recognition and treatment. Lesions can be found in other arteries throughout the body, including the aorta (giant cell aortitis).

Temporal arteritis is most common in older individuals and rare before age 50 years. Symptoms are either just vague and constitutional (fever, fatigue, weight loss) without localising signs or symptoms, or comprise facial pain or headache, often most intense along the course of the superficial temporal artery, which can be painful to palpation. More serious are the ocular symptoms (associated with involvement of the ophthalmic artery), which appear quite abruptly in about half of patients and range from diplopia to transient or complete vision loss. The diagnosis depends on biopsy and histological confirmation, but because of the segmental nature of the involvement, adequate biopsy requires at least a 2- to 3-cm length of artery, and negative or atypical findings on biopsy do not rule out the condition. Treatment with anti-inflammatory agents is generally very effective.

## 7.4

*Answer: B*    Atrial fibrillation

Atrial fibrillation (AF) is one of the most common arrhythmias. The incidence is higher in men than in women and it is also more common in white people than it is in black people. The prevalence increases with age, and almost 10% of people over the age of 80 years are affected. It tends to occur in patients with a heart disorder, sometimes precipitating heart failure because cardiac output decreases in the absence of atrial contraction. The absent atrial contractions also predispose to thrombus formation, and the annual risk of cerebrovascular embolic events is about 7%. The risk of stroke is higher in patients with a rheumatic valvular disorder, hyperthyroidism, hypertension, diabetes, left ventricular systolic dysfunction or previous thromboembolic events. Systemic emboli can also cause malfunction or necrosis of other organs (eg heart, kidneys, gastrointestinal tract, eye) or of a limb.

AF is often asymptomatic, but many patients have palpitations, vague chest discomfort, or symptoms of heart failure (eg weakness, light-headedness, dyspnoea), particularly when the ventricular rate is very rapid (it is often 140–160/minute). Patients can also present with symptoms and signs of acute stroke or of other organ damage due to systemic emboli. The pulse is irregularly irregular with loss of *a* waves in the jugular venous pulse. A pulse deficit (the apical ventricular rate is faster than the rate palpated at the wrist) might be present because the left ventricular stroke volume is not always sufficient to produce a peripheral pressure wave at fast ventricular rates.

The diagnosis is made by electrocardiography (ECG). Findings include the absence of P waves, f waves ('fibrillatory' waves) between QRS complexes (irregular in timing, irregular in morphology; baseline undulations at rates >300/minute but not always apparent in all leads), and irregularly irregular R–R intervals. Other irregular rhythms can resemble AF on ECG but can be distinguished by the presence of discrete P waves or flutter waves, which can sometimes be made more visible with vagal manoeuvres.

## 7.5

*Answer:* C    ST-segment elevation

Electrocardiography (ECG) is the most important test and should be done within 10 minutes of presentation in a patient suspected of having a myocardial infarction (MI). It is the centre of the decision-making pathway because fibrinolytics benefit patients with ST-segment-elevation MI (STEMI) but can increase the risk for those with non-ST-segment-elevation MI (NSTEMI). For STEMI, the initial ECG is usually diagnostic, showing ST-segment elevation of 1 mm or more in two or more contiguous leads subtending the damaged area. Pathological Q waves are not necessary for the diagnosis. The ECG must be read carefully because ST-segment elevation can be subtle, particularly in the inferior leads (II, III, aVF); sometimes the reader's attention is mistakenly focused on leads with ST-segment depression. If symptoms are characteristic, ST-segment elevation on ECG has a specificity of 90% and a sensitivity of 45% for diagnosing MI. Serial tracings (obtained q 8 h for 1 day, then daily) showing a gradual evolution towards a stable, more normal pattern or the development of abnormal Q waves over a few days tends to confirm the diagnosis.

Because non-transmural (non-Q-wave) infarcts are usually in the subendocardial or mid-myocardial layers, they do not produce diagnostic Q waves or distinct ST-segment elevation on the ECG. Instead, they commonly produce only varying degrees of ST-T abnormalities that are less striking, variable, or non-specific and sometimes difficult to interpret (ie NSTEMI). If such abnormalities resolve (or worsen) on repeat ECGs, ischaemia is very likely. However, when repeat ECGs are unchanged, acute MI is unlikely and, if still suspected clinically, requires other evidence to make the diagnosis. A normal ECG taken when a patient is pain-free does not rule out unstable angina; a normal ECG taken during pain, although it does not rule out angina, suggests that the pain is not ischaemic.

If right ventricular infarction is suspected, a 15-lead ECG is usually recorded; additional leads are placed at $V_4R$ and, to detect posterior infarction, at $V_8$ and $V_9$. ECG diagnosis of MI is more difficult when a left bundle branch block configuration is present because it resembles STEMI changes. ST-segment elevation concordant with the QRS complex strongly suggests MI, as does an ST-segment elevation of more than 5 mm in at least two precordial leads. But generally, any patient with suspect symptoms and new-onset (or not known to be old) left bundle branch block is treated as for STEMI.

## 7.6

*Answer: D*   Stasis of blood

Pulmonary embolism (PE) nearly always arises from thrombus in the lower extremity or pelvic veins (deep venous thrombosis, or DVT). Thrombi in either system can be occult. Thromboemboli can also originate in upper extremity veins or in the right cardiac chambers. Risk factors for DVT and PE are similar in children and adults and include conditions that impair venous return or that cause endothelial injury or dysfunction, particularly in patients with an underlying baseline hypercoagulable state. Bedrest and confinement without walking, even for a few hours, are common precipitators as a result of stasis of blood (the most likely mechanism in this case).

Once a DVT develops, the clot can dislodge and travel through the venous system and right heart to lodge in the pulmonary arteries, where it partially or completely occludes one or more vessels. The consequences depend on the size and number of emboli, the pulmonary reaction, and the ability of the body's intrinsic thrombolytic system to dissolve the clot. Small emboli might have no acute physiological effects; many begin to lyse immediately and resolve within hours or days. Larger emboli can cause a reflex increase in ventilation (tachypnoea); hypoxaemia from ventilation/perfusion mismatch and shunting; atelectasis from alveolar hypocapnia and abnormalities in surfactant; and an increase in pulmonary vascular resistance caused by mechanical obstruction and vasoconstriction. Endogenous lysis reduces most emboli, even those of moderate size, without treatment, and physiological alterations decrease over hours or days. Some emboli resist lysis and can organise and persist. Occasionally, chronic residual obstruction leads to pulmonary hypertension (chronic thromboembolic pulmonary hypertension) that can develop over years and result in chronic right heart failure. When large emboli occlude major arteries, or when several small emboli occlude over 50% of the distal arterial system, the right ventricular pressure increases, causing acute right ventricular failure, failure with shock (massive PE), or sudden death in severe cases. The risk of death depends on the degree and rate of rise of right-sided pressures and on the patient's underlying cardiopulmonary status; higher pressures occur more commonly in patients with pre-existing cardiopulmonary disease. Healthy patients may survive a PE that occludes more than 50% of the pulmonary vascular bed.

Pulmonary infarction occurs in fewer than 10% of patients diagnosed with PE. This low rate has been attributed to the dual blood supply to the lung (ie bronchial and pulmonary). Infarction is typically characterised by a radiographic infiltrate, chest pain, fever and, occasionally, haemoptysis.

## 7.7

*Answer: D*   Fat embolism

Fat embolism is caused by the introduction of fat or bone marrow particles into the systemic venous system and then to the pulmonary arteries. Causes include long-bone fractures (as in this case), orthopaedic procedures, microvascular occlusion or necrosis of bone marrow in patients with sickle cell crisis and, rarely, toxic modification of native or parenteral serum lipids. Fat embolism causes a pulmonary syndrome similar to the acute respiratory distress syndrome, with severe hypoxaemia of rapid onset, often accompanied by neurological changes and a petechial rash.

## 7.8

*Answer: D*    Marantic endocarditis

In patients with chronic wasting diseases, disseminated intravascular coagulation, mucin-producing metastatic carcinomas (of lung, stomach or pancreas) or chronic infections (eg tuberculosis, pneumonia, osteomyelitis), large thrombotic vegetations can form on valves and produce significant emboli to the brain, kidneys, spleen, mesentery, extremities and coronary arteries. These vegetations tend to form on congenitally abnormal cardiac valves or on those damaged by rheumatic fever. The clinical condition is known as 'marantic endocarditis'.

## 7.9

*Answer: E*    Thromboangiitis obliterans

Thromboangiitis obliterans is an inflammatory thrombosis of small and medium-sized arteries and some superficial veins, causing arterial ischaemia in distal extremities and superficial thrombophlebitis. Tobacco use is the primary risk factor. Symptoms and signs include claudication, non-healing foot ulcers, rest pain and gangrene. Diagnosis is by clinical findings, non-invasive vascular testing, angiography, and exclusion of other causes. Treatment is cessation of tobacco use. The prognosis is excellent when tobacco use is stopped, but if the patient does not stop smoking the disorder inevitably progresses, and amputation is often required.

## 7.10

*Answer: B*    Benign neoplasm of the adrenal medulla

A phaeochromocytoma is a catecholamine-secreting tumour of chromaffin cells typically located in the adrenals. It causes persistent or paroxysmal hypertension. Diagnosis is by measuring catecholamine products in blood or urine. Imaging tests, especially computed tomography and magnetic resonance imaging, help to localise tumours.

The catecholamines secreted include noradrenaline (norepinephrine), adrenaline (epinephrine), dopamine and dopa in varying proportions.

About 90% of phaeochromocytomas are in the adrenal medulla, but they can also be located in other tissues derived from neural crest cells, and possible sites include: the paraganglia of the sympathetic chain, retroperitoneally along the course of the aorta, the carotid body, the organ of Zuckerkandl (at the aortic bifurcation), the genitourinary system, the brain, the pericardial sac, and in dermoid cysts.

Phaeochromocytomas in the adrenal medulla occur equally in both sexes, are bilateral in 10% of cases (in 20% in children), and are malignant in fewer than 10% of cases. Of extra-adrenal tumours, 30% are malignant. Although phaeochromocytomas occur at any age, the peak incidence is between the twenties and forties. Phaeochromocytomas vary in size but are on average 5–6 cm in diameter. They weigh 50–200 g, but tumours weighing several kilograms have been reported. Rarely, they are large enough to be palpated or cause symptoms due to pressure or obstruction. Regardless of the histological appearance, the tumour is considered to be benign if it has not invaded the capsule and no metastases are found, although exceptions occur.

Phaeochromocytomas are sometimes part of the syndrome of familial multiple endocrine neoplasia (MEN), types IIA or IIB, in which other endocrine tumours (parathyroid or medullary carcinoma of the thyroid) coexist or develop subsequently. Phaeochromocytoma develops in 1% of patients with neurofibromatosis (von Recklinghausen's disease) and can occur with haemangiomas and renal cell carcinoma, as in von Hippel–Lindau disease. Familial phaeochromocytomas and carotid body tumours may be due to mutations of the enzyme, succinate dehydrogenase.

## 7.11

*Answer: D*   Pulmonary embolism

Pulmonary embolism (PE) is the occlusion of one or more pulmonary arteries by thrombi that originate elsewhere, typically in the large veins of the lower extremities or pelvis. Risk factors are conditions that impair venous return and that cause endothelial injury or dysfunction, especially in patients with an underlying hypercoagulable state.

Most PEs are small, physiologically insignificant, and asymptomatic. Even when present, symptoms are nonspecific and vary in frequency and intensity, depending on the extent of pulmonary vascular occlusion and pre-existing cardiopulmonary function. Larger emboli cause acute dyspnoea and pleuritic chest pain and, less commonly, cough and/or haemoptysis. Massive PE presents with hypotension, tachycardia, syncope or cardiac arrest.

The most common signs of PE are tachycardia and tachypnoea. Less commonly, patients have hypotension, a loud second heart sound ($S_2$) due to a loud pulmonary component ($P_2$) and/or crackles or wheezing. In the presence of right ventricular failure, distended internal jugular veins and a right ventricular heave may be evident, and right ventricular gallop (third and fourth heart sounds [$S_3$ and $S_4$]), with or without tricuspid regurgitation, may be audible. Fever can occur, and in fact deep venous thrombosis and PE are often overlooked causes of fever. Chronic thromboembolic pulmonary hypertension causes symptoms and signs of right heart failure, including exertional dyspnoea, easy fatigue, and peripheral oedema that develops over a period of months to years.

The diagnosis of PE is challenging, because symptoms and signs are non-specific and diagnostic tests are either imperfect or invasive. Diagnosis starts by including PE in the differential diagnosis of a large number of conditions with similar symptoms, including cardiac ischaemia, heart failure, chronic obstructive pulmonary disease (COPD) exacerbation, pneumothorax, pneumonia, sepsis, acute chest syndrome (in sickle cell patients) and acute anxiety with hyperventilation. Initial evaluation should include pulse oximetry, electrocardiography (ECG) and chest X-ray. The chest X-ray usually is non-specific but might show atelectasis, focal infiltrates, an elevated hemidiaphragm and/or a pleural effusion. The classic findings of focal loss of vascular markings (Westermark's sign), a peripheral wedge-shaped density (Hampton's hump) or enlargement of the right descending pulmonary artery (Palla's sign) are suggestive but very insensitive.

Pulse oximetry provides a quick way to assess oxygenation; hypoxaemia is one sign of PE, and other significant disorders must be investigated. ECG most often shows tachycardia and various ST-T-wave abnormalities, which are not specific for PE. An $S_1Q_3T_3$ or a new right bundle branch block might indicate the effect of an abrupt rise in right ventricular pressure on right ventricular conduction. These are specific but insensitive signs, occurring in only about 5% of patients. Right axis deviation (R > S in $V_1$) and P-pulmonale can be present. T-wave inversion in leads $V_1$ to $V_4$ also occurs.

## 7.12

*Answer: A*    Acute aortic dissection

Acute aortic dissection is the surging of blood through a tear in the aortic intima, with separation of the intima and media and creation of a false lumen. The intimal tear can be a primary event or can be secondary to haemorrhage within the media. The dissection can occur anywhere along the aorta and extend proximally or distally into other arteries. Hypertension is an important contributor. Symptoms and signs include abrupt onset of tearing chest or back pain, and dissection can result in aortic regurgitation and compromised circulation in branch arteries. Diagnosis is by imaging tests (eg transoesophageal echocardiography, computed tomographic angiography, magnetic resonance imaging, contrast aortography).

Treatment always involves aggressive blood pressure control and serial imaging to monitor progression of the dissection; surgical repair of the aorta and placement of a synthetic graft is needed for ascending aortic dissections and for certain descending aortic dissections. One fifth of patients die before reaching the hospital, and up to a third die of operative or perioperative complications.

## 7.13

*Answer: C*    Echocardiography

In this clinical scenario the clinical features are suggestive of a valvular lesion which can best be assessed by echocardiography. Echocardiography uses ultrasound waves to produce an image of the heart and great vessels. It helps assess heart wall thickness (eg in hypertrophy or atrophy) and motion, and provides information about ischaemia and infarction and valvular function and structure. It can be used to assess diastolic filling patterns of the left ventricle, which can help in the diagnosis of left ventricular hypertrophy, hypertrophic or restrictive cardiomyopathy, severe heart failure, constrictive pericarditis, and severe aortic regurgitation.

## 7.14

*Answer: B*    Duplex scan

The clinical features in this case are suggestive of deep venous thrombosis. Duplex ultrasonography is a safe, non-invasive, portable technique for detecting lower extremity (primarily femoral vein) thrombi. A clot can be detected in up to three ways: by visualising the lining of the vein, by demonstrating lack of compressibility of the vein, and by demonstrating reduced flow by Doppler. The test has a sensitivity of over 90% and a specificity of over 95% for thrombus. It cannot reliably detect a clot in calf or iliac veins. The absence of thrombi in the femoral veins does not exclude the possibility of thrombus from other sources, but patients with negative duplex test results have an event-free survival rate of over 95% because thrombi from other sources are so much less common. Ultrasonography has been incorporated into many diagnostic algorithms because an ultrasound positive for femoral vein thrombosis indicates the need for anticoagulation, which may make further testing for pulmonary embolism or other thrombi unnecessary.

## 7.15

*Answer: A*    Acute pericarditis

Acute pericarditis can result from infection, autoimmune and inflammatory disorders, uraemia, trauma, myocardial infarction (MI) or certain drugs. Infectious pericarditis is most often viral. Purulent bacterial pericarditis is uncommon but can follow infective endocarditis, pneumonia, septicaemia, penetrating trauma or cardiac surgery. Often, the cause cannot be identified (non-specific or idiopathic pericarditis) but many of these cases are probably viral. Overall, the most common causes are viral and idiopathic. Acute MI causes 10%–15% of cases of acute pericarditis. Post-MI syndrome (Dressler syndrome) is a less common cause now, occurring mainly when reperfusion with percutaneous transluminal coronary angioplasty (PTCA) or thrombolytic drugs are ineffective in patients with transmural infarction. Pericarditis occurs after pericardiotomy (post-pericardiotomy syndrome) in 5%–30% of cardiac operations.

Pericarditis causes chest pain and a pericardial rub, sometimes with dyspnoea. The first evidence can be tamponade, with hypotension, shock or pulmonary oedema. Because the innervation of the pericardium and myocardium is the same, the chest pain of pericarditis is sometimes similar to that of myocardial inflammation or ischaemia: Dull or sharp precordial or substernal pain can radiate to the neck, trapezius ridge (especially on the left) or shoulders. Pain ranges from mild to severe. Unlike ischaemic chest pain, pain due to pericarditis is usually aggravated by thoracic movement, cough, breathing or swallowing food; it can be relieved by sitting up and leaning forwards. There can be tachypnoea and non-productive cough, and fever, chills and weakness are common. In 15%–25% of patients with idiopathic pericarditis, symptoms recur intermittently for months or years.

The most important physical finding is a triphasic or a systolic and diastolic precordial friction rub. However, the rub is often intermittent and evanescent; it might be present only during systole or, less frequently, only during diastole. If no rub is heard with the patient seated and leaning forwards, auscultation could be attempted with the patient 'on all fours' and listening with the diaphragm of the stethoscope. Sometimes, a pleural component to the rub is noted during breathing, which is due to inflammation of the pleura adjacent to the pericardium. Considerable amounts of pericardial fluid can muffle the heart sounds, increase the area of cardiac dullness and change the size and shape of the cardiac silhouette.

If acute pericarditis is suspected, hospitalisation is sometimes required for initial evaluation. Electrocardiography (ECG) and chest X-rays are done. If symptoms or signs of elevated right-sided pressure, tamponade or an enlarged cardiac silhouette are present, echocardiography should also be performed to check for effusions and cardiac filling abnormalities. Blood tests can show leucocytosis and an elevated erythrocyte sedimentation rate (ESR) but these findings are non-specific.

cardiovascular

The diagnosis is based on the presence of typical clinical findings and ECG abnormalities. Serial ECGs may be needed to show abnormalities. The ECG in acute pericarditis might show abnormalities confined to the ST segments and T waves, usually in most of the leads. The ST segments in two or three of the standard leads become elevated but subsequently return to baseline. Unlike MI, acute pericarditis does not cause reciprocal depression in the ST segments (except in leads aVR and $V_1$), and there are no pathological Q waves. The PR segment can be depressed. After several days or longer, the T waves can become flattened and then inverted throughout the ECG, except in lead aVR; T-wave inversion occurs after the ST segment has returned to baseline, in contrast to the pattern seen in acute ischaemia or MI.

## 7.16

*Answer: B*    Creatine kinase-MB

Cardiac markers or cardiac enzymes are proteins from cardiac tissue found in the blood. These proteins are released into the bloodstream when damage to the heart occurs, as in myocardial infarction. Until the 1980s, the enzymes serum aspartate aminotransferase (AST) and lactate dehydrogenase (LDH) were used to assess cardiac injury. It was then found that a disproportional elevation of the MB subtype of the enzyme creatine kinase (CK) was very specific for myocardial injury. Current guidelines are generally in favour of troponin subunits I or T, which are very specific for the heart muscle and are thought to rise before permanent injury develops. The CK enzyme consists of two subunits, which can be either 'B' (brain-type) or 'M' (muscle-type). There are, therefore, three different isoenzymes: CK-MM, CK-BB and CK-MB. The genes for these subunits are located on different chromosomes: B on 14q32 and M on 19q13. In addition to those, there are two mitochondrial creatine kinases, the ubiquitous and sarcomeric forms. Isoenzyme patterns differ in tissues. CK-BB occurs mainly in tissues, and its levels rarely have any significance in the bloodstream. Skeletal muscle expresses CK-MM (98%) and CK-MB at low levels (1%). The myocardium, in contrast, expresses CK-MM at 70% and CK-MB at 30%.

## 7.17

*Answer:* C    Coronary atherosclerosis

Long-term survival of cardiac transplant recipients is primarily limited by the development of allograft coronary artery disease (ACAD), the leading cause of death after the first post-transplantation year. Angiographically detectable ACAD is reported in approximately 50% of patients 5 years after transplantation. The aetiology of this allograft vasculopathy is multifactorial and involves both immunological and non-immunological factors. Recently, it has been shown that immune-related risk factors appear to be more significant in the development of ACAD. Non-immune-associated related risk factors have also been implicated in ACAD, including increased donor age, hyperlipidaemia and cytomegalovirus (CMV) infection. These immune and non-immune risk factors lead to a unique coronary pathology characterised by diffuse, concentric intimal proliferation, with infiltration by smooth muscle cells and macrophages, leading to narrowing along the entire length of the vessel. Furthermore, collateral vessels are notably absent. ACAD can begin within a few weeks after the transplant and progress insidiously to complete obliteration of the coronary lumen, with allograft failure secondary to ischaemia.

## 7.18

*Answer:* D    Persistent truncus arteriosus

Persistent truncus arteriosus (or truncus arteriosus) is a rare form of congenital heart disease that presents at birth. It derives its name from the embryological structure it is derived from, also known as the 'truncus arteriosus'. In this condition, the vessel never properly divides into the pulmonary artery and aorta

Usually, this defect occurs spontaneously. Genetic disorders and teratogens (viruses, metabolic imbalance and industrial or pharmacological agents) have been associated as possible causes. Up to 50% of cases are associated with chromosome 22q11 deletions. The neural crest, specifically a population of cells known as the 'cardiac neural crest', directly contributes to the aorticopulmonary septum. Microablation of the cardiac neural crest in developing chick embryos and genetic anomalies affecting this population of cells in rodents results in persistent truncus arteriosus. Numerous abnormalities affecting the cardiac neural crest have been associated with persistent truncus arteriosus, including abnormalities of growth factors (fibroblast growth factor 8 and bone morphogenetic protein), transcription factors (T-box, Pax, Nkx2-5, GATA-6 and Forkhead) and gap junction proteins (connexin).The cardiac neural crest also contributes the smooth muscle of the great arteries.

## 7.19

*Answer: B* Endocarditis with *Staphylococcus aureus*

A mycotic aneurysm is a focal dilatation of an artery that occurs as a result of infection, necrosis and weakening of the arterial wall. Because it is usually associated with bacterial endocarditis, the term is inappropriate as the causative agents are usually bacteria and not a fungus. In this case it should be called 'bacterial endocarditis' and not 'mycotic endocarditis'. The bacteria most commonly involved are *Staphylococcus aureus*, *Pneumococcus* and group A streptococci. Bacterial aneurysms are believed to start when an infected embolus lodges in the vessel wall; infection, inflammation and necrosis lead to weakening of the wall and focal aneurysmal dilatation that follows pulsations.

## 7.20

*Answer: E* Reversal of the shunt

Eisenmenger syndrome (or Eisenmenger's reaction) is defined as the process in which a left-to-right shunt in the heart causes increased flow through the pulmonary vasculature, causing pulmonary hypertension, which in turn causes increased pressures in the right side of the heart and reversal of the shunt into a right-to-left shunt. Defining conditions that are required for the diagnosis of Eisenmenger syndrome are:

- An underlying heart defect that allows blood to pass between the left and right sides of the heart

- Pulmonary hypertension, or elevated blood pressure in the lungs

- Polycythaemia, an increase in the number of red blood cells

- Reversal of the shunt.

The left side of the heart supplies blood to the whole body and as a result has higher pressures than the right side, which supplies only deoxygenated blood to the lungs. If a large anatomical defect exists between the sides of the heart, blood will flow from the left side to the right side. This results in high blood flow and pressure travelling through the lungs. The increased pressure causes damage to delicate capillaries, which are then replaced with scar tissue. Scar tissue does not contribute to oxygen transfer, leading to a decrease in the useful volume of the pulmonary vasculature. The scar tissue is also less flexible than normal lung tissue, and this causes further increases in blood pressure, so that the heart must pump harder to continue supplying the lungs, leading to further capillary damage.

The reduction in oxygen transfer reduces oxygen saturation in the blood, leading to increased production of red blood cells in an attempt to bring the oxygen saturation up. The excess of red blood cells is called 'polycythaemia'. Desperate for enough circulating oxygen, the body begins to dump immature red cells into the bloodstream. Immature red cells are not as efficient at carrying oxygen as mature red cells and they are less flexible and less able to squeeze easily through tiny capillaries in the lungs, and so contribute to the death of pulmonary capillary beds. The increase in red blood cells also causes hyperviscosity syndrome.

A person with Eisenmenger syndrome is paradoxically subject to the possibility of both uncontrolled bleeding due to damaged capillaries and high pressure and the development of random clots due to hyperviscosity and stasis of blood. The rough places in the heart lining at the site of the septal defects/shunts tend to gather platelets and keep them out of circulation, and can become the source of random clots. Eventually, due to increased resistance, pulmonary pressures can increase sufficiently to cause a reversal of blood flow, so blood begins to travel from the right side of the heart to the left side, and the body is supplied with deoxygenated blood, leading to cyanosis and organ damage.

cardiovascular

# SECTION 8:
# PULMONARY PATHOLOGY —
# ANSWERS

## 8.1

*Answer: B*   Bronchiectasis

Cystic fibrosis is one of the most common life-shortening, childhood-onset inherited diseases. In the United States the incidence is 1 in 1000. In Victoria, Australia the incidence is 1 in 3600. In northern Italy the incidence is 1 in 4300. It is most common among Europeans and Ashkenazi Jews; 1 in 22 people of European descent carry one gene for cystic fibrosis, making it the most common genetic disease among this population.

Individuals with cystic fibrosis can be diagnosed prior to birth by genetic testing or in early childhood by a sweat test. Newborn screening tests are increasingly common and effective. There is no cure for cystic fibrosis, and most people with cystic fibrosis will die young (many in their twenties and thirties) from respiratory failure, although with many new treatments being introduced, the life expectancy is increasing. Ultimately, lung transplantation is often necessary as the cystic fibrosis worsens.

CF is caused by a mutation in a gene called the 'cystic fibrosis transmembrane conductance regulator' (*CFTR*). The product of this gene helps to make sweat, digestive juices and mucus. Although most people without cystic fibrosis have two working copies of *CFTR*, only one is needed to prevent cystic fibrosis. Cystic fibrosis is an autososmal recessive disease and only develops when neither gene works normally. The name 'cystic fibrosis' refers to the characteristic 'fibrosis' and cyst formation within the pancreas, first recognized in the 1930s.

Cystic fibrosis affects the entire body and affects growth, breathing, digestion and reproduction. The newborn period can be marked by poor weight gain and intestinal blockage caused by thick faeces. Other symptoms of cystic fibrosis appear during the remainder of

pulmonary

childhood and early adulthood. These include continued problems with growth, the onset of lung disease, and increasing difficulties with poor absorption of vitamins and nutrients by the gastrointestinal tract. In addition, difficulties with fertility will manifest.

Lung disease in cystic fibrosis results from clogging of airways due to inflammation. Inflammation and infection cause injury to the lungs and structural changes that lead to a variety of symptoms. In the early stages, incessant coughing, copious phlegm production and reduced ability to exercise are common. Many of these symptoms occur when bacteria that normally inhabit the thick mucus grow out of control and cause pneumonia. In the later stages of cystic fibrosis, changes in the architecture of the lung further exacerbate chronic difficulties in breathing.

Bronchiectasis is defined as a chronic dilatation of bronchi or bronchioles, occurring as a sequel to inflammatory disease or obstruction, and is a debilitating complication of cystic fibrosis. Infection is the mechanism by which the bronchiectasis progresses. The disease, left untreated, will continue to damage lung tissue and airways and cause emphysema and severe breathing difficulties. Dilatation of the bronchial walls results in airflow obstruction and impaired clearance of secretions because the dilated areas interrupt normal air pressure of the bronchial tubes, causing sputum to pool inside the dilated areas instead of being pushed upwards. The pooled sputum provides an environment that is conducive to the growth of infectious pathogens, and these areas of the lungs are therefore very vulnerable to infection. The more the lungs experience infections, the more lung tissue and alveoli are damaged, and the more inelastic and dilated the bronchial tubes become, perpetuating the cycle of the disease.

## 8.2

*Answer: B*    Community-acquired, *Streptococcus pneumoniae* infection, alcoholism

Lobar pneumonia is the result of alveolar wall injury with severe haemorrhagic oedema and is caused by inhaled infectious organisms that reach the subpleural zone of the lung. This injury is followed by a rapid multiplication of organisms and invasion of the infected oedematous fluid by polynuclear leukocytes. The process spreads rapidly through the pores of Kohn, leading to consolidation of an entire lobe or segment.

Community-acquired pneumonia develops in people with limited or no contact with medical institutions or settings. The most commonly identified pathogens are *Streptococcus pneumoniae*, *Haemophilus influenzae* and atypical organisms (eg *Chlamydia pneumoniae*, *Mycoplasma pneumoniae*, *Legionella* species). The symptoms and signs comprise fever, cough, dyspnoea, tachypnoea and tachycardia and the diagnosis is based on the clinical presentation and the chest X-ray.

The typical radiological pattern is one of air-space consolidation involving an entire lobe containing air bronchograms. Because of the use of antibiotics, the pneumonia is limited to one or more segments within a lobe. Necrosis and cavitation are potential complications of lobar pneumonia. Pulmonary gangrene can occur (rarely).

pulmonary

## 8.3

*Answer:* C   Primary tuberculosis

This is a description of the typical 'Ghon complex' of an initial, or primary, tuberculosis (TB) infection. Air-borne droplet nuclei lodge in subpleural terminal air spaces, predominantly in the lower lung, usually in only one site. Tubercle bacilli replicate inside macrophages, ultimately killing them; inflammatory cells are attracted to the area, causing a tubercle and sometimes pneumonitis. In the early weeks of infection some infected macrophages are borne to regional lymph nodes (eg hilar, mediastinal). Haematogenous spread to any part of the body, particularly the apical-posterior portion of the lungs, epiphyses of the long bones, kidneys, vertebral bodies or meninges can occur. In 95% of cases, after about 3 weeks of uninhibited growth, the immune system suppresses bacillary replication before symptoms or signs develop. Foci of infection in the lung or other sites resolve into epithelioid-cell granulomas, which can have caseous and necrotic centres; tubercle bacilli can survive in this material for years, the host's resistance determining whether the infection ultimately resolves without treatment, remains dormant or becomes active.

Foci can leave nodular scars in the apices of one or both lungs ('Simon foci'), calcified scars from the primary infection (the Ghon foci) or calcified hilar lymph nodes. The tuberculin skin test is positive.

Rarely, the primary focus immediately progresses, causing acute illness with pneumonia (sometimes cavitary), pleural effusion and marked mediastinal or hilar lymph node enlargement (which can compress bronchi in children). Small pleural effusions are predominantly lymphocytic, typically contain few organisms, and clear within a few weeks. Primary extrapulmonary TB at any site can sometimes present without any evidence of lung involvement. TB lymphadenopathy is the most common extrapulmonary presentation; meningitis is the most feared complication because of its high mortality in the very young and very old.

## 8.4

*Answer: D*   Pulmonary embolus

Clinical features of pulmonary embolism (PE) are sudden-onset dyspnoea, tachypnoea, chest pain of 'pleuritic' nature (worsened by breathing), cough, haemoptysis, and, in severe cases, cyanosis, tachycardia, hypotension, shock, loss of consciousness and death. Although in most cases there is no clinical evidence of deep venous thrombosis (DVT) in the legs, findings that indicate DVT may aid in the diagnosis.

The most common sources of embolism are proximal leg deep venous thrombosis or pelvic vein thromboses. Any risk factor for DVT also increases the risk that the venous clot will dislodge and migrate to the lung circulation, which happens in up to 15% of all DVTs. The conditions are generally regarded as a continuum called 'venous thromboembolism'.

The development of thrombosis is classically associated with a group of factors known as 'Virchow's triad' (alterations in blood flow, factors in the vessel wall and factors affecting the properties of the blood); more than one risk factor is commonly present:

- **Alterations in blood flow:** immobilisation (after surgery, injury or long-distance air travel), pregnancy (also pro-coagulant), obesity (also pro-coagulant)

- **Factors in the vessel wall** (of limited direct relevance in venous thromboembolism)

- **Factors affecting the properties of the blood** (pro-coagulant state):

  o oestrogen-containing hormonal contraception

  o genetic thrombophilia (factor V Leiden, prothrombin mutation G20210A, protein C deficiency, protein S deficiency, antithrombin deficiency, hyperhomocysteinaemia and plasminogen/fibrinolysis disorders

  o acquired thrombophilia (antiphospholipid syndrome, nephrotic syndrome, paroxysmal nocturnal haemoglobinuria).

## 8.5

*Answer: B*    Alpha$_1$-antitrypsin deficiency

Alpha$_1$-antitrypsin deficiency is congenital lack of a primary lung antiprotease, alpha$_1$-antitrypsin, which leads to increased protease-mediated tissue destruction and emphysema in adults. Hepatic accumulation of abnormal alpha$_1$-antitrypsin can cause liver disease (cirrhosis) in both children and adults. A serum alpha$_1$-antitrypsin level of less than 11 $\mu$mol/l (<80 mg/dl) confirms the diagnosis.

## 8.6

*Answer: A*    Lung abscess

Most lung abscesses develop after aspiration of oral secretions by patients with gingivitis or poor oral hygiene who are unconscious or obtunded from alcohol, illicit drugs, anaesthesia, sedatives or opioids. Older patients and those unable to handle their oral secretions, often because of neurological disease, are also at risk. Lung abscess less commonly complicates necrotising pneumonia that may have developed from haematogenous seeding of the lungs due to septic embolism from intravenous drug use or suppurative thromboembolism.

pulmonary

In contrast to aspiration, these conditions typically cause multiple rather than isolated lung abscesses.

The most common pathogens are anaerobic bacteria, but about a half of all cases involve both anaerobic and aerobic organisms. The most common aerobic pathogens are streptococci. Immunocompromised patients with lung abscess are more likely to have infection with *Nocardia*, mycobacteria or fungi. People from developing countries are at risk of abscess due to *Mycobacterium tuberculosis*, amoebic infection (*Entamoeba histolytica*), paragonimiasis or *Burkholderia pseudomallei*.

Lung abscess is suspected on the basis of the history, physical examination and chest X-ray. In anaerobic infection due to aspiration, the chest X-ray classically shows consolidation, with a single cavity containing an air–fluid level in portions of the lung that are dependent when the patient is recumbent (eg the posterior segment of the upper lobe or the superior segment of the lower lobe). This pattern helps to distinguish anaerobic abscess from other causes of cavitary pulmonary disease, such as diffuse or embolic pulmonary disease, which may cause multiple cavitations, or tuberculosis, which involves the apices. Computed tomography is not required routinely, but can be useful when the X-ray suggests a cavitating lesion or when an underlying pulmonary mass obstructing the drainage of a lung segment is suspected.

## 8.7

*Answer: A*   Asbestosis

Asbestosis, a form of interstitial pulmonary fibrosis, is much more common than malignant disease. Shipbuilders, textile and construction workers, workers who work with asbestos removal, and miners exposed to asbestos fibres are among the many categories of workers at risk of the disease. Second-hand exposure can occur among family members of exposed workers and among those who live close to mines. The pathophysiology is similar to that of other pneumoconioses – alveolar macrophages attempting to engulf inhaled fibres release cytokines and growth factors that stimulate inflammation, collagen deposition and ultimately fibrosis – in addition to the fact that asbestos fibres themselves can also be directly toxic to lung tissue. The risk of disease is generally related to duration and intensity of exposure and the type, length and thickness of the inhaled fibres.

Asbestosis is initially asymptomatic but can cause progressive dyspnoea, non-productive cough and fatigue. The disease progresses in over 10% of patients after exposure ceases. Advanced asbestosis can cause clubbing, dry bibasilar crackles and, in severe cases, symptoms and signs of right ventricular failure (cor pulmonale). The diagnosis is based on the history of exposure and chest X-ray or computed tomography (CT). Chest X-rays show linear reticular or nodular opacities suggestive of fibrosis, usually in the peripheral lower lobes, often accompanied by pleural changes. Honeycombing signifies more advanced disease, which can involve the mid-lung fields. As with silicosis, the severity is graded on the International Labor Organization scale on the basis of size, shape, location and profusion of opacities. In contrast to silicosis, however, asbestosis produces reticular opacities with a lower lobe predominance. Hilar and mediastinal adenopathy are uncharacteristic and suggest a different diagnosis. Chest X-ray is insensitive; high-resolution chest CT (HRCT) is useful when asbestosis is a likely diagnosis. HRCT is also superior to the chest X-ray in identifying the pleural abnormalities. Pulmonary function tests, which might show reduced lung volumes, and the diffusing capacity of the lung for carbon monoxide ($D_{LCO}$) are non-specific but help to characterise changes in lung function over time once the diagnosis has been made. Bronchoalveolar lavage or lung biopsy is indicated only when non-invasive measures fail to provide a conclusive diagnosis; the demonstration of asbestos fibres indicates asbestosis in people with pulmonary fibrosis, although such fibres can occasionally be found in the lungs of exposed people without disease.

## 8.8

*Answer: E*    Squamous cell carcinoma

Squamous cell carcinoma accounts for 25%–30% of all lung cancers. The classic manifestation is a cavitary lesion in a proximal bronchus. Histologically, this tumour is characterised by the presence of keratinisation and/or intercellular bridges. Keratinisation can take the form of squamous pearls or individual cells with markedly eosinophilic (pink), dense cytoplasm. These features are prominent in the well-differentiated tumours.

pulmonary

**8.9**

*Answer: A*    Adult respiratory distress syndrome

Adult respiratory distress syndrome (ARDS) is a diffuse pulmonary parenchymal injury associated with non-cardiogenic pulmonary oedema, which results in severe respiratory distress and hypoxaemic respiratory failure. The pathological hallmark is diffuse alveolar damage, but lung tissue is rarely available for a pathological diagnosis so the diagnosis is therefore made on clinical grounds according to the following criteria, which were laid down by the American-European Consensus Conference:

- Acute onset

- Bilateral infiltrates

- Pulmonary artery wedge pressure less than 19 mmHg (or no clinical signs of congestive heart failure)

- $p(O_2)/Fi(O_2)$ ratio less than 200 (ARDS) or less than 300 (acute lung injury, a milder clinical expression of the injury of ARDS that may or may not progress to ARDS).

Several conditions have been found to precipitate ARDS, though in some cases a predisposing condition cannot be identified. The following is a list of the most common predisposing conditions:

- Infection: pneumonia of any cause (especially viral) and systemic sepsis (especially Gram-negative)

- Shock: any type, particularly septic and traumatic shock

- Aspiration: gastric contents, near drowning, toxic inhalation

- Trauma: pulmonary contusion, fat embolisation, multiple trauma

- Other: systemic inflammatory response syndrome, pancreatitis, post-cardiopulmonary bypass, massive blood transfusion, drug ingestion (eg heroin, methadone, barbiturates, salicylates).

pulmonary

ARDS is thought to develop when pulmonary or systemic inflammation leads to systemic release of cytokines and other pro-inflammatory molecules. The cytokines activate alveolar macrophages and recruit neutrophils to the lungs, which in turn release leukotrienes, oxidants, platelet-activating factor and proteases. These substances damage capillary endothelium and alveolar epithelium, disrupting the barriers between capillaries and air spaces. Oedema fluid, protein, and cellular debris flood the air spaces and interstitium, causing disruption of surfactant, air-space collapse, ventilation–perfusion mismatch, shunting, stiffening of the lungs with decreased compliance and pulmonary hypertension. The injury is distributed heterogeneously but mainly affects dependent lung zones. Histopathologically, diffuse alveolar damage results, with intra-alveolar neutrophils, red blood cells and cellular debris, and denuded epithelial basement membranes with formation of hyaline membranes.

## 8.10

*Answer: A*  Bronchoalveolar carcinoma

Bronchoalveolar carcinoma is a distinct subtype of adenocarcinoma which classically manifests as an interstitial lung disease on chest X-ray. Bronchoalveolar carcinoma arises from type II pneumocytes and grows along alveolar septa. This subtype can manifest as a solitary peripheral nodule, as multifocal disease or as a rapidly progressing pneumonic form. A characteristic finding in people with advanced disease is voluminous watery sputum.

## 8.11

*Answer: C*  Sarcoidosis

Sarcoidosis is characterised by non-caseating granulomas in one or more organs and tissues. The aetiology of sarcoidosis is unknown. Sarcoidosis primarily affects people between the ages of 20 years and 40 years but occasionally affects children and older adults. The lungs and lymphatic system are most often affected, but sarcoidosis can affect any organ. Pulmonary symptoms range from none (limited disease) to exertional dyspnoea and, rarely, respiratory or other organ failure (advanced disease). Diagnosis usually is first suspected because of pulmonary involvement and is confirmed by chest X-ray, biopsy and exclusion of other causes of granulomatous inflammation.

## 8.12

*Answer: D*  Small-cell anaplastic carcinoma

Small cell lung cancers (SCLCs) are considered to be distinct from the other lung cancers, the non-small-cell lung cancers (NSCLCs), because of their clinical and biological characteristics. SCLCs exhibit aggressive behaviour, with rapid growth, early spread to distant sites, exquisite sensitivity to chemotherapy and radiation and frequent association with distinct paraneoplastic syndromes (see table below). Surgery usually plays no role in its management, except in rare situations (<5% of patients) in which it presents at a very early stage as a solitary pulmonary nodule. Even then, adjuvant chemotherapy after surgical resection is recommended, because SCLC should always be considered to be a systemic disease.

In this scenario the patient has features of Cushing syndrome secondary to ectopic ACTH production.

Paraneoplastic syndromes associated with small-cell lung cancers:

| Organ system | Syndrome | Mechanism | Frequency |
|---|---|---|---|
| Endocrine | SIADH | Antidiuretic hormone | 5%–10% |
| | Ectopic secretion of ACTH | Adrenocorticotropic hormone | 5% |
| | Atrial natriuretic factor | | — |
| Neurological | Eaton–Lambert reverse myasthenic syndrome | — | 5%–6% |
| | Subacute cerebellar degeneration | — | — |
| | Subacute sensory neuropathy | — | — |
| | Limbic encephalopathy | Anti-Hu, Anti-Yo antibodies | — |

SIADH, syndrome of inappropriate ADH secretion; ACTH, adrenocorticotrophic hormone.

## 8.13

*Answer: B*    Pulmonary metastases

The lung is the most common site for metastatic neoplasms. Pulmonary metastases occur most frequently with tumours that have rich systemic venous drainage. Examples of such metastases include renal cancers, bone sarcomas, choriocarcinomas, melanomas, testicular teratomas and thyroid carcinomas. Most pulmonary metastases arise from common tumours, such as breast, colorectal, prostate, bronchial, head and neck, and renal cancers.

## 8.14

*Answer: B*    Congestive heart failure

Transudates are ultrafiltrates of plasma in the pleura caused by a small, defined group of underlying conditions:

- Congestive heart failure
- Cirrhosis (hepatic hydrothorax)
- Atelectasis (due to malignancy or pulmonary embolism)
- Hypoalbuminaemia
- Nephrotic syndrome
- Peritoneal dialysis
- Myxoedema
- Constrictive pericarditis.

Laboratory testing helps to distinguish pleural fluid transudates from exudates. However, certain types of exudative pleural effusions might be suspected simply by observing the quality of the fluid obtained during thoracentesis:

- Frankly purulent fluid indicates an empyema.
- A putrid odour suggests an anaerobic empyema.
- A milky, opalescent fluid suggests a chylothorax, resulting most often from lymphatic obstruction

*pulmonary*

423

by malignancy or thoracic duct injury by trauma or surgical procedures.

- Grossly bloody fluid indicates the need for a spun haematocrit test of the sample. A pleural fluid haematocrit level of more than 50% of the peripheral hematocrit level defines a haemothorax, which often requires tube thoracostomy.

The initial diagnostic consideration is distinguishing transudate from exudate. The fluid is considered an exudate if any of the following apply:

- Pleural fluid to serum protein ratio more than 0.5

- Pleural fluid to serum lactate dehydrogenase (LDH) ratio more than 0.6

- Pleural fluid LDH more than two-thirds of the upper limits of normal serum value.

## 8.15

*Answer: B*     Mediastinal malignant lymphoma

'Chylothorax' refers to the presence of lymphatic fluid in the pleural space, secondary to leakage from the thoracic duct or one of its main tributaries. A chylothorax can be non-traumatic or traumatic, or can be a pseudochylothorax.

### Non-traumatic chylothorax:

- Malignant causes account for more than 50% of chylothorax diagnoses and are separated into lymphomatous and non-lymphomatous. Lymphoma is the most common cause, representing about 60% of all cases, with non-Hodgkin's lymphoma more likely than Hodgkin's lymphoma to cause a chylothorax. In contrast, non-lymphomatous causes are rare.

- Non-malignant causes are separated into idiopathic, congenital and miscellaneous. Clinicians must rule out all possible malignant causes before designating the chylothorax as idiopathic.

- Congenital chylothorax is the leading cause of pleural effusion in neonates.

- Miscellaneous causes include cirrhosis, tuberculosis, sarcoidosis, amyloidosis and filariasis.

**Traumatic chylothorax:**

- Trauma is the second leading cause of chylothorax (25%). Iatrogenic injury to the thoracic duct has been reported with most thoracic procedures. In particular, cardiothoracic surgery has been associated with 69%–85% of cases of chylothorax in children.

- Non-surgical traumatic injury is a rare cause, and usually secondary to penetrating trauma.

**Pseudochylothorax:**

- Chylothorax must be distinguished from pseudochylothorax, or cholesterol pleurisy, which results from accumulation of cholesterol crystals in a chronic existing effusion.

- The most common cause of pseudochylothorax is chronic rheumatoid pleurisy, followed by tuberculosis and poorly treated empyema.

### 8.16

*Answer: A*  Sputum cytology

Sputum cytology consists of the microscopic examination of a sample of sputum in order to determine whether abnormal cells are present. Sputum has some normal lung cells in it. Sputum cytology can be done as the first diagnostic test to help detect lung cancer and certain non-cancerous lung conditions. A sputum sample can be collected by coughing up mucus, by breathing in a saline mist and then coughing, or during bronchoscopy.

**8.17**

*Answer: C   Nocardia asteroides*

Several *Nocardia* species (family Actinomycetaceae) cause human disease. The most common human pathogen is *N. asteroides*, which usually causes pulmonary and disseminated infection. *N. brasiliensis* most commonly causes skin infection, particularly in tropical climates. Infection is via inhalation or by direct inoculation of the skin. Nocardiosis occurs worldwide in all age groups, but the incidence is greater among older adults, especially men. Person-to-person spread is rare. Lymphoreticular malignancies, organ transplantation, high-dose corticosteroid or other immunosuppressive therapy and underlying pulmonary disease are predisposing factors, but about 50% of patients have no pre-existing disease. Nocardiosis is also an opportunistic infection in patients with advanced human immunodeficiency virus (HIV) infection.

**8.18**

*Answer: E   Pneumothorax*

The risk of pneumothorax is 20%–40%, but it is rarely significant enough to require insertion of a chest tube. Although it is impossible to predict which patients will experience this complication, pneumothorax is more frequent and more serious in patients with severe emphysema and in patients in whom the biopsy was difficult to perform.

**8.19**

*Answer: A   Bronchial carcinoid*

Bronchial carcinoids are rare, slow-growing neuroendocrine tumours arising from bronchial mucosa that affect patients in their forties to sixties. Half the patients with these tumours are asymptomatic, and half present with symptoms of airway obstruction, including dyspnoea, wheezing and cough, which often leads to a misdiagnosis of asthma. Recurrent pneumonia, haemoptysis and chest pain are also common. Paraneoplastic syndromes, including Cushing's syndrome due to ectopic adrenocorticotrophic hormone (ACTH), acromegaly due to ectopic growth hormone-releasing factor and Zollinger–Ellison syndrome due to ectopic gastrin production, are more common than carcinoid syndrome, which occurs in fewer than 3% of patients with the tumour. A left-sided heart murmur (mitral stenosis or regurgitation) occurs rarely, due to serotonin-induced valvular damage (in contrast to the right-sided valvular lesions associated with gastrointestinal carcinoids). Diagnosis is based on bronchoscopic biopsy, but evaluation often initially involves computed tomography of the chest, which reveals tumour calcifications in up to a third of patients. Indium[111]-labelled octreotide scans are useful for determining regional and metastatic spread. Increased urinary serotonin and 5-hydroxyindoleacetic acid levels support the diagnosis but are not commonly present.

## 8.20

*Answer: E*    Pulmonary hamartoma

The size of the lesion and the fact that the patient is healthy, asymptomatic and a non-smoker all point towards a benign lung lesion. Hamartomas are the third most common cause of a solitary pulmonary nodule and the most common benign tumour of the lung, accounting for 75% of all benign lung tumours. They are composed of tissues that are normally present in the lung, including fat, epithelial tissue, fibrous tissue and cartilage, but they exhibit disorganised growth. Although most hamartomas are asymptomatic and although they have no malignant potential, bronchogenic carcinoma is an important differential diagnosis, and an accurate imaging interpretation and diagnosis is important. Peripheral tumours are usually simply observed after the definitive diagnosis, while central tumours might be excised. The prognosis is excellent.

pulmonary

# SECTION 9:
# RENAL PATHOLOGY — ANSWERS

## 9.1

*Answer: E*    Transitional cell carcinoma of renal pelvis

The lack of findings in the bladder but the presence of atypical cells suggests that the lesion is located higher up, possibly in the renal pelvis or ureter. Transitional cell carcinoma (TCC) of the renal pelvis accounts for about 7% of all kidney tumours; TCC of the ureters accounts for about 4% of upper tract tumours. Risk factors are the same as those for bladder cancer. Also, inhabitants of the Balkans with endemic familial nephropathy are inexplicably predisposed to develop upper tract TCC.

Most patients present with haematuria; dysuria and frequency can occur if the bladder is also involved. Colicky pain can accompany obstruction. Uncommonly, hydronephrosis results from a renal pelvic tumour. Evaluation typically includes ultrasound or computed tomography with contrast. Diagnosis must be confirmed by cytological or histological analysis. Ureteroscopy, nephroscopy or both are done when biopsy of the upper tract is needed or when urine cytology is positive but no source of the malignant cells is obvious. Staging for obviously superficial tumours is probably unnecessary. For other tumours, abdominal and pelvic computed tomography and chest X-ray are done to determine tumour extent and to check for metastases. The standard TNM staging system is used.

## 9.2

*Answer: D*    Multiple myeloma

The patient has Bence Jones protein. The dipstick is most sensitive for albumin, not globulins such as seen in patients with multiple myeloma. Multiple myeloma is a malignancy of plasma cells that produce monoclonal immunoglobulin and invade and destroy adjacent bone tissue. Common manifestations include bone pain, renal insufficiency, hypercalcaemia, anaemia and recurrent infections. Diagnosis requires demonstration of M-protein (sometimes present in urine and not serum) and either lytic bone lesions, light-chain proteinuria or excessive marrow plasma cells. A bone marrow biopsy is usually needed.

The incidence of multiple myeloma is 2–4 per 100,000 population, the male to female ratio is 1.6 to 1, and most patients are aged over 40 years. The prevalence in blacks is twice that in whites. The aetiology is unknown, although chromosomal and genetic factors, radiation, and chemicals have been suggested.

Plasma cell tumours (plasmacytomas) produce IgG in about 55% of myeloma patients and IgA in about 20%; of these patients, 40% also have Bence Jones proteinuria, which is free monoclonal kappa or lamda light chains in the urine. In 15%–20% of patients, plasma cells secrete only Bence Jones protein. These patients tend to have a higher incidence of lytic bone lesions, hypercalcaemia, renal failure and amyloidosis than do other myeloma patients. IgD myeloma accounts for about 1% of cases.

## 9.3

*Answer: D*    Squamous epithelium

Squamous epithelium is normally not seen above the outer urethra. All the other structures are present.

## 9.4

*Answer: D*    Proteinuria of >3 g/24 hours

Nephrotic syndrome is defined by the urinary excretion of over 3 g of protein per day due to glomerular disease. Nephrotic syndrome occurs at any age but is more prevalent in children, mostly between the ages of 18 months and 4 years. At younger ages, boys are affected more often than girls, but both are affected equally at older ages. Causes differ by age. The most common primary causes are minimal-change disease, focal segmental glomerulosclerosis and membranous nephropathy. Secondary causes account for fewer than 10% of childhood cases but over 50% of adult cases, most commonly diabetic nephropathy and pre-eclampsia. Amyloidosis is an under-recognised cause in 4% of cases.

Proteinuria occurs because of changes to capillary endothelial cells, the glomerular basement membrane or podocytes, which normally filter serum protein selectively by size and charge. The mechanism of damage to these structures is unknown in primary glomerular disease, but evidence suggests that T cells up-regulate a circulating permeability factor or down-regulate an inhibitor of permeability factor in response to unidentified immunogens and cytokines. The result is urinary loss of macromolecular proteins, primarily albumin but also opsonins, immunoglobulins, erythropoietin, transferrin, hormone-binding proteins and antithrombin III in conditions that cause non-selective proteinuria. As a result, patients with nephrotic syndrome develop peripheral oedema, ascites and effusions, and are at increased risk of infection (especially cellulitis and, in 2%–6%, spontaneous bacterial peritonitis), anaemia, abnormal thyroid function and thromboembolism (especially renal vein thrombosis and pulmonary embolism in up to 5% of children and 40% of adults). Thromboembolism can develop not only because of urinary loss of antithrombin III but also because of increased hepatic synthesis of clotting factors, platelet abnormalities and hyperviscosity from hypovolaemia.

Chronic complications of nephrotic syndrome include malnutrition in children, coronary artery disease in adults, chronic renal failure and bone disease. Malnutrition can mimic kwashiorkor, with brittle hair and nails, alopecia and stunted growth. Coronary artery disease develops because nephrotic syndrome causes hyperlipidaemia, hypertension and hypercoagulability. Bone disease develops because of vitamin D deficiency and corticosteroid use. Other chronic complications include hypothyroidism, from loss of thyroid-binding globulin, and proximal tubular dysfunction, which causes glucosuria, aminoaciduria, potassium depletion, phosphaturia and renal tubular acidosis.

Renal failure is rarely a presenting finding but can occur after a prolonged illness. However, patients with nephrotic syndrome due to a secondary cause frequently have renal insufficiency at onset or soon thereafter.

### 9.5

*Answer: B*   Concentration

Renal concentrating ability is reflected by the specific gravity. In humans, normal specific gravity values range from 1.002 g/ml to 1.028 g/ml. Increased specific gravity (ie increased concentration of solutes in the urine) is associated with dehydration, diarrhoea, vomiting, excessive sweating, glucosuria and the syndrome of inappropriate antidiuretic hormone secretion (SIADH). Decreased specific gravity (ie decreased concentration of solutes in urine) is associated with renal failure, pyelonephritis, diabetes insipidus, acute tubular necrosis, interstitial nephritis and excessive fluid intake.

### 9.6

*Answer: E*   A 45-year-old woman with scleroderma

The diffuse form of scleroderma can be associated with hyperplastic arteriolosclerosis and malignant hypertension. Post-streptococcal glomerulonephritis produces glomerular hypercellularity. End-stage kidneys all look alike: thickened arteries, globally sclerotic glomeruli and interstitial scarring with chronic inflammation. The child is most likely to have minimal-change disease and the kidney will be grossly normal, will be normal on light microscopy, and will show only fusion of foot processes on electron microscopy. An acute myocardial infarction could cause decreased cardiac output with decreased renal perfusion and ischaemia, leading to acute tubular necrosis.

### 9.7

*Answer: E*   Wilms' tumour

Wilms' tumour, an embryonal cancer of the kidney composed of blastemal, stromal and epithelial elements, usually presents in children under the age of 5 years but occasionally presents in older children and rarely in adults. Wilms' tumour accounts for about 6% of cancers in children aged under 15 years. Bilateral synchronous tumours occur in about 4% of cases, with bilateral disease more common in very young children, especially in girls. A chromosomal deletion of *WT1*, the Wilms' tumour suppressor gene, on chromosome 11 has been identified in some cases. Other associated genetic abnormalities include deletion of *WT2* (another Wilms' tumour suppressor gene), deletion of chromosome 16 and duplication of chromosome 12.

About 10% of cases manifest other congenital abnormalities, especially genitourinary abnormalities, but also commonly hemihypertrophy (asymmetry of the body). 'WAGR syndrome' is the combination of **W**ilms' tumour (with the *WT1* deletion), **a**niridia, **g**enitourinary malformations (eg renal hypoplasia, cystic disease, hypospadias, cryptorchidism) and mental **r**etardation.

The most common presentation is a painless, palpable abdominal mass. Less common findings include abdominal pain, haematuria, fever, anorexia, nausea and vomiting. Haematuria (occurring in 15%–20%) indicates invasion of the collecting system. Hypertension can occur if compression of the renal pedicle or renal parenchyma causes ischaemia.

## 9.8

*Answer: E*   Minimal-change disease

Minimal-change disease (MCD) is the most common cause of nephrotic syndrome in children aged 4–8 years (80%–90% of cases of childhood nephrotic syndrome), but it also occurs in adults (20% of cases of adult nephrotic syndrome). The cause is almost always unknown, although rarely it occurs secondary to drug use (especially non-steroidal anti-inflammatory drugs) and haematological malignancies (especially Hodgkin's lymphoma).

MCD causes nephrotic syndrome without hypertension or azotaemia; microscopic haematuria occurs in about 20% of patients. Azotaemia can occur in non-idiopathic cases and in patients aged over 60 years. Albumin is lost in the urine of patients with MCD to a greater extent than larger serum proteins, probably because MCD causes changes in the charge barrier rather than the size barrier in the glomerular capillary wall.

renal

Diagnosis in children is most often clinical, but biopsy is required in atypical cases and in adults. Electron microscopy demonstrates oedema with diffuse swelling (effacement) of foot processes of the epithelial podocytes. Although effacement is not observed in the absence of proteinuria, heavy proteinuria can occur with normal foot processes.

**9.9**

*Answer: C*   Acute tubular necrosis

The ethylene glycol causes toxic injury to renal tubules and this is called 'acute tubular necrosis' (ATN). ATN is characterised by acute tubular cell injury and dysfunction and causes renal insufficiency or failure. The most common causes of ATN are hypotension and nephrotoxins. Common agents include aminoglycoside antibiotics, amphotericin, cisplatin and radiocontrast (particularly at volume greater than 100 ml). Major surgery and advanced hepatobiliary disease, poor perfusion states and advanced age all increase the risk of aminoglycoside toxicity. Less common causes include haem pigments (myoglobin and haemoglobin), poisons (ethylene glycol) and herbal and folk remedies (eg ingestion of fish gallbladder in Southeast Asia). Certain drug combinations (eg aminoglycosides with amphotericin B) can be especially nephrotoxic. Toxic exposures cause patchy, segmental, tubular luminal occlusion with casts and cellular debris or segmental tubular necrosis. ATN is more likely to develop in those with a baseline creatinine clearance <47 ml/ minute, diabetes mellitus and pre-existing hypovolaemia or poor renal perfusion.

**9.10**

*Answer: E*   Systemic lupus erythematosus and acute renal failure

Therapy may depend on determination of the severity and nature of the renal disease with systemic lupus erythematosus (SLE) and so a percutaneous needle biopsy is appropriate and helpful in this situation. You should treat the acute infection. A urinalysis with microscopic examination and urine culture is indicated if you suspect a urinary tract infection. Clinical examination with palpation of the prostate can help confirm a diagnosis of prostatic hyperplasia, and an ultrasound of the prostate would also be useful. Hydronephrosis can be assessed with an intravenous pyelogram. Ultrasonography can help determine whether the kidneys are cystic. A family history also helps. Renal cysts should not be biopsied. They are incidental findings

## 9.11

*Answer: D*    Transitional cell carcinoma

Transitional cell carcinomas can occur anywhere in the urothelium and multicentricity and recurrence are common. There is only one prostate gland. Adenocarcinomas in the prostate can spread within the prostate, and most arise in the posterior lobe. Renal cell carcinomas are sometimes bilateral or multicentric, but not often. Generally, penile carcinomas are solitary (but infiltrative) mass lesions. Wilms' tumour usually presents as a solitary mass, though about 10% are bilateral or multicentric at the time of diagnosis (see also *Answer* to **9.1**).

## 9.12

*Answer: A*    Glomerular crescents

Rapidly progressive glomerulonephritis manifests pathologically as extensive glomerular crescent formation. If untreated this progresses to end-stage renal disease over weeks to months. It is relatively uncommon, affecting 10%–15% of patients with glomerulonephritis, and occurs predominantly in patients aged 20–50 years. The types and causes are classified on the basis of the immunofluorescence microscopy findings.

The presentation is usually insidious, with weakness, fatigue, fever, nausea and vomiting, anorexia, arthralgia and abdominal pain. About 50% of patients have oedema and a history of an acute influenza-like illness within 4 weeks of the onset of renal failure, usually followed by severe oliguria. Nephrotic syndrome is present in 10%–30%. Hypertension is uncommon and rarely severe. Patients with anti-glomerular basement membrane antibody disease can

renal

have pulmonary haemorrhage, which can present with haemoptysis or might be detectable only by the presence of diffuse alveolar infiltrates on chest X-ray.

### 9.13

*Answer: B*    Membranous glomerulonephritis

Membranous glomerulonephritis (MGN), also known as 'membranous nephropathy', is a slowly progressive disease of the kidney that mainly affects people between ages of 30 years and 50 years. In 85% of cases the condition is classified as primary or idiopathic. The remaining 15% of cases are secondary to:

- Autoimmune conditions (eg systemic lupus erythematosus)
- Infections (eg syphilis, malaria, hepatitis B)
- Drugs (eg captopril, non-steroidal anti-inflammatory drugs)
- Inorganic salts
- Malignant tumours (particularly carcinoma of the lung and colon, and melanoma).

MGN is caused by circulating immune complex. Current research indicates that the majority of the immune complexes are formed via binding of antibodies to antigens in situ to the glomerular basement membrane. The antigens can be endogenous to the basement membrane, or 'planted' from systemic circulation.

The immune complex serves as an activator that triggers a response from the C5b–C9 complements, which form a membrane attack complex (MAC) on the glomerular epithelial cells. This in turn stimulates the release of proteases and oxidants by the mesangial and epithelial cells, damaging the capillary walls and causing them to become 'leaky'. In addition, the epithelial cells also seem to secrete an unknown mediator that reduces nephrin synthesis and distribution.

## 9.14

*Answer: A*    Acute tubular necrosis

Ischaemia, typically in hypotensive hospitalised patients, is the most frequent antecedent to acute tubular necrosis (see also *Answer* to **9.9**).

## 9.15

*Answer: E*    White blood cell casts

The white blood cell casts are most characteristic of an acute tubulointerstitial nephritis (acute pyelonephritis). Tubulointerstitial nephritis is a primary injury to renal tubules and interstitium that results in decreased renal function. The acute form is most often due to allergic drug reactions or to infections.

## 9.16

*Answer: E*    Ureteric calculus

The features in this case are suggestive of a ureteric calculus. During passage through the ureter a calculus irritates the ureter and can become lodged, obstructing urine flow and causing hydroureter and sometimes hydronephrosis. Common sites for stones to become stuck include the ureteropelvic junction, the distal ureter (at the level of the iliac vessels) and the ureterovesical junction. Typically, a calculus must have a diameter of >5 mm to become lodged; calculi with a diameter of ≤5 mm are likely to pass spontaneously.

Even partial obstruction causes decreased glomerular filtration, which can persist briefly after the calculus has passed. With hydronephrosis and elevated glomerular pressure, renal blood flow declines, which further worsens renal function. Generally, however, permanent renal dysfunction occurs only after about 28 days of complete obstruction. Secondary infection can occur with long-standing obstruction.

renal

**9.17**

*Answer: B*     Bladder exstrophy

In bladder exstrophy the bladder is open suprapubically, and urine drips from the opening rather than through the urethra. The bladder mucosa is continuous with the abdominal skin and the pubic bones are separated. Despite the seriousness of the deformity, normal renal function is usually maintained. The bladder can usually be reconstructed and returned to the pelvis, although vesicoureteral reflux invariably occurs. Continent urinary diversion can be used to treat a bladder reservoir that fails to expand sufficiently or has sphincter insufficiency. Reconstruction of the genitals is required.

**9.18**

*Answer: A*     Chlamydia

Sexually transmitted urethritis, cervicitis, proctitis and pharyngitis infections that are not due to gonorrhoea are caused predominantly by *Chlamydia* and infrequently by *Mycoplasma* or *Ureaplasma* organisms. Because the organisms that cause most cases of non-gonococcal, sexually transmitted cervicitis in women and most cases of urethritis, proctitis and pharyngitis in both sexes have been identified, the previously used terms 'non-specific urethritis' and 'non-gonococcal urethritis' are imprecise. Causal agents include *Chlamydia trachomatis* (responsible for about 50% of such cases of urethritis and most such cases of mucopurulent cervicitis), *Mycoplasma genitalium*, *Ureaplasma urealyticum*, and *Trichomonas vaginalis*.

**9.19**

*Answer: C*     Nephrotic syndrome

Oval fat bodies appear with pronounced proteinuria and lipiduria, as seen in nephrotic syndrome.

## 9.20

*Answer: A*    Myoglobinuria

Myoglobinuria is the presence of myoglobin in the urine, usually associated with rhabdomyolysis or muscle destruction. Trauma, including electrical injuries and burns, vascular problems, venoms and certain drugs can destroy or damage the muscle, releasing myoglobin into the circulation and thus to the kidneys. Under ideal situations myoglobin will be filtered and excreted with the urine, but if too much myoglobin is released into the circulation or where there are renal problems, it can occlude the renal filtration system, leading to acute tubular necrosis and acute renal insufficiency.

renal

# SECTION 10:
# GASTROINTESTINAL AND
# HEPATOBILIARY PATHOLOGY —
# ANSWERS

## 10.1

*Answer: D*    Normal architecture

Hepatitis A virus is a single-stranded RNA picornavirus. It is the most common cause of acute viral hepatitis and is particularly common in children and young adults. In some countries more than 75% of adults have been exposed. Hepatitis A virus spreads primarily by faecal–oral contact and so can occur in areas of poor hygiene. Water-borne and food-borne epidemics occur, especially in underdeveloped countries. Eating contaminated raw shellfish is sometimes responsible. Sporadic cases are also common, usually as a result of person-to-person contact. Faecal shedding of the virus occurs before symptoms develop and usually ceases a few days after symptoms begin. This means that infectivity often has already ceased when the hepatitis becomes clinically evident. Hepatitis A virus has no known chronic carrier state and does not lead to chronic hepatitis or cirrhosis. If a liver biopsy is performed after the patient has completely recovered from this infection it will therefore show normal architecture.

## 10.2

*Answer: A*    Alcoholic hepatitis

Mallory bodies (also known as 'alcoholic hyaline' or 'Mallory's hyaline') are pathological inclusions found in the cytoplasm of liver cells. They are most commonly found in the livers of people suffering from alcoholic hepatitis. They are highly eosinophilic and appear pink on haematoxylin and eosin staining. The bodies themselves are made up of intermediate keratin filament proteins that have been ubiquinated, or bound by other proteins such as heat shock proteins or p62. Mallory bodies are also seen in Wilson's disease.

## 10.3

*Answer: B*    Crohn's disease

Crohn's disease is a chronic transmural inflammatory disease that usually affects the distal ileum and colon but which can occur in any part of the gastrointestinal tract. The most common initial presentation is chronic diarrhoea with abdominal pain, fever, anorexia and weight loss. The abdomen is tender, and a mass or fullness might be palpable. Gross rectal bleeding is unusual except in isolated colonic disease, which can manifest similarly to ulcerative colitis. Some patients present with an acute abdomen that simulates acute appendicitis or intestinal obstruction. About 33% of patients have perianal disease (especially fissures and fistulas), which is sometimes the most prominent or even the initial complaint. In children, extraintestinal manifestations frequently predominate over gastrointestinal symptoms: arthritis, pyrexia of unknown origin, anaemia or growth retardation can be the presenting symptoms, whereas abdominal pain or diarrhoea might be absent.

Crohn's disease begins with crypt inflammation and abscesses, which progress to tiny focal aphthoid ulcers. These mucosal lesions can develop into deep longitudinal and transverse ulcers with intervening mucosal oedema, creating a characteristic cobblestoned appearance in the bowel. Transmural spread of inflammation leads to lymphoedema and thickening of the bowel wall and mesentery. Mesenteric fat typically extends onto the serosal surface of the bowel. Mesenteric lymph nodes often enlarge. Extensive inflammation can result in hypertrophy of the muscularis mucosae, fibrosis and stricture formation, which can lead to bowel obstruction. Abscesses are common, and fistulas often penetrate into adjoining structures, including other loops of bowel, the bladder or psoas muscle. Fistulas can even extend to the skin of the anterior abdomen or flanks. Independently of intra-abdominal disease activity, perianal fistulas and abscesses occur in 25%–33% of cases; these complications are frequently the most troublesome aspects of Crohn's disease.

Non-caseating granulomas can occur in lymph nodes, the peritoneum, the liver and in all layers of the bowel wall. Although pathognomonic when present, granulomas are not detected in about half of patients with Crohn's disease. The presence of granulomas does not seem to be related to the clinical course.

Segments of diseased bowel are sharply demarcated from adjacent normal bowel ('skip areas'). In about 35% of patients with Crohn's disease only the ileum is involved (ileitis); in around 45% the ileum and colon are involved (ileocolitis), with a predilection for the right side of the colon; and in about 20% only the colon is involved (granulomatous colitis), in most cases sparing the rectum (unlike ulcerative colitis). Occasionally, the entire small bowel is involved (jejunoileitis). The stomach, duodenum and oesophagus are rarely affected clinically, although microscopic evidence of disease is often detectable in the gastric antrum, especially in younger patients. In the absence of surgical intervention, the disease almost never extends into areas of small bowel that are not involved at first diagnosis.

There is an increased risk of cancer in affected small-bowel segments. Patients with colonic involvement have a long-term risk of colorectal cancer equal to that of patients with ulcerative colitis, given the same extent and duration of disease.

## 10.4

*Answer: A   AFP*

Alpha-fetoprotein (AFP), a glycoprotein normally synthesised by the yolk sac in the embryo and then the fetal liver, is elevated in the newborn and therefore also in the pregnant woman. AFP decreases rapidly during the first year of life, reaching adult values (normally <20 ng/ml) by the age of 1 year. Marked elevations (>500 ng/ml) in a high-risk patient (for example a patient with a liver mass detected on ultrasound) is diagnostic of primary hepatocellular carcinoma, although not all hepatocellular carcinomas produce AFP. Because small tumours can have low levels of AFP, rising values suggest the presence of hepatocellular carcinoma. The degree of AFP elevation, however, is not prognostic. In populations in which chronic hepatitis B infection and hepatocellular carcinoma are common (eg

gastrointestinal

sub-Saharan Africans, ethnic Chinese), AFP can reach levels as high as 100,000 ng/ml, whereas regions with lower frequencies of the tumour have more modest levels (about 3000 ng/ml).

A few other conditions (eg embryonic teratocarcinomas, hepatoblastomas, some hepatic metastases from gastrointestinal tract cancers, some cholangiocarcinomas) cause levels to rise to 500 ng/ml or above. In fulminant hepatitis, AFP can occasionally rise to 500 ng/ml; lesser elevations occur in acute and chronic hepatitis. These levels probably reflect liver regeneration. The sensitivity and specificity of AFP therefore vary according to population, but values of ≥20 ng/mL have a sensitivity range of 39%–64% and a specificity range of 76%–91%. Because values of ≤500 ng/ml are non-specific, 500 ng/ml has been suggested as the diagnostic cut-off level.

## 10.5

*Answer: D* Leucocytosis

The clinical features in this case are typical of acute appendicitis. Appendicitis is thought to result from obstruction of the appendiceal lumen, typically by lymphoid hyperplasia, but occasionally by a faecolith, foreign body or even worms. The obstruction leads to distension, bacterial overgrowth, ischaemia and inflammation. If untreated, necrosis, gangrene and perforation occur. If the perforation is contained by the omentum, an appendiceal abscess results.

Over 5% of the population develop appendicitis at some point. It is most common in the teens and twenties but can occur at any age. The classic symptoms of acute appendicitis are epigastric or periumbilical pain, followed by brief nausea, vomiting and anorexia; after a few hours the pain shifts to the right lower quadrant. Pain increases with cough and movement. The classic signs are right lower quadrant direct and rebound tenderness located at McBurney's point (the junction of the middle and outer thirds of the line joining the umbilicus to the anterior superior spine). Additional signs are pain felt in the right lower quadrant with palpation of the left lower quadrant (Rovsing's sign), an increase in pain on passive extension of the right hip joint (this stretches the iliopsoas muscle and the sign is known as the 'psoas sign') and pain on passive internal rotation of the flexed thigh (obturator sign). Low-grade fever (rectal temperature 37.7 °C to 38.3 °C) is common.

Unfortunately, these classic findings appear in fewer than 50% of patients. Many variations in symptoms and signs occur. Pain may not be localised, particularly in infants and children. Tenderness can be diffuse or, in rare instances, absent. Bowel movements are usually less frequent or absent; if diarrhoea is a sign, a retrocaecal appendix should be suspected. Red blood cells or white blood cells might be found in the urine. Atypical symptoms are common in elderly patients and in pregnant women; in particular, pain is less severe and local tenderness is less marked.

When classic signs and symptoms are present, the diagnosis is clinical. In such patients, delaying laparotomy in order to perform imaging tests only increases the likelihood of perforation and subsequent complications. In patients with atypical or equivocal findings, imaging studies should be performed without delay. Contrast-enhanced computed tomography is reasonably accurate for diagnosing appendicitis and can also reveal other causes of an acute abdomen. Graded compression ultrasound can usually be obtained more quickly than computed tomography but is occasionally limited by the presence of bowel gas and is less useful for recognising non-appendiceal causes of pain. The use of these studies has reduced the rate of negative laparotomy.

Laparoscopy can be used for diagnosis; it can be especially helpful in women with lower abdominal pain of unclear aetiology. Laboratory studies typically show leucocytosis ($12–15 \times 10^9/l$), but this finding is highly variable; a normal white blood cell count should not be used to exclude appendicitis.

## 10.6

*Answer: B*   Hyperplastic polyp

Non-adenomatous (non-neoplastic) colonic polyps include hyperplastic polyps, hamartomas, juvenile polyps, pseudopolyps, lipomas, leiomyomas and other rarer tumours. Peutz–Jeghers syndrome is an autosomal dominant disease with multiple hamartomatous polyps in the stomach, small bowel and colon. Symptoms include melanotic pigmentation of the skin and mucous

gastrointestinal

membranes, especially of the lips and gums. Juvenile polyps occur in children, typically outgrow their blood supply and auto-amputate some time during or after puberty. Treatment is required only for uncontrollable bleeding or intussusception. Inflammatory polyps and pseudopolyps occur in chronic ulcerative colitis and in Crohn's disease of the colon. Multiple juvenile polyps (but not sporadic ones) carry an increased cancer risk. The exact number of polyps required to increase the risk is not known.

## 10.7

*Answer: D*  Hirschsprung's disease

Hirschsprung's disease is caused by congenital absence of Meissner's and Auerbach's autonomic plexus in the intestinal wall. It is usually limited to the distal colon but can involve the entire colon or even the entire large and small bowel. Peristalsis in the involved segment is absent or abnormal, resulting in continuous smooth-muscle spasm and partial or complete obstruction, with accumulation of intestinal contents and massive dilatation of the more proximal, normally innervated intestine. 'Skip lesions' almost never occur.

Patients most commonly present early in life: 15% in the first month, 60% by the age of 1 year, and 85% by the age of 4 years. The infant presents with obstipation, abdominal distension and finally vomiting, as in other forms of distal bowel obstruction. Occasionally, infants with ultra-short segment aganglionosis have only mild or intermittent constipation, often with intervening bouts of mild diarrhoea, resulting in a delay in making the diagnosis. In older infants, symptoms and signs can include anorexia, lack of a physiological urge to defecate and, on examination, an empty rectum with stool palpable higher up in the colon. The child might also fail to thrive. A diagnosis should be made as soon as possible. The longer the disease goes untreated, the greater the chance of developing Hirschsprung's enterocolitis (toxic megacolon), which can be fulminant and fatal. Most cases can be diagnosed in early infancy.

The initial approach is typically with a barium enema or sometimes a rectal suction biopsy. Barium enema can show a transition in diameter between the dilated, normally innervated colon proximal to the narrowed distal segment (which lacks normal innervation). Barium enema should be done without prior preparation, which can dilate the abnormal segment, rendering the test non-diagnostic. Because characteristic findings might not be present in the neonatal period, a 24-hour post-evacuation film should be obtained: if the colon is still filled with barium, Hirschsprung's disease is likely. A rectal suction biopsy can reveal the absence of ganglion cells. Acetylcholinesterase staining can be performed to highlight the enlarged nerve trunks. Some centres also have the facility to perform rectal manometrics, which can reveal abnormal innervation. Definitive diagnosis requires a full-thickness biopsy of the rectum.

## 10.8

*Answer: B*    Haemolysis

Hyperbilirubinaemia results from increased bilirubin production, decreased liver uptake or conjugation, or decreased biliary excretion. Total bilirubin normally is mostly unconjugated, with values of <1.2 mg/dl (<20 µmol/l). Fractionation can measure the proportion of bilirubin that is conjugated (or direct, ie measured directly). Fractionation is required only in neonatal jaundice or if the bilirubin is elevated, but the other liver test results are normal, suggesting that hepatobiliary disease is not the cause.

Unconjugated hyperbilirubinaemia (indirect bilirubin fraction >85%) reflects increased bilirubin production (for example when haemolysis is the case, as in this scenario) or defective liver uptake or conjugation (eg in Gilbert syndrome). Such increases in unconjugated bilirubin are generally less than five-fold (<6 mg/dl or <100 µmol/l) unless there is concurrent liver disease.

## 10.9

*Answer: B*    Hepatocellular carcinoma

Hepatocellular carcinoma (hepatoma) usually occurs in patients with cirrhosis and is common in areas where infection with hepatitis B and hepatitis C viruses is prevalent. Symptoms and signs are usually non-specific. The diagnosis is based on alpha-fetoprotein (AFP) levels,

gastrointestinal

imaging tests, and sometimes liver biopsy. Screening with periodic AFP measurement and ultrasound is sometimes recommended for high-risk patients. The prognosis is grim, but small localised tumours can sometimes be cured by surgical resection or liver transplantation (see also *Answer* to **10.4**).

## 10.10

*Answer: D*   Pseudopolyps

The presence of sclerosing cholangitis (an extraintestinal manifestation) along with the bloody diarrhoea in this scenario is indicative of ulcerative colitis, which affects the mucosa and submucosa of the rectum and colon, with a sharp border between normal and affected tissue. Only in severe disease is the muscularis layer involved. In early cases, the mucous membrane is erythematous, finely granular and friable, with loss of the normal vascular pattern and often with scattered haemorrhagic areas. Large mucosal ulcers with copious purulent exudate are characteristic of severe disease. Islands of relatively normal or hyperplastic inflammatory mucosa (pseudopolyps) project above areas of ulcerated mucosa. Fistulas and abscesses do not occur.

## 10.11

*Answer: C*   Extension to the serosa

Extension of the cancer to the serosa suggests a poor prognosis.

## 10.12

*Answer: A*   Aflatoxin

Aflatoxins are naturally occurring mycotoxins that are produced by many species of the *Aspergillus* fungus, most notably *A. flavus* and *A. parasiticus*. Aflatoxins are toxic and carcinogenic. After entering the body, aflatoxins are metabolised by the liver to a reactive intermediate, aflatoxin $M_1$, an epoxide. Aflatoxin-producing *Aspergillus* organisms are common and widespread in nature. They can colonise and contaminate grain before harvest or during storage. Host crops are particularly susceptible to infection by *Aspergillus* after prolonged exposure to a high-humidity environment or after damage resulting from stressful conditions such as drought. The native habitat of *Aspergillus* is soil, decaying vegetation, hay and grains undergoing microbiological deterioration, and it invades all types of organic substrates, whenever conditions are favourable for its growth. Favourable conditions include high moisture content (at least 7%) and high temperature.

High-level aflatoxin exposure causes acute necrosis, cirrhosis and carcinoma of the liver. There can be haemorrhage, acute liver damage, oedema, and alteration in digestion and in absorption and/ or metabolism of nutrients. No animal species is immune to the acute toxic effects of aflatoxins, including humans. However, humans have an extraordinarily high tolerance for aflatoxin exposure and rarely succumb to acute aflatoxicosis. Chronic, subclinical exposure does not lead to symptoms that are as dramatic as the symptoms of acute aflatoxicosis. Children, however, are particularly affected by aflatoxin exposure, which leads to stunted growth and delayed development. Chronic exposure also carries a high risk of developing liver cancer, as the metabolite aflatoxin $M_1$ can intercalate into DNA and alkylate the bases through its epoxide moiety.

## 10.13

*Answer: E*   Pancreatic carcinoma

Increased levels of alkaline phosphatase, a hepatocyte enzyme, suggest cholestasis. However, alkaline phosphatase consists of several isoenzymes and originates in various tissues, particularly in bone. Alkaline phosphatase levels increase four-fold or higher 1–2 days after the onset of biliary obstruction, regardless of the site of the obstruction. Levels can remain elevated for several days after the obstruction resolves because the half-life of alkaline phosphatase is about 7 days. Increases of up to three times normal occur in many liver disorders, including hepatitis, cirrhosis, space-occupying lesions and infiltrative disorders. Isolated elevations (ie when other liver test results are normal) often occur with focal liver lesions (eg abscess, tumour) or in partial or intermittent bile duct obstruction. Isolated elevations also occur in the absence of liver or biliary disease, for example in some malignancies (bronchogenic carcinoma, Hodgkin's lymphoma, renal cell carcinoma), after fatty

gastrointestinal

meals (from the small intestine), in pregnancy (from the placenta), in growing children and adolescents (from bone growth) and in chronic renal failure (from intestine and bone). Fractionating these alkaline phosphatases is technically difficult. Elevation of enzymes more specific to the liver, 5-nucleotidase or gamma-glutamyltransferase (GGT), can help to differentiate between hepatic and extrahepatic sources of alkaline phosphatase. An isolated alkaline phosphatase elevation in an otherwise asymptomatic elderly person usually originates from bone (eg Paget's disease) and does not require further investigation.

In this scenario the presence of jaundice accompanied by pale stools, weight loss and a raised alkaline phosphatase suggests obstructive jaundice, most probably due to pancreatic carcinoma.

## 10.14

*Answer: D*   Primary biliary cirrhosis

Primary biliary cirrhosis is an autoimmune liver disease that is characterised by the progressive destruction of intrahepatic bile ducts, leading to cholestasis, cirrhosis and liver failure. Patients are usually asymptomatic at presentation but can experience fatigue, symptoms of cholestasis (eg pruritus, steatorrhoea), or symptoms of cirrhosis (eg portal hypertension, ascites). Laboratory tests reveal cholestasis, increased IgM and, characteristically, antimitochondrial antibodies in the serum. Liver biopsy is usually required for diagnosis and staging.

## 10.15

*Answer: E*   Sclerosing cholangitis

Primary sclerosing cholangitis is a chronic cholestatic syndrome characterised by patchy inflammation, fibrosis and strictures of the intrahepatic and extrahepatic bile ducts. Around 80% of patients have inflammatory bowel disease, often ulcerative colitis. Symptoms of fatigue and pruritus develop late. The diagnosis is based on contrast cholangiography (with endoscopic retrograde cholangiopancreatography) or magnetic resonance cholangiopancreatography. The disease leads to eventual obliteration of the bile ducts, with cirrhosis, hepatic failure, and sometimes cholangiocarcinoma.

## 10.16

*Answer: A*   Duodenal ulcer

Duodenal ulcers tend to be associated with a fairly consistent pattern of pain. Pain is absent when the patient awakens but appears mid-morning, is relieved by food, but recurs 2–3 hours after a meal. Pain that awakens a patient at night is common and is highly suggestive of duodenal ulcer.

## 10.17

*Answer: E*   Oesophageal stricture

These findings point to scleroderma, probably CREST syndrome, in which the 'e' represents (o)esophageal dysmotility. Scleroderma varies in severity and progression, ranging from generalised skin thickening with rapidly progressive and often fatal visceral involvement to isolated skin involvement (often just the fingers and face) and slow progression (often several decades) before the development of serious visceral disease. The latter form is known as 'limited cutaneous scleroderma' or 'CREST syndrome' (**c**alcinosis cutis, **R**aynaud's phenomenon, (o)**e**sophageal dysmotility, **s**clerodactyly, and **t**elangiectasia).

## 10.18

*Answer: D*   Micronodular cirrhosis

Cirrhosis is fibrosis that progresses to produce diffuse disorganisation of normal hepatic structure, characterised by regenerative nodules surrounded by dense fibrotic tissue. Symptoms might not develop for years and are often non-specific, for example anorexia, fatigue and weight loss. Late manifestations include portal hypertension, ascites and liver failure.

gastrointestinal

Cirrhosis can be micronodular or macronodular. Micronodular cirrhosis is characterised by uniformly small nodules (<3 mm in diameter) and thick regular bands of connective tissue. Typically, nodules lack lobular organisation; terminal (central) hepatic venules and portal triads are distorted. With time, macronodular cirrhosis often develops, in which nodules vary in size (3 mm to 5 cm in diameter) and contain some rather normal lobular organisation of portal triads and terminal hepatic venules. Broad fibrous bands of varying thickness surround the large nodules. Collapse of the normal liver architecture is suggested by the concentration of portal triads within the fibrous scars. Mixed cirrhosis (incomplete septal cirrhosis) combines elements of both micronodular and macronodular cirrhosis.

## 10.19

*Answer: E*    Ulceration of mucosa by ectopic gastric tissue

A Meckel's diverticulum is present at birth, unlike colonic diverticula, which are acquired in adulthood. There can be ectopic tissue in the Meckel's diverticulum, most likely pancreatic tissue, but sometimes gastric mucosa, which can cause ulceration and bleeding, as is the case in this scenario. In early fetal life the vitelline duct that runs from the terminal ileum to the umbilicus and yolk sac is normally obliterated by the seventh week. If the portion connecting to the ileum fails to atrophy, a Meckel's diverticulum results. This congenital diverticulum arises from the antimesenteric margin of the intestine and contains all layers of the normal bowel. About 50% of diverticula also contain heterotopic tissue of the stomach (and so contain parietal cells that secrete hydrochloric acid), pancreas or both.

Only about 2% of people with Meckel's diverticulum develop complications. Although diverticula are equally common in males and females, males are two to three times more likely to have complications. Complications include bleeding, obstruction, diverticulitis and tumours. Bleeding is more common in young children (<5 years) and occurs when acid secreted from ectopic gastric mucosa in the diverticulum ulcerates the adjacent ileum. Obstruction can occur at any age but is more common in older children and adults. In children, intussusception of the diverticulum is the most likely cause. Obstruction can also result from adhesions, volvulus, retained foreign bodies, tumours or incarceration in a hernia (Littre's hernia). Acute Meckel's diverticulitis can occur at any age, but its incidence peaks in older children. Tumours, including carcinoids, are rare and occur mainly in adults.

## 10.20

*Answer: A*    Adhesions from previous surgery

The findings point to an acute bowel obstruction. The abdominal scar indicates prior surgery and suggests the development of peritoneal adhesions that have predisposed to obstruction. Hepatitis can cause vague abdominal pain, and there can be distension from ascites with liver dysfunction, but not dilated loops of bowel. Amoebiasis can cause an inflammatory bowel disease that mainly affects the colon, with diarrhoea that can be positive for occult blood. Primary adenocarcinoma of the ileum is rare. A Meckel's diverticulum is a small focal lesion that can cause obstruction, but the clinical features and radiological findings are more consistent with obstruction due to adhesions from previous surgery.

gastrointestinal

# SECTION 11: HAEMATOPATHOLOGY — ANSWERS

## 11.1

*Answer: A*    A 5-year-old boy with a sore throat and runny nose

This is the appearance of a benign, reactive lymph node. Lymphadenopathy is common in children.

## 11.2

*Answer: B*    Acute myelogenous leukaemia

Acute myeloid leukaemia (AML), also known as 'acute myelogenous leukaemia', is a cancer of the myeloid line of white blood cells, characterised by the rapid proliferation of abnormal cells which accumulate in the bone marrow and interfere with the production of normal blood cells. AML is the most common acute leukaemia in adults, and its incidence increases with age. While AML is a relatively rare disease overall, its incidence is expected to increase as the population ages.

The symptoms of AML are caused by replacement of normal bone marrow with leukaemic cells, resulting in a drop in red blood cells, platelets and normal white blood cells. These symptoms include fatigue, shortness of breath, easy bruising and bleeding and increased risk of infection. While a number of risk factors for AML have been elucidated, the specific cause of AML remains unclear. AML progresses rapidly and is typically fatal in weeks to months if left untreated.

Auer rods can be seen in the leukaemic blasts of acute myeloid leukaemia. Auer rods are clumps of azurophilic granular material that form elongated needles seen in the cytoplasm of leukaemic blasts. They are composed of fused lysosomes and contain peroxidase, lysosomal enzymes and large crystalline inclusions. Auer rods are classically seen in myeloid blasts of M1, M2, M3 and M4 acute leukaemias. They are also used to distinguish the preleukaemia myelodysplastic syndromes.

## 11.3

*Answer: B*    Chronic lymphocytic leukaemia

The most common type of leukaemia in the Western world, chronic lymphocytic leukaemia (CLL) involves mature-appearing but defective neoplastic lymphocytes with an abnormally long life span. The peripheral blood, bone marrow, spleen and lymph nodes undergo leukaemic infiltration. The incidence of CLL increases with age: 75% of cases are diagnosed in patients aged over 60 years. CLL is twice as common in men. Although the cause is unknown, some cases are familial. CLL is rare in Japan and China and does not seem to increase among Japanese expatriates in the United States, suggesting a genetic factor. CLL is more common among Jews of Eastern European descent.

In about 98% of cases, CD5+ B cells undergo malignant transformation, with lymphocytes initially accumulating in the bone marrow and then spreading to lymph nodes and other lymphoid tissues, eventually inducing splenomegaly and hepatomegaly. As the disease progresses, abnormal haematopoiesis results in anaemia, neutropenia, thrombocytopenia and decreased immunoglobulin production. Many patients develop hypogammaglobulinaemia and impaired antibody response, perhaps related to increased T-suppressor cell activity. Patients have increased susceptibility to autoimmune disease, characterized by immunohaemolytic anaemias (usually Coombs' test-positive) or thrombocytopenia, and a modest increase in the risk of developing other cancers.

In 2%–3% of cases, the clonal expansion is T-cell in type, and even this group has a subtype (eg large granular lymphocytes with cytopenias). In addition, other chronic leukaemic patterns have been categorised under CLL: prolymphocytic leukaemia, the leukaemic phase of cutaneous T-cell lymphoma (Sézary syndrome), hairy cell leukaemia and lymphoma/leukaemia (ie the leukaemic changes seen in the advanced stages of malignant lymphoma). Differentiation of these subtypes from typical CLL is usually straightforward.

haem

The onset is usually insidious and CLL is often diagnosed incidentally during routine blood tests or on investigation of asymptomatic lymphadenopathy. The symptomatic patient usually has non-specific complaints of fatigue, anorexia, weight loss, dyspnoea on exertion, or a sense of abdominal fullness (secondary to an enlarged spleen). Initial findings include generalised lymphadenopathy and minimal-to-moderate hepatomegaly and splenomegaly. With progressive disease, there might be pallor due to anaemia. Skin infiltration, either maculopapular or diffuse, can be a feature of T-cell CLL. Hypogammaglobulinaemia and granulocytopenia in late CLL can predispose to bacterial, viral and fungal infection, especially pneumonia. Herpes zoster is common and usually dermatomic.

CLL is confirmed by examining the peripheral blood smear and bone marrow; the hallmark is a sustained, absolute peripheral lymphocytosis (>5 10$^9$/l) and an increased proportion of lymphocytes in the bone marrow (>30%). The differential diagnosis is simplified by immunophenotyping. Other findings at diagnosis can include hypogammaglobulinaemia (<15% of cases) and, rarely, an elevated lactate dehydrogenase (LDH). Only 10% of patients present with moderate anaemia (sometimes immunohaemolytic) and/or thrombocytopenia. A monoclonal serum immunoglobulin spike of the same type might be found on the leukaemic cell surface in 2%–4% of cases.

## 11.4

*Answer: D*  Serum vitamin B$_{12}$ and folate

The markedly elevated mean corpuscular volume (MCV) suggests a megaloblastic anaemia, and the hypersegmented neutrophils are consistent with this. Either a B$_{12}$ or a folate deficiency is the likely cause. Megaloblastic states result from defective DNA synthesis. RNA synthesis continues, resulting in a large cell with a large nucleus. All cell lines have dyspoiesis, in which cytoplasmic maturity is greater than nuclear maturity. This produces megaloblasts in the marrow before they appear in the peripheral blood. Dyspoiesis results in intramedullary cell death, making erythropoiesis ineffective and causing indirect hyperbilirubinaemia and hyperuricaemia. Because dyspoiesis affects all cell lines, reticulocytopenia and, during later stages, leukopenia and thrombocytopenia develop. Large,

haem

oval red blood cells (macro-ovalocytes) enter the circulation. Hypersegmentation of polymorphonuclear neutrophils is common; the mechanism of their production is unknown.

## 11.5

*Answer: A*   Atypical lymphocytosis

Epstein–Barr virus infection, causing infectious mononucleosis often leads to the appearance of atypical lymphocytes in the peripheral blood. The symptoms of infectious mononucleosis develop most often in older children and adults. The incubation period is about 30–50 days. Usually, fatigue develops initially, lasting several days to a week or longer, followed by fever, pharyngitis and adenopathy. However, not all of these symptoms will appear. Fatigue can last months, but is usually maximal in the first 2–3 weeks. Fever usually peaks in the afternoon or early evening, with a temperature around 39.5 °C, although it can reach 40.5 °C. When fatigue and fever predominate (the so-called 'typhoidal form'), the onset and resolution can be much slower. The pharyngitis can be severe, painful and exudative, and can resemble streptococcal pharyngitis. Lymphadenopathy is usually symmetric and can involve any group of nodes, particularly the anterior and posterior cervical chains. Adenopathy is sometimes the only manifestation.

Splenomegaly, which occurs in about 50% of cases, is maximal during the second and third weeks and is usually barely palpable. Mild hepatomegaly and hepatic percussion tenderness can occur. Less frequent findings include maculopapular eruptions, jaundice, periorbital oedema and palatal enanthema.

Laboratory diagnosis usually involves a full blood count and a heterophil antibody test. Lymphocytes that are morphologically atypical account for up to 80% of the white blood cells. Although individual lymphocytes can resemble leukaemic lymphocytes, the lymphocytes are heterogeneous, which is unlikely with leukaemia.

haem

## 11.6

*Answer: C*    Metastatic carcinoma

This patient has a leucoerythroblastic picture in the peripheral blood. At this age, prostatic adenocarcinoma or lung cancer are the likely primaries.

## 11.7

*Answer: E*    A 15-year-old boy with haemoglobin SS disease

'Autosplenectomy' is the rule with sickle cell anaemia by late childhood or teenage years. Vaso-occlusive crises are caused by sickle-shaped red blood cells that obstruct capillaries and restrict blood flow to an organ, resulting in ischaemia, pain and organ damage. Because of its narrow vessels and its function in clearing defective red blood cells, the spleen is frequently affected. It is usually infarcted before the end of childhood in individuals suffering from sickle cell anaemia. This autosplenectomy increases the risk of infection with encapsulated organisms, and so prophylactic antibiotics and vaccinations are recommended for people with this type of asplenia.

## 11.8

*Answer: E*    Polycythaemia vera

There is a markedly increased haematocrit. It is possible that this is secondary, but the thrombocytosis and the leucocytosis suggest a myeloproliferative disorder. Polycythaemia vera is the most common of the myeloproliferative disorders, occurring in about 5 in 1 million people, more often in males (about 1.4 to 1). The mean age at diagnosis is 60 years (range 15–90 years, rare in childhood); 5% of patients are aged under 40 years at onset.

Polycythaemia vera involves increased production of all cell lines, including red blood cells, white blood cells and platelets. Increased production confined to the red blood cell line is known as 'primary erythrocytosis'. In people with polycythaemia vera red blood cell production proceeds independently of erythropoietin.

haem

Extramedullary haematopoiesis occurs in the spleen, liver and other sites with the potential for blood cell formation. Peripheral blood cell turnover increases. Eventually, about 25% of patients have reduced red blood cell survival and inadequate erythropoiesis. Anaemia, thrombocytopenia and myelofibrosis can develop, and red blood cell and white blood cell precursors are released into the circulation. Depending on treatment received, the incidence of transformation to acute leukaemia varies between 1.5% and 10%. In polycythaemia vera the blood volume expands and hyperviscosity develops, predisposing to thrombosis. Platelets function abnormally, predisposing to increased bleeding. Patients can become hypermetabolic, and increased cell turnover leads to hyperuricaemia.

Polycythaemia vera itself is often asymptomatic. Occasionally, increased blood volume and viscosity cause weakness, headache, light-headedness, visual disturbances, fatigue and dyspnoea. Pruritus is common, particularly after a hot bath. The face may be red and the retinal veins engorged. The lower extremities can be red, warm and painful, sometimes with digital ischaemia (erythromelalgia). Hepatomegaly is common and more than 75% of patients have splenomegaly, which may be massive. Thrombosis can occur in most vessels, resulting in stroke, transient ischaemic attacks, deep venous thrombosis, myocardial infarction, retinal artery or vein occlusion, splenic infarction (often with a friction rub) or Budd–Chiari syndrome.

Bleeding, typically gastrointestinal, occurs in 10%–20% of patients. Complications of hyperuricaemia (eg gout, renal calculi) tend to occur later in polycythaemia vera. Hypermetabolism can cause low-grade fevers and weight loss.

**11.9**

*Answer: C*  Hodgkin's lymphoma

Hodgkin's lymphoma is a localised or disseminated malignant proliferation of cells of the lymphoreticular system, primarily involving lymph node tissue, spleen, liver and bone marrow. Symptoms include painless lymphadenopathy, sometimes with fever, night sweats, unintentional weight loss, pruritus, splenomegaly and hepatomegaly. Biopsy of enlarged lymph nodes reveals Reed–Sternberg cells (large binucleated cells) in a characteristically heterogeneous cellular infiltrate consisting of histiocytes, lymphocytes, monocytes, plasma cells and eosinophils.

## 11.10

*Answer: E*    Leukaemoid reaction

The leukocyte alkaline phosphatase (LAP) is increased in non-neoplastic leucocytic proliferations. The term 'leukaemoid' is used because there is an increased white blood cell count with immature forms similar to leukaemia. Conventionally, a leucocytosis exceeding $50 \times 10^9/l$ with a significant increase in early neutrophil precursors is referred to as a 'leukaemoid reaction'. The peripheral blood smear might show myelocytes, metamyelocytes, promyelocytes, and even myeloblasts, but there is a mix of early mature neutrophil precursors, in contrast to the immature forms typically seen in acute leukaemia. The bone marrow in a leukaemoid reaction, if examined, might be hypercellular but is otherwise typically unremarkable.

Leukaemoid reactions are generally benign and are not inherently dangerous, although they are often a response to a significant disease state. However, leukaemoid reactions can resemble more serious conditions such as chronic myelogenous leukaemia (CML), which can present with identical findings on peripheral blood smear. Historically, various clues, including the LAP score and the presence of basophilia were used to distinguish CML from a leukaemoid reaction. However, at present the test of choice in adults to distinguish CML from a leukaemoid reaction is an assay for the presence of the Philadelphia chromosome, either using cytogenetics and fluorescent in-situ hybridisation or using a polymerase chain reaction for the Bcr/abl fusion protein. The LAP score is high in reactive states but is low in CML.

Causes of leukemoid reactions include:

- Haemorrhage

- Drugs:

  o glucorticoids

haem

- o granulocyte-colony stimulating factor or related growth factors

  - o all-trans retinoic acid (ATRA).

- Infections (eg tuberculosis, pertussis)

- As a feature of trisomy 21 in infancy (incidence approximately 10%)

- As a paraneoplastic phenomenon (rare).

## 11.11

*Answer: A*   Anaemia of chronic disease

The serum iron, iron-binding capacity and saturation are all low, but there is plenty of storage iron that is not being utilised. This is typical of anaemia of chronic disease. In haemolytic anaemia the haemolysed cells release haemoglobin that is usually not lost from the body and is recycled, so the iron is not usually low. Chronic blood loss can lead to iron deficiency because of the loss of iron, with a low serum iron, high total iron-binding capacity (TIBC) and low ferritin. Malabsorption, particularly in disease processes involving the duodenum, can occasionally explain iron deficiency anaemia, which has a high TIBC and low ferritin. Vitamin $B_{12}$ and folate deficiencies lead to a megaloblastic anaemia that is not associated with abnormalities in iron metabolism.

## 11.12

*Answer: D*   Poorly differentiated lymphocytic lymphoma

Lymphadenopathy with malignant lymphoma is typically non-tender, in contrast to the lymphadenopathy of infections. As with most infections, the lymphadenopathy with Epstein–Barr virus infection (infectious mononucleosis) is usually tender to palpation. In addition, the lymphoid hyperplasia of infectious mononucleosis is benign and polyclonal.

haem

## 11.13

*Answer:* C    Myelofibrosis

Myelofibrosis is known to cause massive splenomegaly. Other causes include:

- Chronic myelogenous leukaemia
- Lymphomas
- Hairy cell leukaemia
- Polycythaemia vera
- Gaucher's disease
- Chronic lymphocytic leukaemia
- Sarcoidosis
- Autoimmune haemolytic anaemia
- Malaria.

## 11.14

*Answer:* C    Thrombotic thrombocytopenic purpura

The hyaline thrombi are typical of thrombotic thrmobocytopenic purpura (TTP). Platelet transfusion is contraindicated. TTP is caused by non-immunological platelet destruction. Loose strands of fibrin are deposited in multiple small vessels, which damage passing platelets and red blood cells. Platelets are also destroyed within the multiple small thrombi. Multiple organs develop bland platelet–fibrin thrombi (without the granulocytic infiltration of the vessel wall that is characteristic of vasculitis) that are localised primarily to arteriocapillary junctions, described as 'thrombotic microangiopathy'. Treatment is by plasma exchange.

haem

## 11.15

*Answer: A* β-Thalassaemia

Beta-thalassaemia results from decreased production of β-polypeptide chains. The inheritance is autosomal. Heterozygotes are carriers and have asymptomatic mild to moderate microcytic anaemia (thalassaemia minor). Homozygotes (β-thalassaemia major, or Cooley's anaemia) develop severe anaemia and bone marrow hyperactivity. Beta-thalassaemia major presents by the age of 1–2 years with symptoms of severe anaemia and transfusional and absorptive iron overload. Patients are jaundiced, and leg ulcers and cholelithiasis occur (as in sickle cell anaemia). Splenomegaly, often massive, is common. Splenic sequestration can develop, accelerating destruction of transfused normal red blood cells. Bone marrow hyperactivity causes thickening of the cranial bones and malar eminences. Long bone involvement predisposes to pathological fractures and impairs growth, possibly delaying or preventing puberty. Iron deposits in heart muscle can cause heart failure. Hepatic siderosis is typical, leading to functional impairment and cirrhosis.

Thalassaemias are suspected in patients with a family history, suggestive symptoms or signs or microcytic haemolytic anaemia. If thalassaemias are suspected, laboratory tests for microcytic and haemolytic anaemias and quantitative haemoglobin studies are performed. Serum bilirubin, iron and ferritin levels are increased.

In β-thalassaemia major the anaemia is severe, often with haemoglobin levels of 6 g/dl or less. The red blood cell count is elevated relative to the haemoglobin because the cells are very microcytic. The blood smear is virtually diagnostic, with many nucleated erythroblasts, target cells, small pale red blood cells, and punctate and diffuse basophilia.

## 11.16

*Answer: D* Increased neutrophil segmentation

Atrophic gastritis can be followed by pernicious anaemia. Megaloblastic changes lead to hypersegmented neutrophils, as well as an increased mean corpuscular volume of the red blood cells. The

haem

term 'pernicious anaemia' is often used synonymously with 'vitamin $B_{12}$ deficiency'. However, pernicious anaemia refers specifically to vitamin $B_{12}$ deficiency caused by an autoimmune gastritis with loss of intrinsic factor. Classic pernicious anaemia, most common in younger adults, is associated with an increased risk of stomach and other gastrointestinal cancers.

## 11.17

*Answer:* C    Plasma cells

The features are suggestive of multiple myeloma. Multiple myeloma is a malignancy of plasma cells that produce monoclonal immunoglobulin and invade and destroy adjacent bone tissue. Common manifestations include bone pain, renal insufficiency, hypercalcaemia, anaemia and recurrent infections. Diagnosis requires the demonstration of M-protein (sometimes present in urine and not serum) and either lytic bone lesions, light-chain proteinuria or excessive marrow plasma cells.

## 11.18

*Answer:* B    Idiopathic thrombocytopenic purpura

Idiopathic thrombocytopenic purpura (ITP) usually results from the development of an antibody directed against a structural platelet antigen (ie an autoantibody). In childhood ITP the autoantibody can be triggered by binding of viral antigen to megakaryocytes. The symptoms and signs are petechiae and mucosal bleeding. Although in ITP there are circulating antibodies to platelets that lead to platelet destruction, the spleen itself is usually not enlarged unless it is enlarged as a result of a coexistent childhood viral infection.

ITP is suspected in patients with unexplained thrombocytopenia. The peripheral blood is normal except for reduced platelet numbers. Bone marrow is examined if blood counts or a blood smear reveal abnormalities in addition to the thrombocytopenia. Bone marrow examination reveals normal or possibly increased numbers of megakaryocytes in an otherwise normal marrow. Because diagnostic findings are non-specific, diagnosis of this condition

haem

requires exclusion of other thrombocytopenic disorders suggested by clinical or laboratory test data.

## 11.19

*Answer: B*   Hypersegmented neutrophils

The mean corpuscular volume points to a macrocytic anaemia such as a megaloblastic anaemia, which can feature hypersegmented neutrophils.

## 11.20

*Answer: D*   Mycosis fungoides

Mycosis fungoides is an uncommon, chronic T-cell lymphoma primarily affecting the skin and occasionally the internal organs. It is rarer than Hodgkin's lymphoma and non-Hodgkin's lymphoma. Unlike most other lymphomas, it is insidious in onset, sometimes appearing as a chronic, pruritic rash that is difficult to diagnose. It begins focally but can spread to involve most of the skin. Lesions are plaque-like but can become nodular or ulcerated. Eventually, systemic involvement of lymph nodes, liver, spleen and lungs occurs, resulting in the advent of symptoms, which include fever, night sweats and unintentional weight loss. Diagnosis is based on skin biopsy, but the histology can be equivocal early in the course of the disease because of insufficient quantities of lymphoma cells. The malignant cells are mature T cells (T4+, T11+, T12+). Characteristic Pautrier's microabscesses are present in the epidermis. In some cases, a leukaemic phase known as 'Sézary syndrome' occurs, characterised by the appearance of malignant T cells with serpentine nuclei in the peripheral blood.

Once mycosis fungoides has been confirmed, the stage is determined by computed tomography of the torso and bone marrow biopsy for blood or lymph node involvement. Positron emission tomography (PET) can also be used for investigation of suspected visceral involvement. Most patients are aged over 50 years at diagnosis, and the average life expectancy is 7–10 years after diagnosis, even without treatment. Survival rates depend on the stage at diagnosis.

# SECTION 12:
# ENDOCRINE PATHOLOGY —
# ANSWERS

## 12.1

*Answer: D*    Calcitonin

Medullary (solid) carcinoma constitutes about 3% of thyroid cancers and is composed of parafollicular cells (C cells) that produce calcitonin. It can be sporadic (usually unilateral), but is often familial, caused by a mutation of the *ret* proto-oncogene. The familial form can occur in isolation or as a component of multiple endocrine neoplasia (MEN) syndromes types IIA and IIB. Although calcitonin can lower the serum calcium and phosphate, the serum calcium is normal because the high level of calcitonin ultimately down-regulates its receptors. Characteristic amyloid deposits that stain with Congo red are also present.

Patients typically present with an asymptomatic thyroid nodule, although in many cases the tumour is now diagnosed during routine screening of affected relatives with MEN IIA or MEN IIB before a palpable tumour develops. Medullary carcinoma can have a dramatic biochemical presentation when associated with ectopic production of other hormones or peptides (eg, adrenocorticotrophic hormone, vasoactive intestinal polypeptide, prostaglandins, kallikreins, serotonin). Metastases spread via the lymphatic system to cervical and mediastinal nodes and sometimes to liver, lungs and bone. The best test is the serum calcitonin, which is greatly elevated. A challenge with calcium (15 mg/kg intravenously over 4 hours) provokes excessive secretion of calcitonin. X-rays may show a dense, homogenous, conglomerate calcification.

CA-125 is a tumour-associated glycoprotein which is frequently expressed by ovarian carcinomas. CA15-3 is a tumour-associated glycoprotein which is frequently expressed by breast carcinomas. Alpha-fetoprotein can be elevated in the serum in association with hepatomas and gonadal tumours. Elevations of human chorionic gonadotrophin in the serum can be seen in normal pregnancies, gonadal tumours, and choriocarcinomas.

## 12.2

*Answer: B*   Exposure to ionising radiation in childhood

Papillary carcinoma accounts for 70%–80% of all thyroid cancers. The female to male ratio is 3 : 1, and is familial in up to 5% of patients. Most patients present between the ages of 30 years and 60 years. The tumour is often more aggressive in elderly patients. It is also the predominant cancer type in children with thyroid cancer, and in patients with thyroid cancer who have had previous radiation to the head and neck (in this group the cancer tends to be multifocal, with early lymphatic spread and a relatively poor prognosis). Thyroglobulin can be used as a tumour marker for well-differentiated papillary thyroid cancer. Many papillary carcinomas contain follicular elements. The tumour spreads via lymphatics to regional lymph nodes in a third of patients and can metastasise to the lungs. Patients aged under 45 years with small tumours that are confined to the thyroid have an excellent prognosis.

Characteristic pathological features:

- Characteristic 'Orphan Annie' eye nuclear inclusions and psammoma bodies on light microscopy.

- Lymphatic spread is more common than haematogenous spread.

- Multifocality is common.

- The so-called 'lateral aberrant thyroid' is actually a lymph node metastasis from papillary thyroid carcinoma.

endocrine

## 12.3

*Answer: D*   Phaeochromocytoma

A phaeochromocytoma is a neuroendocrine tumour of the adrenal medulla originating in the chromaffin cells, which secretes excessive amounts of catecholamines, usually adrenaline (epinephrine) and noradrenaline (norepinephrine). Extra-adrenal paragangliomas (often described as extra-adrenal phaeochromocytomas) are closely related, though less common tumours that originate in the ganglia of the sympathetic nervous system and are named on the basis of the primary anatomical site of origin.

Traditionally the phaeochromocytoma is known as the '10% tumour':

- Bilateral disease is present in approximately 10% of patients.

- Approximately 10% of tumours are malignant.

- Approximately 10% of tumours are located in chromaffin tissue outside the adrenal gland.

Up to 25% of phaeochromocytomas are be familial. Mutations of the genes *VHL, RET, NF1, SDHB* and *SDHD* are all known to cause familial phaeochromocytoma/extra-adrenal paraganglioma. The clinical features of a phaeochromocytoma are those of sympathetic nervous system hyperactivity, which can generally be described as those of 'impending doom', including:

- Tachycardia

- Hypertension (a clue to the presence of phaechromocytoma is orthostatic hypotension, a fall in systolic blood pressure of more than 10 mmHg when the patient stands up)

- Palpitations

- Anxiety, often resembling that of a panic attack

- Excessive sweating

- Headaches

- Pallor

endocrine

- A phaeochromocytoma can also cause resistant arterial hypertension, and can be fatal if it causes malignant hypertension.

The diagnosis can be established by measuring catecholamines and metanephrines in plasma or in a 24-hour urine collection. Care should be taken to rule out other causes of adrenergic excess such as hypoglycaemia, stress, exercise and drugs that affect catecholamine levels (eg methyldopa, dopamine agonists, ganglion-blocking antihypertensives). Various foodstuffs (eg vanilla ice cream) can also affect the levels of urinary metanephrine and vanillylmandelic acid (VMA). Imaging by computed tomography or T2-weighted magnetic resonance imaging of the head, neck, chest and abdomen can help to locate the tumour. Tumours can also be located using iodine-131 meta-iodobenzylguanidine ($I^{131}$ MIBG) imaging. One diagnostic test used in the past for diagnosing phaeochromocytoma was to administer clonidine, a centrally-acting alpha-2 agonist used to treat high blood pressure. Clonidine mimics catecholamines in the brain, reducing the activity of the sympathetic nerves that control the adrenal medulla. A healthy adrenal medulla will respond to clonidine by reducing catecholamine production; the lack of a response is evidence of phaeochromocytoma.

## 12.4

*Answer: A*    Decreased plasma concentration of amino acids

A glucagonoma is a rare tumour of the alpha cells of the pancreas that results in up to a 1000-fold overproduction of the hormone glucagon. Alpha cell tumours are commonly associated with glucagonoma syndrome, though similar symptoms are present in cases of pseudoglucagonoma syndrome in the absence of a glucagon-secreting tumour. The primary physiological effect of glucagonoma is an overproduction of the peptide hormone glucagon, which enhances blood glucose levels through the activation of gluconeogenesis and lipolysis. Gluconeogenesis produces glucose from protein and amino acids. The net result is hyperglucagonaemia, decreased blood levels of amino acids (hypoaminoacidaemia), anaemia, diarrhoea, and weight loss of 5–15 kg.

endocrine

Necrolytic migratory erythema (NME) is a classic symptom observed in patients with glucagonoma and is present in 80% of cases. Associated NME is characterised by the spread of erythematous blisters and swelling across areas subject to greater friction and pressure, including the lower abdomen, buttocks, perineum and groin. Diabetes mellitus also frequently results from the insulin and glucagon imbalance that occurs in glucagonoma. Diabetes mellitus is present in 80%–90% of cases of glucagonoma, and is exacerbated by pre-existing insulin resistance.

A plasma glucagon concentration of 1000 pg/ml or greater is indicative of glucagonoma (the normal range is 50–200 pg/ml). Blood tests can also reveal abnormally low concentrations of amino acids, zinc and essential fatty acids, which are thought to play a role in the development of NME. Skin biopsies can also be taken to confirm the presence of NME. A full blood count can uncover anaemia. The tumour itself can be located by any number of radiographic modalities, including angiography, computed tomography, magnetic resonanace imaging, positron emission tomography and endoscopic ultrasound. Laparotomy/laparoscopy is useful for obtaining histological samples for analysis and confirmation of the glucagonoma.

Heightened glucagon secretion can be treated with octreotide, a somatostatin analogue, which inhibits the release of glucagon. Doxorubicin and streptozotocin have also been used successfully to selectively damage alpha cells of the pancreatic islets. These do not destroy the tumour, but help to minimise progression of symptoms. The only curative therapy for glucagonoma, however, is surgical resection, which has been known to reverse symptoms in some patients.

Fewer than 250 cases of glucagonoma have been described in the literature since their first description by Becker in 1942. Because of its rarity (fewer than one in 20 million worldwide), long-term survival rates are as yet unknown.

endocrine

## 12.5

*Answer: B*    Hyperthyroidism

Hyperthyroidism is a clinical syndrome caused by an excess of circulating free thyroxine (T4) or free triiodothyronine (T3) or both. Major causes in humans are:

- Graves' disease (the most common cause, responsible for 70%–80% cases)

- Toxic thyroid adenoma

- Toxic multinodular goitre.

Excess thyroid hormone intake can also cause hyperthyroidism. Amiodarone, an antiarrhythmic medication, can sometimes cause hyperthyroidism. Other causes of hyperthyroxinaemia (high blood levels of thyroid hormones) are not to be confused with true hyperthyroidism and include subacute and other forms of thyroiditis (inflammation). Thyrotoxicosis (the symptoms caused by hyperthyroxinemia) can occur in both hyperthyroidism and thyroiditis. When the metabolic rate is acutely raised this is sometimes known as a 'thyroid storm'.

The major clinical features include weight loss (often accompanied by a ravenous appetite), intolerance to heat, fatigue, weakness, hyperactivity, irritability, apathy, depression, polyuria and sweating. Patients can present with a variety of symptoms, including palpitations and arrhythmias (notably atrial fibrillation), shortness of breath, loss of libido, nausea, vomiting and diarrhoea. In the elderly these classic symptoms are sometimes absent and they can present with fatigue and weight loss alone, leading to 'apathetic hyperthyroidism'. Neurological manifestations include tremor, chorea, myopathy and periodic paralysis. Stroke of cardioembolic origin due to coexisting atrial fibrillation is one of the most serious complications of hyperthyroidism.

## 12.6

*Answer: A*   Hyperprolactinaemia

Hyperprolactinaemia is the presence of abnormally high levels of prolactin in the blood. Normal levels are less than 580 mIU/l for women and less than 450 mIU/l for men. The hormone prolactin is down-regulated by dopamine and is up-regulated by oestrogen. A falsely high measurement can occur due to the presence of the biologically inactive macroprolactin in the serum. This can show up as a high prolactin in some types of tests, but is asymptomatic.

Hyperprolactinaemia can be caused either by disinhibition (eg compression of the pituitary stalk or reduced dopamine levels) or excess production from a prolactinoma (a pituitary gland adenoma). A prolactin level of 1000–5000 mIU/l could occur with either mechanism, but a level of over 5000 mIU/l is likely to be due to an adenoma, with macroadenomas (large tumours over 10 mm diameter) being associated with levels of up to 100,000 mIU/l. Hyperprolactinaemia inhibits gonadotrophin-releasing hormone (GnRH) by increasing the release of dopamine from the arcuate nucleus of the hypothalamus (dopamine inhibits GnRH secretion), thus inhibiting gonadal steroidogenesis, which is the cause of many of the symptoms associated with hyperprolactinaemia.

In women, a high blood level of prolactin often causes hypo-oestrogenism, with anovulatory infertility and a decrease in menstruation. In some women, menstruation can disappear altogether (amenorrhoea). In others, menstruation can become irregular or the menstrual flow can change. Women who are not pregnant or nursing might begin to produce breast milk. Some women experience loss of libido, and intercourse can become painful because of vaginal dryness. In addition, the hypo-oestrogenism associated with the hyperprolactinaemia can lead to osteoporosis.

In men, the most common symptoms of prolactinoma are impotence, decreased libido, erectile dysfunction and infertility. Because men have no reliable indicator such as menstruation to signal a problem, many men with hyperprolactinoma caused by an adenoma delay going to the doctor until they have headaches or eye problems caused by the enlarged pituitary pressing against the optic chiasma. They may not recognise a gradual loss of sexual function or libido.

endocrine

## 12.7

*Answer: D*    Non-functioning adrenal adenoma

Adrenal adenomas are common (one in 10 people have them), benign and asymptomatic. They are often found as an incidental finding on computed tomography of the abdomen (an 'incidentaloma'). Only about one in 10,000 are malignant (adrenal adenocarcinoma). A biopsy is rarely called for, especially if the lesion is homogeneous and smaller than 3 cm in diameter. Follow-up images taken after 3–6 months can confirm their stability in terms of size. While some adrenal adenomas do not secrete hormones at all (ie non-functional adenomas, often incidentalomas), some secrete cortisol (causing Cushing syndrome), aldosterone (causing Conn syndrome) or androgens (causing hyperandrogenism).

This adrenal gland is an unlikely site for a traumatic lesion such as a haematoma. Granulomatous involvement in *Histoplasma capsulatum* infection is typically bilateral and the granulomas are multiple. Metastases are often multiple and/or larger than 1 cm and the patient will have a primary lesion in the lung. Simple cysts can occur anywhere, but this would be an unusual location.

## 12.8

*Answer: B*    Conn syndrome

Conn syndrome is overproduction of the mineralocorticoid hormone, aldosterone by the adrenal glands. The syndrome is due to either an aldosterone-secreting adrenal adenoma (a benign tumour, 50%–60% of cases) or to hyperplasia of the adrenal gland (40%–50% of cases). Aldosterone causes sodium and water retention and potassium excretion in the kidneys, leading to arterial hypertension. It is a rare but recognised cause of non-essential hypertension, and is the most common form of primary hyperaldosteronism. Apart from hypertension, the symptoms can include muscle cramps and headaches (due to the low potassium) and metabolic alkalosis (due to increased secretion of $H^+$ ions by the kidney). The high pH of the blood makes calcium less available to the tissues and causes symptoms of hypocalcaemia. It can be mimicked by liquorice ingestion and Liddle syndrome.

endocrine

Measuring aldosterone alone is not considered adequate to make a diagnosis of Conn syndrome. Rather, both renin and aldosterone are measured, and it is the ratio of these that is diagnostic. Usually, renin levels are suppressed, leading to a very low renin to aldosterone ratio (<0.05). This test is confounded by antihypertensive drugs, which have to be stopped for up to 6 weeks. If there is biochemical proof of hyperaldosteronism, computed tomographic scanning can confirm the presence of an adrenal adenoma.

Congenital adrenal hyperplasia presents in the paediatric age group and the most common variety, 21-OH deficiency, is associated with salt wasting. Cushing's syndrome does not explain the hypokalaemia and normal blood glucose. Nelson's syndrome is increased adrenocorticotrophic hormone (ACTH) secretion from a pituitary adenoma, which does not fit with the results of the laboratory investigations. A phaeochromocytoma could be part of a MEN IIA or MEN IIB syndrome and asymptomatic, but many episodically secrete catecholamines and can produce hypertension. However, hypokalemia will not be a feature of a phaeochromocytoma.

## 12.9

*Answer: B* Psammoma bodies are a common histological feature

De Quervain's thyroiditis, also known as 'subacute granulomatous thyroiditis' or 'subacute thyroiditis', usually occurs in women aged 30–50 years. It is believed to be have a viral aetiology and is usually preceded by an upper respiratory tract infection. Patients will initially experience a hyperthyroid period (extravasation of colloid), with neck pain and fever, and then will become hypothyroid before becoming euthyroid again. The symptoms are therefore those of hyperthyroidism and hypothyroidism. In addition, patients will also suffer from painful dysphagia. Psammoma bodies are typically seen in papillary carcinoma of the thyroid. De Quervain's thyroiditis is characterised by granulomatous inflammation with giant cells and follicular destruction. It is self-limiting and runs a course of weeks to months.

endocrine

## 12.10

*Answer: C* Craniopharyngioma

Craniopharyngiomas comprise 9% of all paediatric brain tumours and usually occur in children between the ages of 5 years and 10 years. They are very slow-growing tumours. They arise from the cells along the pituitary stalk. Craniopharyngioma is a rare, usually suprasellar neoplasm, which can be cystic. It develops from the nests of epithelium derived from Rathke's pouch. The histological pattern consists of nests of squamous epithelium bordered by radially arranged cells. It is often accompanied by calcium deposition and shows a papillary type of architecture. These tumours are also known as 'Rathke pouch tumours', 'hypophyseal duct tumours' or 'adamantinomas'.

ACTH-secreting adenomas of the anterior pituitary are rare and are often microadenomas. Astrocytomas in the paediatric age range are usually in the posterior fossa. Gliomas are unlikely to erode bone and have calcifications. Null cell adenomas of the anterior pituitary can produce mass effects, with headache and visual field defects but they are not suprasellar. Prolactinomas arise in the anterior pituitary in the sella and are often small and slow-growing, though they are commonly associated with headaches and visual field disturbances.

## 12.11

*Answer: C* Meningococcaemia

The clinical presentation in this scenario is suggestive of Waterhouse–Friderichsen syndrome secondary to meningococcaemia. The annual incidence of Addison's disease is approximately 4/100,000. It occurs in all age groups, has an equal sex distribution, and tends to become clinically apparent during metabolic stress or trauma. The onset of severe symptoms (for example the adrenal crisis seen in this case) can be precipitated by acute infection, usually meningococcal (a common cause, especially with septicaemia). Other causes include trauma, surgery, and sodium loss from excessive sweating.

endocrine

## 12.12

*Answer: B*    Multiple endocrine neoplasia type IIA

The multiple endocrine neoplasia (MEN) syndromes comprise three genetically distinct familial diseases in which adenomatous hyperplasia and malignant tumours are found in several endocrine glands. The clinical features depend on the glandular elements present. Each syndrome is inherited as an autosomal dominant trait with a high degree of penetrance and variable expressivity, with the production of seemingly unrelated effects by a single mutant gene. The specific genetic abnormalities are not always known.

In this scenario the patient has multiple endocrine neoplasia, type IIA (MEN IIA) which is characterised by medullary carcinoma of the thyroid, phaeochromocytoma and hyperparathyroidism. MEN IIA should be suspected in patients with bilateral phaeochromocytoma, a familial history of MEN, or at least two of its characteristic endocrine manifestations. The diagnosis is confirmed by genetic testing. Many cases come to medical attention after bilateral phaeochromocytomas are diagnosed in a relative.

Medullary carcinoma of the thyroid is diagnosed by measuring plasma calcitonin after provocative infusion of pentagastrin and calcium. In most patients with palpable thyroid lesions, basal calcitonin levels are elevated; in early disease, the basal levels may be normal, and the medullary carcinoma can be diagnosed only by an exaggerated response to calcium and pentagastrin. Early diagnosis of medullary carcinoma of the thyroid is important so that the tumour can be removed while still localised.

Because phaeochromocytoma can be asymptomatic, its exclusion can be difficult. The most sensitive tests are plasma free metanephrines and fractionated urinary catecholamines, particularly adrenaline (epinephrine). Computed tomography or magnetic resonance imaging are useful for locating the phaeochromocytoma or establishing the presence of bilateral lesions. Hyperparathyroidism is diagnosed by the presence of hypercalcaemia, hypophosphataemia and an increased parathyroid hormone level.

endocrine

Genetic testing, used to confirm the diagnosis, is highly accurate. First-degree relatives and any symptomatic relatives of the index patient should also undergo genetic testing. Annual screening for hyperparathyroidism and phaeochromocytoma should begin in early childhood and continue indefinitely. Screening for hyperparathyroidism is performed by measuring the serum calcium. Screening for phaeochromocytoma includes a symptom history, measurement of the blood pressure and laboratory testing.

## 12.13

*Answer: A*    Adrenal cortical carcinoma

Adrenocortical carcinoma is a rare malignancy and has a poor prognosis. The reported incidence of adrenal carcinoma is two per million. When identified, tumours are often large, measuring 4–10 cm in diameter. Adrenal carcinomas arise from the adrenal cortex and are bilateral in up to 10% of patients. Approximately 50%–80% are functional tumours, with most causing Cushing syndrome (as is the case in this scenario). Overall, there is an approximately equal sex distribution, but functional tumours are slightly more common in women, while non-functional tumours are slightly more common in men. Men with adrenocortical carcinoma often tend to be older than women who have this tumour and appear to have a worse prognosis.

## 12.14

*Answer: D*    Papillary carcinoma of the thyroid

Papillary carcinoma of the thyroid has the best prognosis. It accounts for 70%–80% of all thyroid cancers. The female to male ratio is 3 : 1, and the tumour is familial in up to 5% of patients. Most patients present between the ages of 30 years and 60 years. The tumour is often more aggressive in elderly patients. Many papillary carcinomas contain follicular elements. The tumour spreads via lymphatics to regional lymph nodes in a third of patients and can metastasise to the lungs. Patients aged under 45 years with small tumours confined to the thyroid have an excellent prognosis. About 10%–20% of patients, mainly the elderly, have recurrent or persistent disease.

endocrine

## 12.15

*Answer:* C    Parathyroid adenoma

The elevated serum calcium and hypophosphataemia point to parathyroid disease, and adenomas are more common than hyperplasia. Metastatic carcinoma would be unusual at this age. Primary hyperparathyroidism is caused by parathyroid adenoma in 80%–85% of patients, by multiple parathyroid adenomas in 2%–3%, by parathyroid hyperplasia in 10%–15% and by parathyroid carcinoma in 2%–3%. Common clinical presentations include nephrolithiasis (stones), bone pain (bones), arthralgias, muscular aches, peptic ulcer disease, pancreatitis (groans), fatigue, depression (moans), anxiety and other mental disturbances.

## 12.16

*Answer:* E    Secondary hyperparathyroidism

Secondary hyperparathyroidism refers to the excessive secretion of parathyroid hormone (PTH) by the parathyroid glands in response to hypocalcaemia. The parathyroid glands show hyperplasia and hypertrophy. This disorder is often seen in patients with chronic renal failure. Bone and joint pain are common, as are limb deformities. The elevated PTH also has pleiotropic effects on the blood, immune system and neurological system. In chronic renal failure the failing kidneys do not convert enough vitamin D to its active form, and they do not excrete phosphorus adequately. When this happens, insoluble calcium phosphate forms in the body, removing calcium from the circulation. Both processes leads to hypocalcaemia and therefore to secondary hyperparathyroidism.

endocrine

## 12.17

*Answer: D*   Prolactinoma

This finding is typical of a pituitary adenoma that is enlarging and compressing the optic chiasma. Prolactinoma is the most common adenoma. The symptoms experienced in women and men are as for hyperprolactinaemia from any cause. In addition, macroprolactinomas, by their very size, can press on surrounding structures, causing headaches or loss of vision from pressure on the optic chiasma. Unlike women, who can observe a disruption of menstruation, men have no reliable indicator to signal a problem and so often delay going to the doctor until they have headaches or eye problems. A craniopharyngioma is an uncommon lesion that usually appears in children and young adults.

## 12.18

*Answer: D*   Small-cell anaplastic (oat cell) carcinoma

These findings point to Cushing syndrome arising from glucocorticoid excess. Ectopic adrenocorticotrophic hormone from an oat cell carcinoma is one possible cause. The presence of tenderness in the lower back could be due to metastatic disease because oat cell carcinoma is the most widely metastatic of all tumours.

## 12.19

*Answer: B*   Serum calcium

The total thyroidectomy might also have damaged or removed the parathyroids. The serum calcium level is requested postoperatively to prevent potential problems associated with hypocalcaemia due to hypoparathyroidism.

endocrine

## 12.20

*Answer: E*    Thyroglossal duct cyst

A thyroglossal duct cyst is a vestigial remnant of thyroid development that can become manifest at any age. It is the most common clinically significant congenital thyroid anomaly. The most common locations for a thyroglossal cyst are midline or slightly off-midline, between the isthmus of the thyroid and the hyoid bone or just above the hyoid bone. A thyroglossal cyst can develop anywhere along the thyroglossal duct, though cysts within the tongue or in the floor of the mouth are rare.

Women are affected more commonly than men. A thyroglossal cyst will move upwards with protrusion of the tongue. Thyroglossal cysts are associated with an increased incidence of ectopic thyroid tissue. Occasionally, a lingual thyroid can be seen as a flattened, strawberry-like lump at the base of the tongue. Very rarely, the persistent duct can become cancerous (thyroglossal duct carcinoma), where the cancerous cells are ectopic thyroid tissue that has been deposited along the thyroglossal duct. This usually follows exposure to radiation.

endocrine

# SECTION 13:
# BREAST AND FEMALE
# REPRODUCIVE PATHOLOGY —
# ANSWERS

## 13.1

*Answer: E*    The opposite breast might also be involved

Lobular carcinoma of the breast can be divided into in-situ and invasive forms, and they both arise from the acini or terminal ductules of the lobule. It accounts for about 10% of breast carcinomas. It tends to be multifocal within the same breast, and is bilateral in 20% of cases. Metastases often seed the peritoneum. In-situ disease progresses to invasive carcinoma at a rate of 15% over a 20-year period.

## 13.2

*Answer: E*    Virginal breast hypertrophy

Virginal breast hypertrophy is also known as 'juvenile macromastia' and 'juvenile gigantomastia'. It causes excessive growth of the breasts during puberty and is much more common than the rare cases of breast hypertrophy in pregnancy. Virginal breast hypertrophy normally starts when puberty starts, soon after the girl's first menstrual period. The breast growth is sometimes not constant and comes in 'growth spurts'. At times, women can have minimal or no breast growth and then experience a growth spurt where the breasts grow very rapidly in a short space of time. These growth spurts cause great physical discomfort, the main symptoms being red, itchy skin and sometimes a general ache in the breasts. At puberty the breasts can also grow continuously at an even pace over several years. This process can overdevelop a completely normal and healthy breast, sometimes to gigantic proportions. Enlargement of the nipples usually also occurs, and the nipples can grow to an enormous size.

## 13.3

*Answer: B*  Fibroadenoma

Fibroadenoma of the breast is a benign tumour that is characterised by proliferation of both glandular and stromal elements. Most often it appears before the age of 30 years, and results from oestrogenic hormonal excess. The tumour is usually solitary and multiple tumours are rare. The tumour is mobile and not adherent to adjacent structures.

Macroscopically, the tumour is round, elastic, nodular and encapsulated (ie well circumscribed), its cut surface being grey-white in colour. Microscopically, the epithelial proliferation describes duct-like spaces surrounded by a fibroblastic stroma. Depending on the amount and the relationship between these two components, there are two main histological types: intracanalicular and pericanalicular. Both types are commonly found in the same tumour. In intracanalicular fibroadenoma the stromal proliferation predominates and compresses the ducts, which are irregular and reduced to slits. In pericanalicular fibroadenoma the fibrous stroma proliferates around the ductal spaces, so that they remain round or oval on cross-section. The basement membrane is intact.

## 13.4

*Answer: A*  Acute mastitis

Acute mastitis is a bacterial infection of the breast, and results in the classic signs of infection – pain (*dolor*), redness (*rubor*), swelling (*turgor*) and warmth (*calor*). Most often it occurs 2–3 weeks after delivery but it can occur at any time. Typical causative organisms include *Staphylococcus aureus*, *Streptococcus* species, and *Escherichia coli*. Prompt treatment can prevent complications such as abscess formation. Antibiotics, continued breastfeeding, and plenty of rest are the treatments of choice. In severe cases intravenous antibiotics can be required.

## 13.5

*Answer: B*  Cyst formation

Breast cysts are very common and are rarely associated with cancer. With a cyst, the lump feels smooth and firm, moves easily, and might be tender. If several cysts are grouped together, any swelling may feel irregular. Cysts often occur in both breasts and can develop anywhere within them. About 10% of women develop recurrent cysts. The fluid within the cyst comes from fluid in the breast which occurs as part of a woman's normal menstrual cycle. Towards the end of the menstrual cycle the cells in the breasts enlarge and swell. After a period the cells shrink and the fluid that is released disappears. But in some cases this fluid remains in the breast and forms a cyst. Cysts are most common in women in their thirties and forties and tend to disappear after the menopause. They are linked to oral contraceptive intake. Women who take hormone replacement therapy can also develop breast cysts because their breasts are similar to those of a younger woman.

## 13.6

*Answer: D*  Phyllodes tumour

Phyllodes tumours are typically large, fast-growing masses that arise from the periductal stroma of the breast. They account for less than 1% of all breast neoplasms. Phyllodes tumours are fibroepithelial tumours that are composed of an epithelial component and a cellular stromal component. They can be benign, borderline or malignant, depending on the histological features (stromal cellularity, infiltration at the tumour's edge, mitotic activity). This is predominantly a tumour of adult women, with very few cases reported in adolescents. Most occur in women between the ages of 40 years and 50 years, prior to the menopause. This is about 15 years older than the typical age of patients with fibroadenoma, a condition with which phyllodes tumours can be confused.

female

## 13.7

*Answer: D*    Pain and contracture

A breast implant is a prosthesis used to enlarge the size of a woman's breasts for cosmetic reasons, to reconstruct the breast (eg after a mastectomy or to correct genetic deformities), or as an aspect of male-to-female sex reassignment surgery. There are two primary types of breast implants, saline-filled and silicone gel-filled implants. Saline implants have a silicone elastomer shell filled with sterile saline liquid. Silicone gel implants have a silicone shell filled with a viscous silicone gel. A variety of other types of breast implant have been developed, such as polypropylene string or soy oil, but these are not seen commonly.

Local complications that can occur with breast implants include postoperative bleeding (haematoma), fluid collections (seroma), surgical site infection, breast pain, alterations in nipple sensation, interference with breastfeeding, visible wrinkling, asymmetric appearance, wound dehiscence (with potential implant exposure), thinning of the breast tissue and synmastia (disruption of the natural plane between breasts).

## 13.8

*Answer: A*    Axillary lymph node metastases

Invasion of the lymphatics is a poor prognostic sign, because it suggests that the carcinoma is spreading. A family history makes breast cancer more likely, but does not predict the prognosis. Aneuploidy, diagnosed with flow cytometry, suggests a worse prognosis. An oestrogen receptor-postitive tumour has a better prognosis because it will respond to certain therapies.In-situ lesions are the lowest stage possible for a carcinoma and carry an excellent prognosis if excised.

**13.9**

*Answer: E* *Staphylococcus aureus* infection

A breast abscess due to staphylococcal infection is the most likely diagnosis. These are most common in the postpartum period when the nipple becomes cracked or fissured with nursing. Fat necrosis is usually caused by trauma and leads to the formation of an ill-defined mass. Ductal carcinomas are ill-defined masses that are not usually tender. They are extremely rare before age 25 years. Sclerosing adenosis is a part of fibrocystic disease, which can lead to a cystic mass that can be tender, but without nipple fissuring. A 'plasma cell mastitis' is the result of inspissated duct secretions and is seen in women in their forties and fifties.

**13.10**

*Answer: E* Paget's disease of the breast

Paget's disease of the breast, also known as 'Paget's disease of the nipple', is a condition that outwardly can resemble eczema, with skin changes involving the nipple of the breast. Because of its seemingly innocuous appearance, it often presents late, but it is a condition that can be fatal. There is typically an underlying carcinoma. It results when malignant cells from an underlying carcinoma that originated in the ducts of the mammary glands spread to the epithelium. It usually affects only one nipple and presents with redness, oozing and crusting, and a sore that does not heal.

**13.11**

*Answer: C* Intraductal papilloma

Intraductal papilloma is a small benign tumour that grows within a milk duct of the breast, and is most common in women aged 35–55 years. The causes and risk factors are unknown. Intraductal papilloma is the most common cause of spontaneous nipple discharge from a single duct. A small lump beneath the nipple might be felt by the examiner, but it is not always palpable. A mammogram often does not show papillomas, but ultrasound and ductography can be helpful. Cytologicical examination of discharge might identify potentially malignant cells, but a breast biopsy is necessary to make a definitive diagnosis and rule out cancer.

## 13.12

*Answer: D*   Medullary carcinoma of breast

Medullary carcinoma of breast is a special type of infiltrating breast cancer that has a rather well-defined, distinct boundary between tumour tissue and normal tissue. It also has some other special features, including the large size of the cancer cells and the presence of lymphoid cells at the edges of the tumour. They can be difficult to distinguish from invasive ductal carcinoma. Medullary carcinoma accounts for about 5% of breast cancers. The prognosis for medullary carcinoma is better than for other types of invasive breast cancer.

## 13.13

*Answer: A*   Hepatic failure

Gynaecomastia is hypertrophy of breast tissue in males. During puberty, enlargement of the male breast is normal. It is usually transient, bilateral, smooth, firm and symmetrically distributed under the areola; the breasts can be tender. Similar changes can occur during old age but are more often unilateral. Most of the enlargement is due to proliferation of stroma, not of breast ducts.

Gynaecomastia can be caused by various disorders (especially hepatic and renal failure; less commonly, endocrine disorders), drugs (eg anabolic steroid abuse, antineoplastic drugs, calcium-channel blockers, cimetidine, digitalis, oestrogens, isoniazid, ketoconazole, methadone, metronidazole, reserpine, spironolactone, theophylline) and marijuana. Gynaecomastia is rarely confused with cancer, which is asymmetric, hard, and often fixed to dermis or fascia. Usually, the only imaging or other diagnostic test needed is mammography. In most cases, no specific treatment is needed because gynaecomastia usually remits spontaneously or disappears after any causative drug (except perhaps anabolic steroids) is stopped or underlying disorder is treated.

## 13.14

*Answer: D*   Microglandular hyperplasia

Microglandular hyperplasia (endocervical polyp) occurs secondary to oral contraceptives (progestagens) and must be distinguished from adenocarcinoma histologically. Cervical polyps are common benign growths of the cervix and endocervix, and originate in the endocervical canal. They occur in about 2%–5% of women. Most cervical polyps are asymptomatic. Endocervical polyps can bleed between menses or after intercourse and can become infected, causing purulent vaginal discharge (leukorrhoea). Endocervical polyps are usually reddish-pink, measure less than 1 cm in all dimensions, and are friable. They are rarely malignant.

## 13.15

*Answer: B*   Fibrothecoma

A fibrothecoma is a benign ovarian tumour. The thecoma component of the neoplasm gives the tumour a yellowish appearance because of the lipid content and can also produce oestrogen, which is responsible for the endometrial hyperplasia. These are tumours that arise from the ovarian stroma. They are bilateral in only about 10% of cases. A right-sided hydrothorax in association with this tumour is known as 'Meigs' syndrome'.

## 13.16

*Answer: B*   It causes dyspareunia

Endometriosis is a non-cancerous disorder in which functioning endometrial tissue is implanted outside the uterine cavity. It is usually confined to the peritoneal or serosal surfaces of abdominal organs, commonly the ovaries, broad ligaments, posterior cul-de-sac and uterosacral ligaments. Less common sites include the serosal surfaces of the small and large intestines, ureters, bladder, vagina, cervix, surgical scars, pleura and pericardium. Bleeding from these peritoneal implants is thought to initiate inflammation, followed by fibrin deposition, adhesion formation and, eventually, scarring, which distorts the peritoneal surfaces of organs and the pelvic anatomy.

female

The most widely accepted pathophysiological hypothesis is that endometrial cells are transported from the uterine cavity and subsequently become implanted at ectopic sites. Retrograde flow of menstrual tissue through the Fallopian tubes could transport endometrial cells intra-abdominally; the lymphatic or circulatory system could transport endometrial cells to distant sites (such as the pleural cavity). Another hypothesis is coelomic metaplasia, where coelomic epithelium is transformed into endometrium-like glands. Microscopically, endometriotic implants consist of glands and stroma identical to intrauterine endometrium. These tissues contain oestrogen and progesterone receptors and so usually grow, differentiate, and bleed in response to changes in hormone levels during the menstrual cycle.

The symptoms depend on the location of the implants and can include dysmenorrhoea, dyspareunia, infertility, dysuria and pain during defecation. The incidence of endometriosis is increased in first-degree relatives of women with endometriosis, suggesting that heredity is a factor. The incidence is also increased in women who delay childbearing, who have shortened menstrual cycles (<27 days) with menses that are abnormally long (>8 days), or who have Müllerian duct anomalies. The reported incidence varies but is probably about 10%–15% in actively menstruating women aged 25–44 years. The average age at diagnosis is 27 years, but endometriosis also occurs in adolescents. About 25%–50% of infertile women have endometriosis. In patients with severe endometriosis and distorted pelvic anatomy, the incidence of infertility is high because mechanisms of ovum pick-up and tubal transport are impaired. Some patients with minimal endometriosis and normal pelvic anatomy can also be infertile: in these patients, fertility might be decreased because the incidence of luteal phase dysfunction or luteinised unruptured ovarian follicle syndrome (trapped oocyte) is increased, because peritoneal prostaglandin production or peritoneal macrophage activity is increased (resulting in phagocytosis), or because the endometrium is non-receptive. Potential protective factors seem to be multiple pregnancies, the use of low-dose oral contraceptives (continuous or cyclic), and regular exercise (especially if begun before the age of 15 years or if undertaken for more than 7 hours per week, or both).

**13.17**

*Answer: E* Ovarian serous cystadenocarcinoma

Ovarian carcinomas are often associated with ascites because they seed throughout the peritoneal cavity. Psammoma body formation is common. Ovarian cancer affects mainly perimenopausal and postmenopausal women. Nulliparity, delayed childbearing and delayed menopause increase the risk; oral contraceptive use decreases the risk. A personal or family history of endometrial, breast or colon cancer also increases the risk. Probably 5%–10% of ovarian cancers are related to mutations in the autosomal dominant *BRCA* gene. XY gonadal dysgenesis predisposes to ovarian germ cell cancer.

Ovarian cancers are histologically diverse. At least 80% originate in the epithelium; 75% of these cancers are serous cystadenocarcinomas, and the rest include mucinous, endometrioid, transitional cell, clear cell and unclassified carcinomas, and Brenner tumours. The remaining 20% of ovarian cancers originate in primary ovarian germ cells or in sex cord and stromal cells, or are metastases to the ovary (most commonly from the breast or gastrointestinal tract). Germ cell cancers usually occur in women under the age of 30 years and include dysgerminomas, immature teratomas, endodermal sinus tumours, embryonal carcinomas, choriocarcinomas and polyembryomas. Stromal (sex cord–stromal) cancers include granulosa-theca cell tumours and Sertoli–Leydig cell tumours.

Ovarian cancer spreads by direct extension, exfoliation of cells into the peritoneal cavity (peritoneal seeding), lymphatic dissemination to the pelvis and around the aorta or, less often, haematogenously to the liver or lungs.

**13.18**

*Answer: D* Human papillomavirus infection

Cervical cancer results from cervical intraepithelial neoplasia (CIN), which appears to be caused by infection with human papillomavirus (HPV) types 16, 18, 31, 33, 35 or 39. Risk factors for cervical cancer include younger age at the time of first intercourse, a high lifetime number of sex partners and intercourse with men whose previous partners had cervical cancer. Other factors, including cigarette smoking and immunodeficiency also appear to contribute to the risk. CIN is graded as grade 1 (mild cervical dysplasia), grade 2 (moderate dysplasia) or grade 3 (severe dysplasia and carcinoma in situ). CIN 3 is unlikely to regress spontaneously; if untreated, it can, over months or years, penetrate the basement membrane, becoming invasive carcinoma. About 80%–85% of all cervical cancers are squamous cell carcinoma; most of the rest are adenocarcinomas. Sarcomas and small-cell neuroendocrine tumours are rare. Invasive cervical cancer usually spreads by direct extension into surrounding tissues or via the lymphatics to the pelvic and para-aortic lymph nodes. Haematogenous spread also occurs.

## 13.19

*Answer: E*    Serum β-hCG

Gestational trophoblastic disease is a tumour originating from the trophoblast, which surrounds the blastocyst and develops into the chorion and amnion. This disease can occur during or after an intrauterine or ectopic pregnancy. If the disease occurs during a pregnancy, spontaneous abortion, eclampsia or fetal death typically occur; the fetus rarely survives. Some forms are malignant; others are benign but behave aggressively.

If gestational trophoblastic disease is suspected, testing includes measurement of serum beta subunit of human chorionic gonadotrophin (β-hCG) and pelvic ultrasonography. A very high β-hCG level might suggest the diagnosis, but a biopsy is required to confirm it. After the tumour has been removed, gestational trophoblastic disease is classified clinically to determine whether additional treatment is needed. (The clinical classification system does not correspond to the morphological classification system.) A chest X-ray is taken and the serum β-hCG is measured. If the β-hCG level does not normalise within 10 weeks, the disease is classified as persistent. Persistent disease requires investigation by computed tomography of the brain, chest, abdomen and pelvis, the results of these dictating whether disease is classified as non-metastatic or metastatic. Persistent disease is usually treated with chemotherapy.

Treatment is considered successful if at least three consecutive serum β-hCG measurements at 1-week intervals are normal. Beta-hCG is used for follow-up.

## 13.20

*Answer: D*   Imperforate hymen

Haematocolpos (accumulation of menstrual blood in the vagina), which can cause the vagina to bulge, and haematometra (accumulation of blood in the uterus), which can cause uterine distension or a mass, are most likely to be associated with an imperforate hymen. In about 1 in 2000 females, the hymen fails to develop any opening at all: this is called an imperforate hymen and if it does not spontaneously resolve itself before puberty a physician will need to make a hole in the hymen to allow menstrual discharge to escape.

female

# SECTION 14:
# MALE REPRODUCTIVE PATHOLOGY
# — ANSWERS

## 14.1

*Answer: D    Staphylococcus aureus*

Balanitis is inflammation of the glans penis. When the foreskin (or prepuce) is also affected, it is called 'balanoposthitis'. Lack of aeration and irritation because of smegma and discharge surrounding the glans penis causes inflammation and oedema. Staphylococcal and streptococcal infections are most likely to be present in this situation. While any man can develop balanitis, the condition is most likely to occur in men who have a tight foreskin that is difficult to pull back, or who have poor hygiene. Diabetes can make balanitis more likely, especially if the blood sugar is poorly controlled.

## 14.2

*Answer: E    Phimosis*

Phimosis is a medical condition in which the foreskin of the penis of an uncircumcised male cannot be fully retracted. In most (but not all) infants phimosis is physiological rather than pathological, whereas in older children and adults phimosis is more often pathological than physiological. It has been suggested that physiological infantile phimosis should be referred to as 'developmental non-retractility of the foreskin' in order to distinguish this normal stage of development more clearly from pathological forms of phimosis.

When phimosis develops in an uncircumcised adult who was previously able to retract his foreskin, it is nearly always due to a pathological cause, and is far more likely to cause problems for the man. An important cause of acquired, pathological phimosis is chronic balanitis xerotica obliterans, a skin condition of unknown origin that causes a whitish ring of indurated tissue (a cicatrix) to form near the tip of the prepuce. This inelastic tissue prevents retraction.

Some evidence suggests that balanitis xerotica obliterans could be the same disease as lichen sclerosus et atrophicus of the vulva in females. Infectious, inflammatory and hormonal factors have all been implicated or proposed as contributing factors. Circumcision is usually recommended, though alternatives have been advocated. Phimosis can also occur after other types of chronic inflammation (eg balanoposthitis), repeated catheterisation, or forceful foreskin retraction.

## 14.3

*Answer: D*  Hypospadias

Hypospadias is a birth defect of the urethra in the male that involves an abnormally placed urethral meatus. Instead of opening at the tip of the glans penis, a hypospadic urethra opens anywhere along a line (the urethral groove) running from the tip, along the underside or ventral aspect of the shaft, to the junction of the penis and scrotum or perineum. A distal hypospadias might be suspected, even in an uncircumcised boy, if there is an abnormally formed foreskin and downward tilt of the glans.

The urethral meatus opens on the glans penis in about 50%–75% of cases; these are categorised as first-degree hypospadias. Second-degree hypospadias (when the urethra opens on the shaft) and third-degree hypospadias (when the urethra opens on the perineum) occur in up to 20% and 30% of cases, respectively. The more severe degrees are more likely to be associated with chordee, in which the phallus is incompletely separated from the perineum or is still tethered downwards by connective tissue, or with undescended testes (cryptorchidism).

Hypospadias is one of the most common birth defects of the male genitalia (second to cryptorchidism), but widely varying incidences have been reported from different countries, from as low as 1 in 4000 to as high as 1 in 125 boys. Most cases of hypospadias are sporadic, without any inheritance pattern or family recurrence. For most cases, no cause can be identified, though a number of hypotheses related to inadequate androgen effect, or environmental agents interfering with androgen effect have been offered.

## 14.4

*Answer: B*    Dark-field microscopic examination of exudate or secretions

Primary syphilis is typically acquired via direct sexual contact with the infectious lesions of a person with syphilis. A skin lesion might be seen on the genitalia approximately 10–90 days after the initial exposure (average 21 days). This lesion, called a 'chancre', is a firm, painless skin ulceration located at the point of initial exposure to the spirochaete, often on the penis, vagina or rectum. Rarely, there can be multiple lesions present, although typically only one lesion is seen. The lesion can persist for 4–6 weeks and usually heals spontaneously. Local lymph node swelling can occur. During the initial incubation period individuals are otherwise asymptomatic. As a result, many patients do not seek medical care immediately.

Microscopy of fluid from the primary or secondary lesion using dark-field illumination can be used to diagnose treponemal disease with high accuracy. As there are other treponemes that may be confused with *Treponema pallidum,* care must be taken in evaluating with microscopy to correlate symptoms with the correct disease. Present-day syphilis screening tests, such as the rapid plasma reagin (RPR) and Venereal Diseases Research Laboratory (VDRL) tests are cheap and fast but not completely specific, as many other conditions can cause a positive result. False positives can be seen in viral infections (Epstein–Barr virus, hepatitis, varicella, measles), lymphoma, tuberculosis, malaria, endocarditis, connective tissue disorders, pregnancy, intravenous drug abuse or with contamination. As a result, these two screening tests should always be followed up by a more specific treponemal test. Tests based on monoclonal antibodies and immunofluorescence, including the *Treponema pallidum* haemagglutination assay (TPHA) and the fluorescent treponemal antibody absorption (FTA-ABS) test are more specific and more expensive. Unfortunately, false positives can still occur in related treponomal infections such as yaws and pinta. Tests based on enzyme-linked immunoassays are also used to confirm the results of simpler screening tests for syphilis.

male

## 14.5

*Answer: A*   Embryonal carcinoma

Embryonal carcinoma is one of the four germ cell tumours, the other three being seminoma, teratoma and choriocarcinoma. Like any cancer, embryonal carcinoma grows because its cells are dividing rapidly and indefinitely. The embryonal carcinoma can spread up the epididymis to the vas deferens and can also spread to the rest of the body, including the lymph nodes that run along the aorta.

Unlike the other types of testicular cancers, an embryonal carcinoma can contain several elements of a maldeveloped fetus, including cartilage. The main tumour is, on average, 2.5 cm in length and can also stem out approximately 9 cm up the testicular cord. Embryonal carcinomas are usually seen in males aged 25–35 years, but have also been found in males in their late teens. The chances of an embryonal carcinoma spreading from one testicle to the other are less than 1%. Embryonal carcinomas account for approximately 25% of testicular tumours. Rarely, embryonal carcinomas are seen in females, in the ovaries.

## 14.6

*Answer: D*   Spermatocoele

Spermatocoele (spermatic cyst) usually occurs at the upper pole of the testis, adjacent to the epididymis, and appears as a cystic scrotal mass. A large spermatocoele might be difficult to differentiate from a hydrocoele, which also is cystic and painless and transilluminates. Ultrasonography can be helpful in reaching a diagnosis. Surgical excision is indicated if the spermatocoele becomes large and bothersome.

## 14.7

*Answer: E*   Varicocoele

A varicocoele is an abnormal enlargement of the veins in the scrotum draining the testis. The testicular blood vessels originate in the abdomen and course down through the inguinal canal as

male

part of the spermatic cord on their way to the testis. Upward flow of blood in the veins is ensured by small one-way valves. Defective valves, or compression of the vein by a nearby structure, can cause dilatation of the veins near the testis, leading to the formation of a varicocoele.

The term 'varicocoele' specifically refers to dilatation and tortuosity of the pampiniform plexus, which is the network of veins that drain the testicle. This plexus travels along the posterior portion of the testicle with the epididymis and vas deferens, and then into the spermatic cord. This network of veins coalesces into the gonadal (or testicular) vein. The right gonadal vein drains into the inferior vena cava, while the left gonadal vein drains into the left renal vein, which then drains into the inferior vena cava. The small vessels of the pampiniform plexus normally range from 0.5–1.5 mm in diameter. A varicocoele is dilatation of these vessels to greater than 2 mm.

**Idiopathic varicocoele** occurs when the valves within the veins along the spermatic cord do not work properly. This is essentially the same process as varicose veins, which are common in the legs. This results in backflow of blood into the pampiniform plexus and causes increased pressures, ultimately leading to damage to the testicular tissue. Varicocoeles usually develop slowly and might not cause any symptoms. They are most commonly diagnosed when a patient is 15–25 years of age, and rarely develop after the age of 40 years. They occur in 15%–20% of all males, and in 40% of infertile males. Approximately 98% of idiopathic varicocoeles occur on the left side, apparently because of the way the left testicular vein runs vertically up to the renal vein rather than directly into the vena cava. In 70% of cases the varicocoele occurs bilaterally. Isolated right-sided varicocoeles are rare, and should prompt evaluation for an abdominal or pelvic mass.

**Secondary varicocoele** is caused by compression of the venous drainage of the testicle. A pelvic or abdominal malignancy is a definite concern when a varicocoele is newly diagnosed in a patient over the age of 40 years. One non-malignant cause of a secondary varicocoele is the so-called 'nutcracker superior mesenteric artery', a condition in which the superior mesenteric artery compresses the left renal vein, causing increased pressures there to be transmitted in retrograde fashion into the left pampiniform plexus.

male

**Symptoms** of varicocoele include the following:

- Pain in the testis
- Feeling of heaviness in the testis
- Infertility
- Atrophy of the testis
- Visible or palpable enlarged vein.

Clinically, palpation of the scrotum will reveal a non-tender, twisted mass along the spermatic cord (classically likened to a bag of worms). The mass might not be obvious, especially when the patient is lying down. The testis on the side of the varicocoele might or might not be smaller compared with the testis on the other side. Varicocoele can be reliably diagnosed with ultrasound, which will show dilatation of the vessels of the pampiniform plexus to more than 2 mm. The patient should undergo a provocative manoeuvre, such as a Valsalva manoeuvre, or stand up during the examination, both of which are designed to increase intra-abdominal venous pressure and increase the dilatation of the veins.

## 14.8

*Answer: A*   Adenocarcinoma

Adenocarcinoma of the prostate is the most common non-dermatological cancer in men aged over 50 years. The incidence increases with each decade of life; autopsy studies show prostate cancer in 15%–60% of men aged 60–90 years, with the incidence increasing with age. The median age at diagnosis is 72 years, and over 75% of prostate cancers are diagnosed in men over the age of 65 years. The risk is highest for black men. Sarcoma of the prostate is rare, occurring primarily in children. Undifferentiated prostate cancer, squamous cell carcinoma, and ductal transitional carcinoma also occur. Hormonal influences contribute to the pathogenesis of adenocarcinoma but almost certainly not to that of other types of prostate cancer. Prostatic intraepithelial neoplasia is a precancerous histological change, and can be either low-grade or high-grade, which is considered to be a precursor of invasive cancer.

### 14.9

*Answer:* C    Peyronie's disease

Peyronie's disease is a connective tissue disorder involving the growth of fibrous plaques in the soft tissue of the penis and affects as many as 1% of men. A French surgeon, François de la Peyronie, first described the disease in 1743. The disease can cause pain, hardened, cord-like lesions (scar tissue known as 'plaques') or abnormal curvature of the penis when erect. In addition, narrowing and/or shortening of the penis can occur. The pain felt in the early stages of the disease often resolves after 12–18 months. Erectile dysfunction, in varying degrees, often accompanies these symptoms in the later stages of the disease process. The condition can also make sexual intercourse painful and/or difficult, though many men report satisfactory intercourse in spite of the disease.

Although it can affect men of any race and age, it is most commonly seen in white men over the age of 40 years. The disease only affects men and is confined to the penis, although about 30% of men with Peyronie's disease develop fibrosis in other elastic tissues of the body, such as on the hand or foot, including Dupuytren's contracture of the hand. An increased incidence in male relatives suggests a genetic component.

### 14.10

*Answer:* C    Seminoma

Germ cell tumours of the testis occur as the following subtypes and with the following frequencies: seminoma (40%), embryonal (25%), teratocarcinoma (25%), teratoma (5%) and choriocarcinoma (pure) (1%).

### 14.11

*Answer:* C    N2

Testicular seminoma is staged according to the American Joint Committee on Cancer (AJCC) 2002 staging guidelines. This is a TNM (tumour-node-metastasis) staging system comprising separate categories for the primary tumour, regional lymph nodes, distant metastases, and serum tumour markers; these four categories are used to determine the stage of the patient's disease. Modern treatment decisions are based in part on the subdivisions of this staging system.

According to the AJCC guidelines, the nodal staging is as follows:

N0: no regional lymph node metastases

N1: metastasis with lymph node(s) 2 cm or less in their greatest dimension or multiple lymph nodes, none more than 2 cm in their greatest dimension

N2: metastasis with lymph node(s) greater than 2 cm but not greater than 5 cm in their greatest dimension, or multiple lymph nodes, any one mass greater than 2 cm, but not more than 5 cm, in its greatest dimension

N3: metastasis with lymph node(s) greater than 5 cm in their greatest dimension

In this scenario, therefore, the patient has N2 disease.

## 14.12

*Answer:* C    T2

According to the AJCC guidelines (see *Answer* to **14.11**), the primary tumour staging for testicular seminoma is as follows:

Tis: intratubular germ cell neoplasia (carcinoma in situ)

T1: tumour limited to testis/epididymis without vascular or lymphatic invasion; the tumour can invade into the tunica albuginea but not the tunica vaginalis

T2: tumour limited to testis/epididymis with vascular or lymphatic invasion or tumour extending through the tunica albuginea with involvement of the tunica vaginalis

T3: tumour invading the spermatic cord, with or without vascular/lymphatic invasion

T4: tumour invading the scrotum, with or without vascular/lymphatic invasion

In this scenario, therefore, the patient has a T2 tumour.

## 14.13

*Answer: B*   S1

According to AJCC guidelines (see *Answer* to **14.11**), the serum tumour marker staging is as follows:

S0: marker studies within normal limits

S1: lactate dehydrogenase (LDH) less than 1.5 times the reference range, beta-human chorionic gonadotrophin (β-hCG) <5000 mIU/ml, and alpha-fetoprotein (AFP) <1000 ng/ml

S2: LDH 1.5–10 times the reference range , β-hCG 5000–50,000 mIU/ml or AFP 1000–10,000 ng/ml

S3: LDH greater than 10 times the reference range, β-hCG >50,000 mIU/ml or AFP >10,000 ng/ml

In this scenario, therefore, the patient has S1 serum tumour marker stage.

## 14.14

*Answer: E*   Stage IIC

According to AJCC guidelines (see *Answer* to 14.11), the clinical staging for testicular seminoma is as follows:

Stage IA: T1 N0 M0 S0

Stage IB: T2/3/4 N0 M0 S0

Stage IC: any T N0 M0 S1/2/3

Stage IIA: any T N1 M0 S0/1

Stage IIB: any T N2 M0 S0/1

Stage IIC: any T N3 M0 S0/1

Stage IIIA: any T any N M1a S0/1

Stage IIIB: any T any N M0/1a S2

Stage IIIC: any T any N M1a/1b S3

In this scenario, therefore, the patient has a T2 N3 M0 S1 seminoma, which fits into stage IIC disease.

male

## 14.15

*Answer: E*    It liquifies gelatinous semen after ejaculation

Prostate-specific antigen (PSA) is an enzyme produced by the prostate. Specifically, PSA is a serine protease similar to kallikrein. Its normal function is to liquify gelatinous semen after ejaculation, allowing spermatozoa to 'swim' more easily through the uterine cervix. PSA levels under 4 ng/ml are generally considered normal, while levels over 4 ng/ml are considered abnormal (although in men over the age of 65 years levels up to 6.5 ng/ml might be acceptable, depending upon each laboratory's reference ranges). PSA levels between 4 ng/ml and 10 ng/ml indicate a risk of prostate cancer that is higher than normal, but the risk does not seem to rise within this six-point range. When the PSA level is above 10 ng/ml, the association with cancer becomes stronger. However, PSA is not a perfect test. Some men with prostate cancer do not have an elevated PSA, and most men with an elevated PSA do not have prostate cancer.

PSA levels can change for many reasons other than cancer. Two common causes of high PSA levels are benign prostatic hyperplasia and prostatitis. It can also be raised for 24 hours after ejaculation and for several days after catheterisation. PSA levels are lowered in men who use medications used to treat benign prostatic hyperplasia or baldness. These medications, finasteride and dutasteride, can decrease the PSA levels by 50% or more.

## 14.16

*Answer: C*    T1c

Prostatic cancer is staged according to the American Joint Committee on Cancer (AJCC) 2002 staging guidelines. This is a TNM staging system comprising separate categories for the primary tumour, regional lymph nodes and distant metastases. It also uses histological grade information in conjunction with TNM status to group cases into four overall stages. According to AJCC guidelines, the primary tumour staging for prostatic cancer is as follows:

TX: cannot evaluate the primary tumour

T0: no evidence of tumour

T1: tumour present, but not detectable clinically or with imaging

T1a: tumour was incidentally found in less than 5% of prostate tissue resected (for other reasons)

T1b: tumour was incidentally found in more than 5% of prostate tissue resected

T1c: tumour was found in a needle biopsy performed due to an elevated serum prostate-specific antigen

T2: the tumour can be felt (palpated) on examination, but has not spread outside the prostate

T2a: the tumour is in half or less than half of one of the prostate gland's two lobes

T2b: the tumour is in more than half of one lobe, but not both

T2c: the tumour is in both lobes

T3: the tumour has spread through the prostatic capsule (if it is only part-way through, it is still T2)

T3a: the tumour has spread through the capsule on one or both sides

T3b: the tumour has invaded one or both seminal vesicles

T4: the tumour has invaded other nearby structures

It should be stressed that the designation 'T2c' implies a tumour which is palpable in both lobes of the prostate. Tumours which are found to be bilateral on biopsy only but which are not palpable bilaterally should not be staged as T2c. In this scenario, therefore, the patient has a T1c tumour.

## 14.17

*Answer:* C  Stage II

According to the AJCC guidelines (see *Answer* to **14.16**), the overall staging for prostatic cancer is summarised as in the following table:

| Stage | Tumour | Node | Metastasis | Grade |
|-------|--------|------|------------|-------|
| Stage I | T1a | N0 | M0 | G1 |
| Stage II | T1a | N0 | M0 | G2–4 |
| | T1b | N0 | M0 | any G |
| | T1c | N0 | M0 | any G |
| | T1 | N0 | M0 | any G |
| | T2 | N0 | M0 | any G |
| Stage III | T3 | N0 | M0 | any G |
| | T4 | N0 | M0 | any G |
| Stage IV | any T | N1 | M0 | any G |
| | any T | any N | M1 | any G |

In this scenario, therefore, the patient has a T2 N0 M0 G2 tumour, which makes it a stage II cancer.

## 14.18

*Answer: D*   It is a 5-alpha-reductase inhibitor

Finasteride is an anti-androgen which acts by inhibiting type 2 5-alpha reductase, the enzyme that converts testosterone to dihydrotestosterone. It is used as a treatment in benign prostatic hyperplasia in low doses, and in prostate cancer in higher doses. It is also indicated for use in combination with doxazosin therapy to reduce the risk of symptomatic progression of benign prostatic hyperplasia. Additionally, it is registered in many countries for male-pattern baldness.

## 14.19

*Answer: B*    T1

The TNM (tumour-node-metastasis) classification of the primary tumour of the penis is given below:

TX: primary tumour cannot be assessed

T0: primary tumour is not evident

Tis: carcinoma in situ is present

Ta: non-invasive verrucous carcinoma is present

T1: tumour is invading subepithelial connective tissue

T2: tumour is invading the corpora spongiosum or cavernosum

T3: tumour invading the urethra or prostate

T4: tumour invading other adjacent structures

In this scenario, therefore, the patient has a T1 primary tumour of the penis.


## 14.20

*Answer: E*    Teratoma

Testicular teratomas occur in both children and adults, but their incidence and natural history are quite different. Pure teratomas are fairly common in children, comprising nearly half of all germ cell tumours. They are relatively rare after puberty and comprise only 2%–3% of germ cell tumours in this age group. In children, they behave as a benign tumour, whereas in adults and adolescents they are invariably malignant.

Childhood testicular teratomas are uniformly benign, with no documented cases of retroperitoneal or lung metastasis in differentiated lesions. Most morbidity results from surgical or postoperative complications, such as haemorrhage or infection. The mortality is less than one per million. During and after puberty, all teratomas are regarded as malignant because even mature teratomas (composed of entirely mature histological elements) can metastasise to retroperitoneal lymph nodes or to other systems. Morbidity is associated with the growth of the tumour, which can invade or obstruct local structures and become unresectable.

male

Malignant transformation is significantly more common in testicular teratomas than in their ovarian counterparts, and the risk of recurrence is around 20% in both mature and immature testicular teratomas.

Testicular teratomas usually present as a painless scrotal mass, but sometimes present as testicular torsion. The masses are firm or hard in 83% of cases. Most are not tender and do not transilluminate. Testicular pain and scrotal swelling occasionally are reported with teratomas, but these are non-specific symptoms and simply indicate torsion until proved otherwise. Hydrocoele is often associated with teratoma in childhood. On examination, the testis is diffusely enlarged, rather than nodular, although a discrete nodule in the upper or lower pole can sometimes be palpated.

# SECTION 15:
# BONE AND JOINT PATHOLOGY
# — ANSWERS

## 15.1

*Answer: A*    Gout

Gout is precipitation of monosodium urate crystals into tissue, usually in and around joints. This usually causes recurrent acute or chronic arthritis. Acute arthritis is initially monoarticular and often involves the first metatarsophalangeal joint. Symptoms include acute pain, tenderness, warmth, redness and swelling. Diagnosis requires identification of crystals in synovial fluid.

Patients suspected of acute gouty arthritis should have arthrocentesis and synovial fluid analysis on initial presentation. Synovial fluid analysis can confirm the diagnosis by identifying needle-shaped, strongly negatively birefringent urate crystals that are either free in the fluid or engulfed by phagocytes. During attacks, synovial fluid shows inflammatory characteristics. The table below summarises the findings of microscopic examination of crystals in joints.

Microscopic Examination of Crystals in Joints

| Crystal Type | Birefringence | Elongation* | Shape | Length (μm) |
|---|---|---|---|---|
| Monosodium urate | Strong | Negative | Needle- or rod-shaped | 2–15 |
| Ca pyrophosphate dihydrate | Weak | Positive | Rhomboid- or rod- shaped | 2–15 |
| Ca oxalate† | Weak or strong | Positive or indeterminate | Bipyramidal | 5–30 |
| Basic Ca phosphate | Not birefringent with polarized light | — | Shiny, coinlike, or slightly irregular | 3–65 |

*Crystals that have negative elongation are yellow parallel to the axis of slow vibration marked on the compensator; positive elongation appears blue in the same direction.
†Occur primarily in patients with renal failure.

bone and joint

## 15.2

*Answer: D*    Paget's disease of bone

Paget's disease of bone is a chronic disorder of the adult skeleton in which bone turnover is accelerated in localised areas. Normal matrix is replaced with softened and enlarged bone. The disease can be asymptomatic or can cause gradual onset of bone pain or deformity. The cause of this disorder is unknown. The appearance of involved bone on electron microscopy suggests a viral infection, but a viral cause has not been established. Paget's disease is sometimes familial, but a specific genetic pattern has been suggested. About 1% of adults in the US aged over 40 years have Paget's disease, with a 3 : 2 male predominance. The disease is most common in Europe (except Scandinavia), Australia, and New Zealand.

Any bone can be involved. The bones most commonly affected are, in decreasing order: the pelvis, femur, skull, tibia, vertebrae, clavicle and humerus. Bone turnover is accelerated at involved sites. Pagetic lesions are metabolically active and highly vascular. Excessively active osteoclasts are often large and contain many nuclei. Osteoblastic repair is also hyperactive, producing coarsely woven, thickened lamellae and trabeculae. This abnormal structure weakens the bone, despite bony enlargement and heavy calcification. Overgrown bone can compress nerves and other structures passing through small foramina. Osteoarthritis can develop in joints adjacent to involved bone.

Paget's disease should be suspected in patients with unexplained bone pain or deformity. It should also be suspected in patients who have suggestive findings on X-ray, in patients who have an unexplained elevation of serum alkaline phosphatase on laboratory tests performed for other reasons, or in older patients who develop hypercalcaemia during bedrest.

If Paget's disease is suspected, plain X-rays and serum alkaline phosphatase, calcium, and phosphate levels should be obtained. Characteristic X-ray findings include increased bone density, abnormal architecture with coarse cortical trabeculation or cortical thickening, bowing and bony enlargement; there might also be stress microfractures of the tibia or femur. Characteristic laboratory findings include elevated serum alkaline phosphatase (due to the increased anabolic activity of the bone) but usually normal serum phosphate levels. The serum calcium is usually normal but can increase due to immobilisation or hyperparathyroidism. If the alkaline phosphatase is not elevated or if it is unclear whether the increased serum alkaline phosphatase is of bony origin, a bone-specific fraction can be measured.

## 15.3

*Answer: D*    Osteoid osteoma

Osteoid osteoma, which tends to affect young adults, can occur in any bone but is most common in long bones. It can cause pain (usually worse at night) that is typically relieved by mild analgesics, particularly aspirin. Physical examination can show atrophy of regional muscles. The characteristic appearance on X-ray is a small radiolucent zone surrounded by a larger sclerotic zone. If a tumour is suspected, a technetium-99m bone scan should be performed; an osteoid osteoma appears as an area of increased uptake.

## 15.4

*Answer: C*    Polymyalgia rheumatica

Polymyalgia rheumatica (PMR) is a syndrome closely associated with temporal arteritis. It affects older adults. The onset can be acute or subacute. PMR is characterised by severe pain and stiffness of the neck and pectoral and pelvic girdles; the stiffness is particularly severe in the morning or after a period of inactivity. Pain is most often localised to the proximal muscles rather than the joints, and symptoms are usually bilateral. Systemic symptoms, such as weight loss, malaise, fever and depression are common. PMR does not cause muscle weakness, although pain might limit muscular effort.

PMR should be suspected in older adults with the typical symptoms. Establishing the diagnosis requires the presence of characteristic symptoms and signs and the exclusion of alternative diagnoses. The erythrocyte sedimentation rate (ESR), full blood count, thyroid-stimulating hormone levels and creatine kinase are usually obtained. In most people, the ESR is elevated, often to over 100 mm/hour and usually to over 50 mm/hour (Westergren method). Normochromic

bone and joint

normocytic anaemia can be present. Electromyography, biopsy and other tests (eg rheumatoid factor) are normal in PMR but are sometimes performed in order to rule out alternative diagnoses.

## 15.5

*Answer: A*    Benign giant-cell tumour

These tumours, which most commonly affect people in their twenties and thirties, occur in the epiphyses and can erode the rest of the bone and extend into the soft tissues. Giant-cell tumours are notorious for their tendency to recur. Rarely, a giant-cell tumour can metastasise, even though it remains histologically benign. Benign giant-cell tumours appear lytic on X-ray.

## 15.6

*Answer: C*    Osteoarthritis

Osteoarthritis is a chronic arthropathy of an entire joint, with disruption and potential loss of joint cartilage, along with other joint changes, including bone hypertrophy (osteophyte formation). This most common joint disorder often becomes symptomatic in the forties and fifties and is nearly universal by the age of 80 years. Only half of those with the pathological changes of osteoarthritis have symptoms. Below the age of 40 years, most osteoarthritis occurs in men and results from trauma. Women predominate between the ages of 40 years and 70 years, after which men and women are affected equally.

Symptoms include gradually developing pain that is aggravated or triggered by activity, with stiffness relieved less than 30 minutes after activity, and occasional joint swelling. The joints most often affected in generalised osteoarthritis include the distal interphalangeal and proximal interphalangeal joints (producing Heberden's and Bouchard's nodes), the thumb carpometacarpal joint, the intervertebral discs and zygapophyseal joints in the cervical and lumbar vertebrae, the first metatarsophalangeal joint, the hips and the knees.

Osteoarthritis should be suspected in patients with gradual onset of

bone and joint

symptoms and signs, particularly in older adults. If osteoarthritis is suspected, plain X-rays should be obtained of the most symptomatic joints. X-rays generally reveal marginal osteophytes, narrowing of the joint space, increased density of the subchondral bone, subchondral cyst formation, bony remodelling and joint effusions. Standing X-rays of the knees are more sensitive to joint-space narrowing.

Laboratory studies are normal in osteoarthritis but might be required to rule out other disorders (eg rheumatoid arthritis) or to diagnose an underlying disorder causing secondary osteoarthritis. If osteoarthritis causes joint effusions, synovial fluid analysis can sometimes be used to differentiate it from inflammatory arthritides; in osteoarthritis, synovial fluid is usually clear, viscous, and contains 2000 white blood cells per microlitre or less.

Osteoarthritic involvement outside the usual joints suggests secondary OA; further evaluation might be required to determine the underlying primary disorder (endocrine, metabolic, neoplastic or biomechanical disorders).

## 15.7

*Answer: C*    It sometimes arises in benign cartilagenous tumours

The features in this scenario are characteristic of chondrosarcoma. Chondrosarcomas are malignant tumours of cartilage. They differ from osteosarcomas clinically, therapeutically and prognostically. Around 90% of chondrosarcomas are primary tumours. Rarely, chondrosarcomas arise in other, pre-existing conditions, particularly multiple osteochondromas. Chondrosarcomas tend to occur in older adults. They often develop in flat bones (eg pelvis, scapula) but can develop in any portion of any bone and can implant in surrounding soft tissues.

Plain X-rays often reveal punctate calcifications. Primary chondrosarcomas also often exhibit cortical bone destruction and loss of normal bone trabeculae. The appearance of punctate calcifications or an increase in size of an osteochondroma are findings that are suggestive of secondary chondrosarcoma. Technetium-99m bone scintigraphy is an accurate method for screening. Biopsy is required for diagnosis and can also determine the grade of the tumour (ie the probability of metastasis).

bone and joint

## 15.8

*Answer: E*     Plasma cells

The features in this case are suggestive of multiple myeloma. Multiple myeloma is the most common primary malignant bone tumour and is of haematopoietic derivation. It occurs mostly in older adults. The neoplastic process is usually multicentric and often involves the bone marrow so diffusely that bone marrow aspiration is diagnostic. Aspiration reveals sheets or clusters of plasma cells that are diagnostic of myeloma. X-rays usually show sharply circumscribed lytic lesions or diffuse demineralisation.

## 15.9

*Answer: B*     Ewing's sarcoma

A 'small, round, blue cell' tumour of bone is Ewing's sarcoma, commonly seen at this age. Most develop in the extremities, but any bone can be involved. Ewing's tumour tends to be extensive, sometimes involving the entire bone shaft. Pain and swelling are the most common symptoms. Lytic destruction is the most common X-ray finding, but multiple layers of subperiosteal reactive new bone formation may produce an 'onion skin' appearance. Plain X-rays do not usually reveal the full extent of bone involvement. Computed tomography and magnetic resonance imaging are better for defining the extent of disease, and can help guide treatment. Many other benign and malignant tumours can have identical appearances, so diagnosis is made by biopsy.

## 15.10

*Answer: C*     Serum prostate-specific antigen of 35 ng/ml

A prostatic adenocarcinoma should be the first guess (particularly in a man!) with osteoblastic (bone-forming) tumour metastases. Extensive metastases can act in a myelophthisic manner that leads to peripheral blood leucoerythroblastosis.

## 15.11

*Answer: A*    Aneurysmal bone cyst

An aneurysmal bone cyst is idiopathic and usually develops before the age of 20 years. This cystic lesion usually occurs in the metaphyseal region of the long bones, but almost any bone can be affected. It tends to grow slowly. Periosteal new bone formation tends to limit the periphery of the mass. Pain and swelling are common. The lesion can be present for anything between a few weeks and a few years before diagnosis. The appearance on X-ray is often characteristic: the rarefied area is usually well circumscribed and eccentric; its periosteum bulges, extending into the soft tissues, and might be surrounded by new bone formation.

## 15.12

*Answer: C*    Osteoporosis

Osteoporosis is one of the complications of long-term therapy with corticosteroids. Corticosteroid-induced osteoporosis is likely to lead to rib fractures and exuberant callus formation at sites of healing fractures.

## 15.13

*Answer: D*    Osteochondroma

Osteochondromas (osteocartilaginous exostoses), the most common benign bone tumours, can arise from any bone but tend to occur near the ends of long bones. They occur most often in people aged 10–20 years and can be single or multiple. Multiple osteochondromas tend to run in families. Secondary malignant chondrosarcoma develops in about 10% of patients with multiple osteochondromas but in fewer than 1% of those with single lesions.

bone and joint

**15.14**

*Answer: B* HA-B27

Ankylosing spondylitis is three times more frequent in men than in women and usually begins between the ages of 20 years and 40 years. It is 10 to 20 times more common in first-degree relatives of patients with ankylosing spondylitis than in the general population. The risk of ankylosing spondylitis in first-degree relatives with the HLA-B27 allele is about 20%. The increased prevalence of HLA-B27 in white people or HLA-B7 in black people supports a genetic predisposition. However, the concordance rate in identical twins is only about 50%, suggesting that environmental factors must also contribute. The pathophysiology probably involves immune-mediated inflammation.

**15.15**

*Answer: A* Bursitis

A bursa is a sac-like cavity or potential cavity that contains fluid, and is found where friction occurs (eg where tendons or muscles pass over bony prominences). Bursas minimise friction between moving parts and facilitate movement. They can communicate with joints. Bursitis can occur in the shoulder (subacromial or subdeltoid bursitis), secondary to rotator cuff tendinitis, which is usually the primary lesion in the shoulder. Other commonly affected bursas include the olecranon bursa (miner's elbow), the prepatellar bursa (housemaid's knee), the suprapatellar bursa, the retrocalcaneal (Achilles) bursa, the iliopectineal (iliopsoas) bursa, the ischial bursa (tailor's or weaver's bottom), the greater trochanteric bursa, the anserine bursa and the first metatarsal head bursa (bunion).

Bursitis can be caused by injury, chronic overuse, inflammatory arthritis (eg due to gout or rheumatoid arthritis) or acute or chronic infection (for example with pyogenic organisms, particularly *Staphylococcus aureus*). Infection is the most common cause in the olecranon and prepatellar bursas. Acute bursitis might occur following unusual exercise or strain and usually causes bursal effusion. Chronic bursitis can follow previous attacks of bursitis or repeated trauma. The bursal wall is thickened, with proliferation of its synovial lining; bursal adhesions, villi, tags and chalky deposits can form. Bursitis occasionally causes inflammation in a communicating joint.

Acute bursitis causes pain, particularly on movement, and localised tenderness. Swelling, sometimes with other signs of inflammation, is common if the bursa is superficial (eg prepatellar bursa, olecranon bursa). Crystal-induced or bacterial-induced bursitis is usually erythematous as well as painful and warm. Bursitis should be suspected in patients with swelling or signs of inflammation over bursas. It can generally be diagnosed clinically. If the swelling is particularly painful, red or warm, or if bursitis involves the olecranon bursa or the prepatellar bursa, then infection and crystal-induced disease should be excluded by bursal puncture. Using local anaesthesia and sterile technique, fluid is withdrawn from the bursa and analysed for cell count, Gram staining and culture, and microscopy for the detection of crystals. Gram staining is not sensitive, however, and white blood cell counts in infection can be lower than those found in septic joints. Urate crystals are easily seen with polarised light, but the apatite crystals typical of calcific tendinitis appear only as shiny, non-birefringent chunks. X-rays should be obtained if the bursitis is persistent or if infection or calcification is suspected.

## 15.16

*Answer: A* Herniated nucleus pulposus

This cricketer has a herniated disc which is impinging on spinal nerve root L5 to produce sensory disturbances. Pain radiates along the course of the sciatic nerve, most often down the buttocks and the posterior aspect of the leg to below the knee. The pain is typically burning, lancinating or stabbing. It can occur with or without low back pain. Performing a Valsalva manoeuvre can exacerbate the pain.

Nerve root compression can produce sensory, motor or (the most objective finding) reflex deficits. L5–S1 disc herniation can affect the ankle jerk reflex, whereas L3–L4 herniation can affect the knee jerk. Straight-leg raising can produce pain that radiates down the leg when the leg is raised above 60° (and sometimes when the

bone and joint

leg is raised even less than this). This is sensitive for sciatica; pain radiating down the involved leg with lifting of the contralateral leg (crossed straight-leg raising) is more specific for sciatica.

## 15.17

*Answer: B*    Fibromatosis

The description is suggestive of Dupuytren's contracture due to palmar fibromatosis. This is one of the more common hand deformities; the incidence is higher in men and increases after the age of 45 years. This autosomal dominant condition with variable penetrance occurs more commonly in patients with diabetes, alcoholism or epilepsy. However, the specific factor that causes the palmar fascia to thicken and contract is unknown. The earliest manifestation is usually a tender nodule in the palm, most often near the middle or ring finger; it gradually becomes painless. Next, a superficial cord forms and contracts the metacarpophalangeal joints and interphalangeal joints of the fingers. The hand eventually becomes arched. The disease is occasionally associated with fibrous thickening of the dorsum of the proximal interphalangeal joints (Garrod's pads), Peyronie's disease (penile fibromatosis) in about 7%–10% of patients and, rarely, with nodules on the plantar surface of the feet (plantar fibromatosis). Other types of flexion deformities of the fingers can also occur in diabetes, in systemic sclerosis, and in chronic reflex sympathetic dystrophy.

## 15.18

*Answer: A*    Carpal tunnel syndrome

Carpal tunnel syndrome is very common and usually occurs in women aged 30–50 years. Risk factors include rheumatoid arthritis or other types of wrist arthritis (sometimes this is the presenting manifestation), diabetes mellitus, hypothyroidism, acromegaly, amyloidosis and pregnancy-induced oedema in the carpal tunnel. Activities or jobs that require repetitive flexion and extension of the wrist can also be contributory factors. Most cases are idiopathic.

Symptoms include pain in the hand and wrist, associated with tingling and numbness, classically distributed along the median nerve (the palmar side of the thumb, the index and middle fingers, and the radial half of the ring finger) but sometimes involving the whole hand. Typically, the patient wakes at night with burning or aching pain and with numbness and tingling, and shakes the hand to obtain relief and restore sensation. Thenar atrophy and weakness of thumb opposition and abduction can also develop later on.

The diagnosis is strongly suggested by Tinel's sign, in which median nerve paraesthesiae are reproduced by tapping at the volar surface of the wrist over the site of the median nerve in the carpal tunnel. Reproduction of tingling with wrist flexion (Phalen's sign) is also suggestive. However, clinical differentiation from other types of peripheral neuropathy can sometimes be difficult. If symptoms are severe or the diagnosis is uncertain, conduction testing of the median nerve should be performed.

## 15.19

*Answer: E*    Positive rheumatoid factor

This is a rheumatoid nodule, a peculiar form of granulomatous inflammation that can be seen in the soft tissues of people with rheumatoid arthritis. Rheumatoid nodules develop in about 30% of patients with rheumatoid arthritis. They consist of a central necrotic area surrounded by palisaded histiocytic macrophages, all enveloped by lymphocytes, plasma cells and fibroblasts. Nodules and vasculitis can also develop in many of the visceral organs.

## 15.20

*Answer: D*    Pseudogout

Pseudogout involves intra-articular and/or extra-articular deposition of calcium pyrophosphate dihydrate (CPPD) crystals. The cause is unknown. Its frequent association with other conditions, such as trauma (including surgery), amyloidosis, myxoedema, hypomagnesaemia, hyperparathyroidism, gout, haemochromatosis and old age, suggests that CPPD crystal deposits are secondary to

bone and joint

degenerative or metabolic changes in the affected tissues. Some cases are familial, usually transmitted in an autosomal dominant pattern, with complete penetration by the age of 40 years. Both symptomatic and asymptomatic CPPD crystal deposition (chondrocalcinosis) are common with ageing.

The incidence of radiological (usually asymptomatic) chondrocalcinosis is about 3% at the age of 70 years, reaching nearly 50% in 90-year-olds. Asymptomatic chondrocalcinosis is common in the knee, hip, annulus fibrosus and symphysis pubis. Men and women are affected equally. Acute, subacute or chronic arthritis can occur, usually in the knee or other large peripheral joints, which can mimic many other forms of arthritis. Attacks are sometimes similar to gout but are usually less severe. There might be no symptoms between attacks or there can be continuous low-grade symptoms in multiple joints, similar to rheumatoid arthritis or osteoarthritis. These patterns tend to persist for life.

CPPD deposition disease should be suspected in older patients with arthritis, particularly inflammatory arthritis. The diagnosis is established by identifying rhomboid or rod-shaped, weakly positively birefringent crystals on polarised light microscopy of synovial fluid. Coincident infectious arthritis must be ruled out by Gram staining and culture. X-rays are indicated if synovial fluid cannot be obtained for analysis: findings of multiple linear or punctate calcification in articular cartilages, especially fibrocartilages, support the diagnosis.

# SECTION 16:
# CENTRAL NERVOUS SYSTEM
# PATHOLOGY — ANSWERS

## 16.1

*Answer:* C    Thromboembolism

The appearance of the infarction in a major blood flow distribution and the previous history of heart disease suggests embolic disease. This patient probably had a large left atrium filled with mural thrombus.

## 16.2

*Answer:* C    Meningioma

Meningiomas, particularly those less than 2 cm in diameter, are among the most common intracranial tumours. Meningioma is the only brain tumour that is more common in women. They tend to occur between the ages of 40 years and 60 years but can occur during childhood. These benign tumours can develop wherever there is dura, most commonly over the convexities near the venous sinuses, along the base of the skull, in the posterior fossa and, rarely, within the ventricles. Multiple meningiomas can develop. Meningiomas compress but do not invade brain parenchyma. They can invade and distort adjacent bone. There are many histological types, but they all follow a similar clinical course, and some become malignant.

Symptoms depend on which part of the brain is compressed and so on the tumour's location. Midline tumours in the elderly can cause dementia with few other focal neurological findings. Diagnosis is similar to that of other brain tumours, usually by magnetic resonance imaging with a paramagnetic contrast agent. Bony abnormalities (eg hyperostosis around the cerebral convexities, changes in the tuberculum sellae) might be seen incidentally on computed tomography or on plain X-rays.

cns

## 16.3

*Answer: B*    Glioblastoma multiforme

Glioblastoma multiforme, also known as 'grade 4 astrocytoma', is the most common and aggressive type of primary brain tumour, accounting for 52% of all primary brain tumours and 20% of all intracranial tumours. Despite being the most prevalent form of primary brain tumour, there are only two to three cases of glioblastoma multiforme per 100,000 people in Europe and North America.

Glioblastoma multiforme tumours are characterised by the presence of small areas of necrotising tissue that are surrounded by highly anaplastic cells. This characteristic differentiates the tumour from grade 3 astrocytomas, which do not have regions of necrotic tissue. Although glioblastoma multiforme can be derived from lower-grade astrocytomas, autopsies have revealed that most do not arise from precursor lesions in the brain.

Unlike oligodendrogliomas, glioblastoma multiforme can form in either the grey matter or the white matter of the brain, but most arise from the deep white matter and quickly infiltrate the brain, often becoming very large before causing any symptoms. The tumour can extend to the meningeal or ventricular wall, leading to a characteristically high protein content of the cerebrospinal fluid (>100 mg/dl), as well as an occasional pleocytosis of 10 to 100 cells, mostly lymphocytes. Malignant cells carried in the cerebrospinal fluid can spread to the spinal cord or cause meningeal gliomatosis. However, metastasis of glioblastoma multiforme beyond the central nervous system is extremely rare. About 50% of these tumours occupy more than one lobe of a hemisphere or are bilateral. Tumours of this type usually arise from the cerebrum, and can exhibit the classic infiltration across the corpus callosum, producing a butterfly (bilateral) glioma.

The tumour can express a variety of appearances, depending on the amount of haemorrhage or necrosis, or on its age. A computed tomographic scan usually shows a non-homogeneous mass with a hypointense centre and a variable ring of enhancement surrounded by oedema. Part of a lateral ventricle is usually deformed and both lateral and third ventricles can be displaced.

Although common symptoms of the disease can include seizures, nausea and vomiting, headache and hemiparesis, the most common symptom is progressive memory, personality or neurological deficit due to temporal and frontal lobe involvement. The kind of symptoms produced depend very much on the location of the tumour, more so than on its pathological properties. These tumours can start producing symptoms quickly, but are occasionally asymptomatic until they reach an enormous size.

## 16.4

*Answer: E*   Liquefactive necrosis

The brain has a high lipid content and typically undergoes liquefaction with ischaemic injury.

## 16.5

*Answer: D*   Increased alpha-fetoprotein

Maternal serum screening during the second trimester is a non-invasive way of identifying women at increased risk of having children with a neural tube defect (usually open spina bifida or anencephaly), Down's syndrome or trisomy 18. Screening should be offered to all pregnant women. When amniocentesis is recommended to test for fetal abnormalities, some women request serum screening before they agree to the procedure, so that risk of such abnormalities can be more precisely defined. Results are most accurate when the initial sample is obtained between 16 weeks' and 18 weeks' gestation, although screening can be done between 15 weeks and 20 weeks; normal values vary with gestational age. Corrections for maternal weight, diabetes mellitus, race and other factors are also necessary.

Maternal alpha-fetoprotein levels are measured first: elevated levels suggest open spina bifida, anencephaly, increased risk of pregnancy complications (eg intrauterine growth restriction, abruptio placentae) or, occasionally, twins or other multiple pregnancy. Closed spina bifida is not usually detected by this test. Designating a cut-off value to determine whether further testing is warranted

cns

involves weighing the risk of missed abnormalities against the risk of complications from unnecessary testing. Usually, a cut-off value in the 95th to 98th percentile or 2.0 to 2.5 times the normal pregnancy median (multiples of the median, or MOM) is used. This value is about 80% sensitive for open spina bifida and 90% sensitive for anencephaly. When this value is used, amniocentesis is eventually required in 1% to 2% of women originally screened. Lower cut-off values increase sensitivity but decrease specificity, resulting in more amniocenteses being performed.

## 16.6

*Answer: A*    Cerebral abscess

A brain abscess can result from direct extension of cranial infections (eg osteomyelitis, mastoiditis, sinusitis, subdural empyema), penetrating head wounds (including neurosurgical procedures), haematogenous spread (bacterial endocarditis, congenital heart disease with right-to-left shunt, intravenous drug abuse) or from unknown causes. The bacteria involved are usually anaerobic and sometimes mixed, often including anaerobic streptococci or *Bacteroides* species. Staphylococci are common after cranial trauma, neurosurgery, or endocarditis. Enterobacteria are common with an ear source. Fungi (eg *Aspergillus*) and protozoa (eg *Toxoplasma gondii*, particularly in HIV-infected patients) can cause cerebral abscesses.

An abscess forms when an area of cerebral inflammation becomes necrotic and encapsulated by glial cells and fibroblasts. Oedema around the abscess can increase the intracranial pressure. Symptoms result from increased intracranial pressure and mass effects. Headache, nausea, vomiting, lethargy, seizures, personality changes, papilloedema and focal neurological deficits develop over days to weeks. Fever, chills and leucocytosis can develop before the infection is encapsulated, and then subside.

When symptoms suggest an abscess, contrast-enhanced computed tomography or magnetic resonance imaging is performed. An abscess appears as an oedematous mass with ring enhancement, which can be difficult to distinguish from a tumour or occasionally infarction; culture and drainage might be necessary. Lumbar puncture is not performed because it could precipitate transtentorial herniation and because the cerebrospinal fluid findings are non-specific.

## 16.7

*Answer: E*    Vestibular neuronitis

Vestibular neuronitis causes a self-limited episode of vertigo, presumably due to inflammation of the vestibular division of cranial nerve VIII; some vestibular dysfunction can persist. Although the cause is unclear, a viral cause is suspected. Symptoms include a single attack of severe vertigo, with nausea and vomiting and persistent nystagmus towards the affected side, which lasts 7–10 days. The nystagmus is unidirectional, horizontal and spontaneous, with fast-beat oscillations in the direction of the unaffected ear. The absence of concomitant tinnitus or hearing loss is a hallmark of vestibular neuronitis. The condition slowly subsides after this initial episode. Some patients have residual disequilibrium, especially with rapid head movements, probably due to permanent vestibular injury.

Patients undergo an audiological assessment, electronystagmography with caloric testing, and gadolinium-enhanced magnetic resonance imaging of the head, paying special attention to the internal auditory canals to exclude other diagnoses, such as cerebellopontine angle tumour, brainstem haemorrhage or infarction. Magnetic resonance imaging might show enhancement of the vestibular nerves, consistent with inflammatory neuritis.

## 16.8

*Answer: D*    Schwannoma

Schwannomas are histologically benign neoplasms that arise from nerve sheaths, most commonly from sensory nerve roots. Schwannomas are clearly delineated from the nerve root and so surgical resection of schwannomas can be accomplished without sacrifice of the associated nerve root. Because they are histologically benign they have an excellent prognosis.

cns

Intracranially, schwannomas most commonly arise from the vestibular nerve. Although the most accurate term for these neoplasms is 'vestibular schwannoma', the term 'acoustic neuroma' is firmly entrenched in the neurosurgical literature. The most common presentation of the acoustic neuroma is progressive, unilateral hearing loss due to compression of the adjacent cochlear nerve. Tinnitus is another common early symptom. As it grows the tumour can compress the adjacent trigeminal nerve and brainstem. Nerve-sheath tumours also occur on other cranial nerves, including the trigeminal and glossopharyngeal nerves.

## 16.9

*Answer: B*   Epidural haematoma

Epidural haematomas (a collection of blood between the skull and the dura mater) are usually caused by arterial bleeding, classically due to damage to the middle meningeal artery by a temporal bone fracture. Without intervention, patients with large or arterial epidural haematomas can deteriorate rapidly and die. Small, venous epidural haematomas are rarely lethal.

Symptoms of epidural haematoma usually develop within minutes to several hours after the injury and consist of increasing headache, decreased level of consciousness, hemiparesis and pupillary dilation with loss of light reactivity. Some patients lose consciousness, followed by a transient lucid interval, then subsequent neurological deterioration.

## 16.10

*Answer: E*   White matter

Brain function can be impaired immediately by direct damage of brain tissue (eg by crush or laceration injuries). Further damage can occur shortly thereafter as a result of the cascade of events triggered by the initial injury. Traumatic brain injury of any sort can cause oedema in the damaged tissues. The greatest amount of salt and water increase with cerebral oedema occurs within the white matter. The cranial vault is fixed in size (constrained by the skull)

cns

and almost completely filled by non-compressible cerebrospinal fluid and minimally compressible brain tissue. Consequently, any swelling from oedema, haemorrhage or haematoma has nowhere to expand into and so increases the intracranial pressure (ICP). Cerebral blood flow is proportional to the cerebral perfusion pressure, which is the difference between mean arterial pressure and the mean ICP. Therefore, as the ICP increases (or the mean arterial pressure decreases), the cerebral perfusion pressue decreases, and when it is below about 50 mmHg, brain tissue can become ischaemic. This mechanism can lead to ischaemia at a local level when compression from focal oedema or haematoma compromises blood flow in the region of the lesion. Ischaemia and oedema then trigger release of excitatory neurotransmitters and free radicals, causing further oedema, which further increases the ICP. Systemic complications from trauma (eg hypotension, hypoxia) can also contribute to cerebral ischaemia and are therefore often called 'secondary brain insults'.

Excessive ICP initially causes global cerebral dysfunction. If excessive ICP is unrelieved, it can push brain tissue across the tentorium or through the foramen magnum, causing herniation, which significantly increases morbidity and mortality risks. Also, if the ICP increases to equal the mean arterial pressure, the cerebral perfusion pressure becomes zero, resulting in complete brain ischaemia, which rapidly leads to brain death; absent cranial blood flow can be used as one criterion for brain death.

## 16.11

*Answer: D*  Ruptured berry aneursym

Subarachnoid haemorrhage is bleeding between the arachnoid mater and the pia mater. In general, head trauma is the most common cause, but traumatic subarachnoid haemorrhage is usually considered as a separate disorder. Spontaneous (primary) subarachnoid haemorrhage usually results from ruptured aneurysms. A congenital intracranial saccular or berry aneurysm is the cause in about 85% of patients. Aneurysmal haemorrhage can occur at any age but is most common between the ages of 40 years and 65 years. Less common causes are mycotic aneurysms, arteriovenous malformations and bleeding disorders.

cns

Blood in the subarachnoid space causes a chemical meningitis that commonly raises the intracranial pressure for several days or even for a few weeks. Secondary vasospasm can cause focal brain ischaemia; about 25% of patients develop signs of a transient ischaemic attack or ischaemic stroke. Brain oedema is maximal and the risk of vasospasm and subsequent infarction (called 'angry brain') is highest between 72 hours and 10 days after the bleed. Secondary acute hydrocephalus is also common. A second rupture (rebleeding) sometimes occurs, most often within about 7 days of the first bleed.

## 16.12

*Answer: B*  Dural bridging vein

A subdural haematoma is blood between the dura mater and the pia-arachnoid mater. Acute subdural haematomas, which are often caused by laceration of brain or cortical veins or avulsion of bridging veins between the cortex and dural sinuses, often occur after falls or motor vehicle crashes. Oedema can occur as the haematoma compresses brain tissue, resulting in signs of increased intracranial pressure. The morbidity and mortality can be significant.

A chronic subdural haematoma can form and cause symptoms gradually, over a period of several weeks after trauma. These haematomas are more common in elderly patients (especially those taking antiplatelet drugs or anticoagulants), who might have thought that the head injury was relatively trivial or might even have forgotten about it. In contrast to acute subdural haematoma, oedema and increased intracranial pressure are unusual.

## 16.13

*Answer: B*  Chronic brain abscess

A brain abscess can result from direct extension of cranial infections (eg osteomyelitis, mastoiditis, sinusitis, subdural empyema), penetrating head wounds (including neurosurgical procedures), haematogenous spread (bacterial endocarditis, congenital heart disease with right-to-left shunt, intravenous drug abuse) or from

cns

unknown causes. The bacteria involved are usually anaerobic and sometimes mixed, often including anaerobic streptococci or *Bacteroides* species. Staphylococci are common after cranial trauma, neurosurgery, or endocarditis. Enterobacteria are common with an ear source. Fungi (eg *Aspergillus*) and protozoa (eg *Toxoplasma gondii*, particularly in HIV-infected patients) can cause cerebral abscesses.

An abscess forms when an area of cerebral inflammation becomes necrotic and encapsulated by glial cells and fibroblasts. Oedema around the abscess can increase the intracranial pressure. Symptoms result from increased intracranial pressure and mass effects. Headache, nausea, vomiting, lethargy, seizures, personality changes, papilloedema and focal neurological deficits develop over days to weeks. Fever, chills and leucocytosis can develop before the infection is encapsulated, and then subside.

When symptoms suggest an abscess, contrast-enhanced computed tomography or magnetic resonance imaging is performed. An abscess appears as an oedematous mass with ring enhancement, which can be difficult to distinguish from a tumour or occasionally infarction; culture and drainage might be necessary. Lumbar puncture is not performed because it could precipitate transtentorial herniation and because the cerebrospinal fluid findings are non-specific.

## 16.14

*Answer: B* Astrocytoma

Astrocytomas are primary intracranial tumours derived from astrocyte cells of the brain. They can arise in the cerebral hemispheres, in the posterior fossa, in the optic nerve and, rarely, in the spinal cord. Well-differentiated astrocytomas comprise 25%–30% of cerebral gliomas. Although astrocytomas have many different histological characteristics, the most common type is the well-differentiated fibrillary astrocytoma. These tumours express glial fibrillary acidic protein (GFAP), which possibly functions as a tumour suppressor, and is a useful diagnostic marker in a tissue biopsy.

In almost half of cases, the first symptom of an astrocytoma is the onset of a focal or generalised seizure. Between 60% and 75% of patients will have recurrent seizures during the course of their illness.

cns

Headache and signs of increased intracranial pressure (headache, vomiting) usually present late in the disease course. In children, the tumour is usually located in the cerebellum and will present with some combination of gait instability, unilateral ataxia and signs of increased intracranial pressure. Children with astrocytoma usually have decreased memory, attention and motor abilities, but unaffected intelligence, language and academic skills. When the tumour metastasises, it can spread via the lymphatic system and cause death even when the primary tumour is well controlled.

Computed tomography (CT) or magnetic resonance imaging is necessary to characterise the anatomy of this tumour (size, location, consistency). CT will usually show distortion of the third and lateral ventricles, with displacement of the anterior and middle cerebral arteries. Histological diagnosis with tissue biopsy will normally reveal an infiltrative character suggestive of the slow growing nature of the tumour. The tumour can be cavitating, pseudocyst-forming or non-cavitating, and is usually white-grey, firm, and almost indistinguishable from normal white matter.

## 16.15

*Answer: B*    Herpes simplex virus

Haemorrhagic lesions of the temporal lobe are typical of herpes simplex virus (HSV) infection. HSV encephalitis occurs at any time of the year, has a bimodal age distribution, tending to affect patients aged under 20 years or over 40 years, and is often fatal if left untreated. In acute encephalitis, cerebral oedema and petechial haemorrhages occur throughout the hemispheres, brainstem, cerebellum and, occasionally, the spinal cord. Direct viral invasion of the brain usually damages neurones, sometimes with visible inclusion bodies. Severe infection, particularly if untreated, can lead to cerebral haemorrhagic necrosis. Magnetic resonance imaging is sensitive for early HSV encephalitis, showing oedema in the orbitofrontal and temporal areas, which HSV typically infects preferentially.

cns

## 16.16

*Answer: B*    Chronic subdural haematoma

The features described in this scenario are consistent with the development of a chronic subdural haematoma, which is more common in men (the male to female ratio is 2 : 1). Most adults with chronic subdural haematoma are aged over 50 years, with two studies reporting average ages of 68 years and 70.5 years. A quarter to a half of patients with chronic subdural haematoma have no identifiable history of head trauma. If a patient does have a history of head trauma, it usually is mild. The average time between head trauma and chronic subdural haematoma diagnosis is 4–5 weeks.

Overall, risk factors for a chronic subdural haematoma include chronic alcoholism, epilepsy, coagulopathy, arachnoid cysts, anticoagulant therapy (including aspirin), cardiovascular disease (hypertension, arteriosclerosis), thrombocytopenia and diabetes. In younger patients, alcoholism, thrombocytopenia, coagulation disorders and oral anticoagulant therapy have been found to be more prevalent. Arachnoid cysts are associated with chronic subdural haematoma more commonly in patients under the age of 40 years. In older patients, cardiovascular disease and arterial hypertension are found to be more prevalent. Severe dehydration is a less commonly associated condition and is found concurrently in only 2% of patients. Clinically, the presentation is often insidious, with symptoms of decreased level of consciousness, balance problems, cognitive dysfunction and memory loss, motor deficit (eg hemiparesis), headache or aphasia. Some patients present acutely, with a seizure for example.

Neurological examination can reveal hemiparesis, papilloedema, hemianopia, or third cranial nerve dysfunction, such as an unreactive dilated pupil or a laterally deviated eye with limited movement. In patients aged 60 years or older, hemiparesis and reflex asymmetry are common presenting signs. In patients younger than 60 years, headache is a common presenting symptom. Chronic subdural haematomas are bilateral in 8.7%–32% of cases.

cns

## 16.17

*Answer: D*   Viral pneumonia

The features described in this scenario are suggestive of Guillain–Barré syndrome, which is the most common acquired inflammatory neuropathy. Although the cause is not fully understood, it is thought to be autoimmune. There are several variants. In some, demyelination predominates; others affect the axons. In about two-thirds of patients, the syndrome begins 5 days to 3 weeks after an infectious disease, surgery or vaccination. Infection is the trigger in over 50% of patients; common pathogens include *Campylobacter jejuni*, enteric viruses, herpesviruses (including cytomegalovirus and those causing infectious mononucleosis) and *Mycoplasma* species.

Flaccid weakness predominates in most patients, which is always more prominent than sensory abnormalities and can be most prominent proximally. Relatively symmetric weakness with paraesthesiae usually begins in the legs and progresses to the arms, but it occasionally begins in the arms or head. In 90% of patients weakness is maximal at 3 weeks. Deep tendon reflexes are lost, but sphincters are usually spared. Facial and oropharyngeal muscles are weak in over 50% of patients with severe disease. Respiratory paralysis severe enough to require endotracheal intubation and mechanical ventilation occurs in 5%–10%.

A few patients (possibly with a variant form) have significant, life-threatening autonomic dysfunction causing fluctuations in the blood pressure, inappropriate antidiuretic hormone secretion, cardiac arrhythmias, gastrointestinal stasis, urinary retention and pupillary changes. An unusual variant (the Fisher variant) causes only ophthalmoparesis, ataxia and areflexia.

If Guillain–Barré syndrome is suspected, patients should be admitted to hospital for electromyography (EMG), analysis of cerebrospinal fluid (CSF), and measurement of forced vital capacity every 6–8 hours. Initial electromyography detects slow nerve conduction velocities and evidence of segmental demyelination in two-thirds of patients; however, a normal EMG does not exclude the diagnosis and should not delay treatment. CSF analysis might detect albuminocytological dissociation (increased protein but a normal white blood cell count), but this sometimes does not appear for up to 1 week and does not develop at all in 10% of patients.

## 16.18

*Answer: B*    Elevated serum glucose of 10.8 mmol/l

Diabetic neuropathy is probably the most common form of peripheral neuropathy in the Western world. This man also has a 'diabetic foot' as a result of severe peripheral vascular atherosclerosis, and the history of myocardial infaction is consistent with severe occlusive coronary atherosclerosis.

## 16.19

*Answer: C*    Metastatic carcinoma

The location of the mass at the grey–white junction is typical of a metastasis. Secondary or metastatic brain tumours originate from malignant tumours located primarily in other organs. Their incidence is higher than that of primary brain tumours. The most frequent types of metastatic brain tumours originate in the lung, skin, kidney, breast and colon. These tumour cells reach the brain via the bloodstream. In this scenario the patient is most likely to have a lung cancer because she is a chronic smoker.

## 16.20

*Answer: A*    Cerebral oedema with uncal herniation

The location of the haemorrhages suggests Duret haemorrhages. Duret haemorrhages are small areas of bleeding in the ventral and paramedian parts of the upper brainstem (midbrain and pons). They occur secondary to raised intracranial pressure with formation of a transtentorial pressure cone in which the cerebellar tonsils are impacted in the foramen magnum by the high pressure. Kernohan's notch is a groove in the cerebral peduncle caused by this displacement of the brainstem against the incisura of the tentorium in some cases. The resulting ipsilateral hemiparesis is a false localising sign, known as the 'Kernohan–Woltman syndrome'. This can either succeed or accompany temporal lobe (uncal) herniation and subfalcial herniation secondary to a supratentorial mass.

cns

The common causes are an acute haematoma, oedema following trauma, abscess or tumour. Duret haemorrhages are demonstrated by computed tomography or magnetic resonance imaging, and they usually indicate a fatal outcome. The mechanism is uncertain but is probably caused by the displacement of the brainstem stretching and lacerating pontine perforating branches of the basilar artery; venous infarction might play a role.

# SECTION 17: PHARMACOLOGY — ANSWERS

## 17.1

*Answer: B*   Competitively inhibits $H_2$ receptors

Cimetidine is a histamine $H_2$-receptor anatgonist that inhibits the production of acid in the stomach. It is largely used in the treatment of heartburn and peptic ulcers. Cimetidine is a known inhibitor of many isozymes of the cytochrome P450 enzyme system (specifically CYP1A2, CYP2C9, CYP2C19, CYP2D6, CYP2E1 and CYP3A4). This inhibition forms the basis of the numerous drug interactions that occur between cimetidine and other drugs. For example, cimetidine can decrease the metabolism of some drugs, such as oral contraceptives. Cimetidine interferes with oestrogen metabolism, enhancing oestrogen activity. This can lead to gynaecomastia. Adverse drug reactions are also found to be relatively common with cimetidine. The development of longer-acting $H_2$-receptor antagonists with fewer adverse effects, such as ranitidine, has proved to be the downfall of cimetidine and, while it is still used, it is not among the more widely used $H_2$-receptor antagonists.

## 17.2

*Answer: E*   Serotonin antagonist

Ondansetron is a serotonin 5-$HT_3$-receptor antagonist used mainly to treat nausea and vomiting caused by chemotherapy. Its effects are thought to be on both peripheral and central nerves: one mechanism is reduction of the activity of the vagus nerve, which is the nerve that activates the vomiting centre in the medulla oblongata; another mechanism is blockage of serotonin receptors in the chemoreceptor trigger zone. It does not have much effect on vomiting due to motion sickness. This drug does not have any effect on dopamine receptors or on muscarinic receptors.

pharmacology

## 17.3

*Answer: D*   Opiate agonist

Diphenoxylate is an opiate agonist used for the treatment of diarrhoea. It acts by slowing down intestinal contractions. It is a congener to the narcotic meperidine. This medication is therefore potentially habit-forming, particularly in high doses or when long-term. Because of this, diphenoxylate is manufactured and marketed as a combination drug with atropine (Lomotil®). This pharmaceutical strategy is designed to discourage abuse, because the anticholinergic effect of atropine will cause severe weakness and nausea if the standard dosage is exceeded.

## 17.4

*Answer: B*   Holds water in the stool

Methylcellulose is a chemical compound derived from cellulose. It is a hydrophilic white powder in pure form and dissolves in cold (but not in hot) water, forming a clear viscous solution or gel. It is sold under a variety of trade names and is used as a thickener and emulsifier in various food and cosmetic products, and also as a treatment of constipation. Like cellulose, it is not digestible, not toxic and not allergenic. When eaten, methylcellulose is not absorbed by the intestines but passes through the digestive tract undisturbed. It attracts large amounts of water into the colon, producing a softer and bulkier stool. It is used to treat constipation, diverticulosis, haemorrhoids and irritable bowel syndrome. It should be taken with sufficient amounts of fluid to prevent dehydration. Because it absorbs water and potentially toxic materials and increases viscosity, it can also be used to treat diarrhoea.

## 17.5

*Answer: B*   Holds water in the stool

Psyllium is a laxative belonging to the subclass of bulk-forming laxatives. It holds water in the stool. Its efficacy is not well documented but it is believed to provide some benefit in irritable bowel syndrome.

pharmacology

## 17.6

*Answer: D*  Irreversibly inhibits H+/K+-ATPase

Lansoprazole is a proton-pump inhibitor. It irreversibly inhibits $H^+/K^+$-ATPase. Proton-pump inhibitors are used to treat stomach and duodenal ulcers, including stomach ulcers caused by taking non-steroidal anti-inflammatory drugs. They are also used to relieve symptoms of oesophagitis and severe gastro-oesophageal reflux.

## 17.7

*Answer: B*  Dopamine antagonist

Metoclopramide is a potent dopamine-receptor antagonist used for its anti-emetic and prokinetic properties. It is therefore primarily used to treat nausea and vomiting, and to facilitate gastric emptying in patients with gastric stasis. It appears to bind to dopamine D2 receptors, where it is a receptor antagonist, and it is also a mixed $5\text{-HT}_3$-receptor antagonist/$5\text{-HT}_4$-receptor agonist. The anti-emetic action of metoclopramide is due to its antagonist activity at D2 receptors in the chemoreceptor trigger zone (CTZ) in the central nervous system. This action prevents nausea and vomiting triggered by most stimuli. At higher doses, $5\text{-HT}_3$-antagonist activity can also contribute to the anti-emetic effect. The prokinetic activity of metoclopramide is mediated by muscarinic activity, D2 receptor-antagonist activity and $5\text{-HT}_4$-receptor agonist activity. The prokinetic effect itself might also contribute to the anti-emetic effect.

## 17.8

*Answer: D*  Lowers the surface tension of the stool, facilitating penetration of water and fats

Docusate sodium (dioctyl sodium sulphosuccinate) surfactant is used as a laxative and stool softener. It is given to make stools softer and easier to pass. It is used to treat constipation due to hard stools, in painful anorectal conditions such as haemorrhoids, and for people who should avoid straining during bowel movements. Of note is that the effect of docusate sodium might not necessarily be exclusively due to its surfactant properties. Perfusion studies have suggested that docusate sodium inhibits fluid absorption or stimulates secretion in the jejunum. While the use of docusate sodium is widespread, data to support its efficacy in treating chronic constipation is lacking. Also, although more research is needed, long-term use of docusate sodium seems to decrease levels of magnesium and potassium in the blood.

## 17.9

*Answer: E*    Opiate agonist

Loperamide is an opioid-receptor agonist and acts on the mu opioid receptors in the myenteric plexus of large intestine; it does not affect the central nervous system, unlike other opioids. It works by decreasing the activity of the myenteric plexus, which decreases the motility of the circular and longitudinal smooth muscles of the intestinal wall. This increases the amount of time substances stay in the intestine, allowing for more water to be absorbed out of the faecal matter. Loperamide also decreases colonic mass movements and suppresses the gastrocolic reflex. Loperamide does not cross the blood–brain barrier and has no analgesic properties or addictive potential. Tolerance in response to long-term use has not been reported.

## 17.10

*Answer: D*    Opiate agonist

Sufentanil is a synthetic opioid analgesic drug that is approximately 5–10 times more potent than fentanyl. The main use of this medication is in operating suites and critical care units, where pain relief is required for a short period of time. It also has sedative properties and this makes it a good analgesic component of anaesthetic regimes during surgery.

pharmacology

## 17.11

*Answer: C*    Modulation of GABAergic, noradrenergic and serotonergic systems

Tramadol is an atypical opioid which is a centrally acting analgesic, and is used for treating moderate to severe pain. It is a synthetic agent, unrelated to other opioids. The mechanism of action of tramadol has yet to be fully elucidated, but it is believed to work through modulation of the GABAergic, noradrenergic and serotonergic systems (where 'GABA' is gamma-aminobutyric acid). The contribution of its non-opioid activity is demonstrated by the analgesic effects of tramadol not being fully antagonised by the mu opioid-receptor antagonist, naloxone.

## 17.12

*Answer: B*    Inhibits cholesterol synthesis

Atorvastatin is a member of the drug class of statins, used for lowering cholesterol (ie a hypolipidaemic agent) in people with hypercholesterolaemia and so for preventing cardiovascular disease. The mode of action of statins is inhibition of 3-hydroxy-3-methylglutaryl-coenzyme A (HMG-CoA) reductase. This enzyme is needed by the body to make cholesterol. Atorvastatin causes cholesterol to be lost from low-density lipoprotein (LDL), but also reduces the concentration of circulating LDL particles. Apolipoprotein B concentration falls substantially during treatment with atorvastatin. Atorvastatin's ability to lower LDL is thought to be due to a reduction in very-low-density lipoprotein (VLDL), which is a precursor of LDL. Also, atorvastatin can increase the number of LDL receptors on the surface of cell membranes, and so increase the breakdown of LDL. Atorvastatin can also produce slight to moderate increases in high-density lipoprotein (HDL), and slight to moderate decreases in triglycerides. Both of these effects are benefical in a patient with a poor lipid profile.

pharmacology

## 17.13

*Answer: A*   Allergic reaction

Streptokinase is an extracellular metallo-enzyme produced by beta-haemolytic streptococci and is used as an effective and cheap clot-dissolving medication in patients with myocardial infarction and pulmonary embolism. It belongs to a group of medications known as 'fibrinolytics', and works by activating plasminogen through cleavage to produce plasmin. The half-life of streptokinase is 6 hours. Plasmin is produced in the blood to break down the major constituent of blood clots, fibrin, therefore dissolving clots once they have fulfilled their purpose of stopping bleeding. Extra production of plasmin caused by streptokinase breaks down unwanted blood clots, for example in the lungs (pulmonary embolism). It is given intravenously as soon as possible in the acute phase of a myocardial infarction to dissolve clots in the coronary arteries. This reduces the amount of damage to the heart muscle.

Because streptokinase is a bacterial product the body will build up an immunity to it. It is recommended that this medication should not be used again after 4 days from the first administration because it might not be as effective and can also cause an allergic reaction. For this reason, it is usually only given for a person's first heart attack.

## 17.14

*Answer: B*   Cataract surgery

Carbachol (carbamylcholine) is a cholinergic agent, a choline ester and a positively charged quaternary ammonium compound. It is not well absorbed in the gastrointestinal tract and does not cross the blood–brain barrier. It is usually administered topically to the eye or through intraocular injection. Carbachol is not easily metabolised by cholinesterase; its duration of action is 4–8 hours with topical administration and 24 hours after intraocular administration. Because carbachol is poorly absorbed through topical administration, benzalkonium chloride is mixed with it to promote absorption. Carbachol is a parasympathomimetic that stimulates both muscarinic and nicotinic receptors. When administered topically in the eye or intraocularly its principal effects are miosis and increased outflow of aqueous humour. It is primarily used topically in the treatment of open-angle glaucoma to reduce the intraocular pressure, but it is also sometimes used intraocularly to constrict the pupils after lens implantation during cataract surgery. Carbachol can also be used to stimulate bladder emptying if the normal emptying mechanism is not working properly.

## 17.15

*Answer: A*   Antifungal

Griseofulvin is an antifungal drug. It is used in both animals and humans to treat ringworm infections of the skin and nails. It is derived from the mould *Penicillium griseofulvum*. It is administered orally. It binds to keratin in keratin precursor cells and makes them resistant to fungal infections. It is only when hair or skin is replaced by the keratin–griseofulvin complex that the drug reaches its site of action. Griseofulvin will then enter the dermatophyte through energy-dependant transport processes and bind to fungal microtubules. This alters the processing for mitosis and also the underlying information for deposition of fungal cell walls. Known side-effects of griseofulvin include hives, skin rashes, confusion, dizziness, diarrhoea, fatigue, headache, impairment of performance of routine activities, inability to fall or stay asleep, nausea, oral thrush, upper abdominal pain, vomiting, swelling, itching, tingling in the hands or feet and loss of taste sensation.

## 17.16

*Answer: E*   Ventricular arrhythmias

Mexiletine belongs to the class IB anti-arrhythmic group of medicines. It is used to treat ventricular arrhythmias. It slows nerve impulses in the heart and makes the heart tissue less sensitive. Dizziness, heartburn, nausea, nervousness, trembling and unsteadiness are common side-effects. It is available in injection and capsule form. Class IB anti-arrhythmics decrease the duration of the action potential by shortening the repolarisation phase. This is achieved by blocking sodium channels.

pharmacology

## 17.17

*Answer: D*    It is poorly lipid-soluble

Nadolol is a non-selective beta-blocker used in the treatment of high blood pressure and angina. Nadolol is non-polar and hydrophobic, with low lipid solubility. It is a beta-specific sympatholytic which non-selectively blocks beta-1 adrenergic receptors, which are mainly located in the heart, inhibiting the effects of the catecholamines adrenaline (epinephrine) and noradrenaline (norepinephrine) and decreasing the heart rate and blood pressure. It also blocks beta-2 adrenergic receptors, which are located in bronchial smooth muscle, causing bronchoconstriction. By binding beta-2 receptors in the juxtaglomerular apparatus, nadolol inhibits the production of renin, thereby inhibiting angiotensin II and aldosterone production. Nadolol therefore inhibits the vasoconstriction and water retention due to angiotensin II and aldosterone, respectively. It also impairs atrioventricular node conduction and decreases the sinus rate. Nadolol can also increase plasma triglycerides and decrease high-density lipoprotein- (HDL-) cholesterol levels.

## 17.18

*Answer: C*    It induces the release of stored factor VIII and
von Willebrand factor

Desmopressin is a synthetic drug that mimics the action of antidiuretic hormone. It can be taken nasally, intravenously or orally as a recently developed pill. Desmopressin is used to reduce urine production in patients with central diabetes insipidus and to promote the release of von Willebrand factor and factor VIII in patients with coagulation disorders such as type I von Willebrand's disease, mild haemophilia A and thrombocytopenia (which occurs after prolonged surgery on cardiopulmonary bypass). Desmopressin is not effective in the treatment of haemophilia B or severe haemophilia A.

## 17.19

*Answer: C*    Anxiolytic

Buspirone is an anxiolytic agent and a serotonin-receptor agonist that belongs to the azaspirodecanedione class of compounds. Its structure is unrelated to that of the benzodiazepines, but it has an efficacy comparable to diazepam. It shows no potential for addiction compared with other drugs commonly prescribed for anxiety, especially the benzodiazepines. The development of tolerance has not been noted. Cross-tolerance to benzodiazepines, barbiturates and alcohol does not occur either. Furthermore, it is non-sedating. It is thought to act by interfering with the function of the neurotransmitter serotonin in the brain, particularly by acting as a 5-HT1A-receptor partial agonist. Additionally, it acts as a mixed agonist/antagonist on postsynaptic dopamine receptors. It has no gamma-aminobutyric acid- (GABA-) mediated effects. Buspirone can also have indirect effects on other neurotransmitters in the brain. The action of a single dose is much longer than the short half-life of 2–3 hours indicates. The bioavailability of buspirone is very low and variable due to extensive first-pass metabolism. The drug is quickly resorbed. Taking the drug together with food can increase the bioavailability, however. The drug is highly plasma-bound (95%). The active metabolite 1-PP is also a 5-HT1A partial agonist with anxiolytic properties, but weaker than those of the mother drug. It is also useful as an augmenting agent, for the treatment of depression, when added to selective serotonin-reuptake inhibitors (SSRIs). Its main disadvantage is that 1–3 weeks elapse before the anxiolytic activity becomes evident, and patients often have to be co-treated with a benzodiazepine for immediate anxiolysis. In general, buspirone works less well than benzodiazepines.

## 17.20

*Answer: B*    Penicillin

Dicloxacillin is a narrow-spectrum beta-lactam antibiotic. It is used to treat infections caused by susceptible Gram-positive bacteria. Notably, it is active against beta-lactamase-producing organisms such as *Staphylococcus aureus* which are resistant to most penicillins. It is very similar to flucloxacillin and these two agents are considered interchangeable. Like other beta-lactam antibiotics, dicloxacillin acts by inhibiting the synthesis of bacterial cell walls. It inhibits cross-linkage between the linear peptidoglycan polymer chains that make up a major component of the cell wall of Gram-positive bacteria. Dicloxacillin is more acid-stable than many other penicillins and can be given orally as well as parenterally. However, like methicillin, it is less potent than benzylpenicillin against non-beta-lactamase-producing Gram-positive bacteria. It is believed to have a lower incidence of severe hepatic adverse effects than flucloxacillin, but a higher incidence of renal adverse effects.

## 17.21

*Answer: E*    Vasodilators

Sodium nitroprusside is a potent peripheral vasodilator that affects both arterioles and venules. It is often administered intravenously to patients who are experiencing a hypertensive emergency. 'Nitroprusside' in fact is an anion that is usually available as the dihydrate of its disodium salt. It reduces both total peripheral resistance as well as venous return, so decreasing both preload and afterload. For this reason it can be used in severe cardiogenic heart failure where this combination of effects can act to increase cardiac output. In situations where cardiac output is normal, the effect is to reduce the blood pressure.

Nitroprusside is light-sensitive and breaks down in sunlight, producing cyanide. Despite its toxicity, however, nitroprusside is still used because it remains an effective drug in certain clinical circumstances such as malignant hypertension or for rapid control of blood pressure during vascular surgery and neurosurgery. Its mechanism of action appears to be liberation of nitric oxide as it is metabolised in the erythrocyte, converting haemoglobin to cyanomethaemaglobin. Nitroprusside also releases cyanide ions, which are converted in the liver to thiocyanate by the enzyme rhodanase, a reaction which requires a sulphur donor such as thiosulphate. Thiocyanate is then excreted by the kidney. In the absence of sufficient thiosulphate, cyanide ions can quickly reach toxic levels. The half-life of nitroprusside is less than 10 minutes, although thiocyanate has an excretion half-life of several days. The duration of treatment should not exceed 72 hours and plasma concentrations of thiocyanate should be monitored.

## 17.22

*Answer: E*    Potassium-sparing diuretics

Spironolactone is a synthetic 17-lactone steroid which is a renal competitive aldosterone antagonist in a class of drugs called 'potassium-sparing diuretics', which are used primarily to treat low-renin hypertension, hypokalaemia and Conn syndrome. On its own, spironolactone is only a weak diuretic, but it can be combined with other diuretics. Spironolactone inhibits the effect of aldosterone by competing for intracellular aldosterone receptors in the distal tubule cells. This increases the secretion of water and sodium, while decreasing the excretion of potassium. Spironolactone has a fairly slow onset of action, this taking several days to develop, and similarly its effect diminishes slowly.

Spironolactone also has anti-androgen activity via binding to the androgen receptor and thus preventing it from interacting with dihydrotestosterone, and so it can also be used to treat hirsutism and is a common component in hormone therapy for male-to-female transgender people. It is also used for treating hair loss and for acne in women.

## 17.23

*Answer: E*    Prevention of re-stenosis after angioplasty

Abciximab (previously known as 'c7E3 Fab') is a platelet aggregation inhibitor that is mainly used during and after coronary artery procedures such as angioplasty to prevent platelets from sticking together and causing thrombus formation in the coronary artery. Its mechanism of action is inhibition of glycoprotein IIb/IIIa. Although abciximab has a short plasma half-life due to its strong affinity for its receptor on the platelets, it can occupy some receptors for weeks. In practice, platelet aggregation gradually returns to normal about 24–48 hours after discontinuation of the drug. Abciximab is made from the Fab fragments of an immunoglobulin that targets

pharmacology

the glycoprotein IIb/IIIa receptor on the platelet membrane. It is indicated for use in people who are undergoing percutaneous coronary intervention (angioplasty, with or without stent placement). The use of abciximab in this setting is associated with a decreased incidence of ischaemic procedure-related complications and a decreased need for repeated coronary artery revascularisation in the first month after the procedure. Many of the side-effects of abciximab are due to its antiplatelet effects. This includes an increased risk of bleeding. The most common type of bleeding due to abciximab is gastrointestinal haemorrhage. Thrombocytopenia is a rare but known serious risk. Abciximab-induced thrombocytopenia can typically be treated with transfusion of platelets. Abciximab has a plasma half-life of about 10 minutes, with a second-phase half-life of about 30 minutes. However, its effects on platelet function can be seen for up to 48 hours after the infusion has finished, and low levels of glycoprotein IIb/IIIa receptor blockade are present for up to 15 days after the infusion is stopped.

## 17.24

*Answer: A*   Inhibits cytochrome P450

Fluconazole is a triazole antifungal drug used in the treatment and prevention of superficial and systemic fungal infections. Like other imidazole- and triazole-class antifungals, fluconazole inhibits the fungal cytochrome P450 enzyme, 14-demethylase. Mammalian demethylase activity is much less sensitive to fluconazole than fungal demethylase. This inhibition prevents the conversion of lanosterol to ergosterol, an essential component of the fungal cell wall, and subsequent accumulation of 14-methyl sterols. Fluconazole is primarily fungistatic, but can be fungicidal against certain organisms in a dose-dependent manner.

## 17.25

*Answer: C*   Third-generation cephalosporins

Ceftriaxone is a third-generation cephalosporin antibiotic. Like other third-generation cephalosporins, it has a broad spectrum of activity against Gram-positive and Gram-negative bacteria. In most cases, it is considered to be equivalent to cefotaxime in terms of safety and efficacy. Ceftriaxone is often used (in combination with macrolide and/or aminoglycoside antibiotics) for the treatment of community-acquired pneumonia. It is also a drug of choice for the treatment of bacterial meningitis. In paediatrics, it is commonly used in febrile infants aged 4–8 weeks who are admitted to hospital to exclude sepsis. It has also been used in the treatment of Lyme disease and gonorrhoea. The usual starting dose is 1g intravenously daily. Doses range from 1g to 2g intravenously or intramuscularly every 12–24 hours, depending on the type and severity or the infection, up to 4g daily. For gonorrhoea the usual adult dose is a single intramuscular injection of 250 mg. Patients treated for gonorrhoea are usually also treated for *Chlamydia*, often with azithromycin. Ceftriaxone is contraindicated in patients with known hypersensitivity to cephalosporins, penicillins and/or carbapenems.

## 17.26

*Answer: D*    Lung cancer

Etoposide phosphate is an inhibitor of the enzyme topoisomerase II. It is used as a form of chemotherapy for malignancies such as lung cancer, testicular cancer, lymphoma, non-lymphocytic leukaemia and glioblastoma multiforme. It is often given in combination with other drugs. Chemically, it is derived from podophyllotoxin, a toxin found in the American mayapple.

## 17.27

*Answer: C*    Peripheral neuropathy

Vincristine (Oncovin®) is an alkaloid derived from the Madagascar periwinkle (*Catharanthus roseus*, formerly *Vinca rosea* and hence its name). It is a chemotherapeutic agent. Tubulin is a structural protein which polymerises to form microtubules. The cell cytoskeleton and mitotic spindle, among other things, are made of microtubules. Vincristine binds to tubulin dimers causing disassembly of microtubule structures. Disruption of the microtubules arrests mitosis in metaphase. The vinca alkaloids therefore affect all

pharmacology

rapidly dividing cell types, including cancer cells, but also intestinal epithelium and bone marrow. The main side-effects of vincristine are peripheral neuropathy and constipation. The latter might require laxative treatment, while the former can be a reason to reduce the dose of vincristine. Accidental intrathecal injection of vinca alkaloids is highly dangerous, with a mortality approaching 100%. Vincristine, injected intravenously only, is used in various types of chemotherapy regimens. Its main uses are in non-Hodgkin's lymphoma as part of the 'CHOP' chemotherapy regimen (cyclophosphamide, hydroxyrubicin, Oncovin® and prednisone), in Hodgkin's lymphoma as part of the Stanford V chemotherapy regimen and in acute lymphoblastic leukaemia.

## 17.28

*Answer: C*    Inhibits dihydrofolate reductase

Trimethoprim is a bacteriostatic antibiotic that is mainly used in the prophylaxis and treatment of urinary tract infections. Trimethoprim acts by interfering with the action of bacterial dihydrofolate reductase, inhibiting synthesis of tetrahydrofolic acid. Tetrahydrofolic acid is an essential precursor in the de novo synthesis of the DNA nucleosides thymidine and uridine. Bacteria are unable to take up folic acid from the environment (ie the infected host) and are thus dependent on their own de novo synthesis. Inhibition of the enzyme starves the bacteria of two bases necessary for DNA replication and transcription.

## 17.29

*Answer: A*    Inhibits beta-lactamase

Tazobactam is a compound which inhibits the action of bacterial beta-lactamases. It is added to the extended-spectrum beta-lactam antibiotic piperacillin to produce Tazocin®. It broadens the spectrum of piperacillin by making it effective against organisms that express beta-lactamase and would normally degrade piperacillin. Tazobactam sodium is a derivative of the penicillin nucleus and is a penicillanic acid sulphone.

pharmacology

## 17.30

*Answer:* C    Hypercalcaemia of malignancy

Mithramycin is a tricyclic pentaglycosidic antibiotic derived from *Streptomyces* strains. It inhibits RNA and protein synthesis by adhering to DNA. It is used as a fluorescent dye and as an antineoplastic agent, especially in bone and testicular tumours. It is also used to reduce hypercalcaemia, especially that caused by malignancy.

## 17.31

*Answer:* C    Inhibits the addition of iodide to thyroglobulin

Methimazole is an antithyroid drug similar in action to propylthiouracil, and is part of the thioamide group. Methimazole is a drug used to treat hyperthyroidism. It is also taken before thyroid surgery or radioactive iodine therapy, to lower thyroid hormone levels and minimise the effects of thyroid manipulation. Thioamides inhibit several steps in the synthesis of thyroid hormones, including the addition of iodide to thyroglobulin by the enzyme thyroperoxidase, a necessary step in the synthesis of thyroxine, and by inhibiting the enzyme 5'-deiodinase which converts T4 to T3. Notably, they do not inhibit the action of the sodium-dependent iodide transporter located on the basolateral membranes of follicular cells. Inhibition of this step requires competitive inhibitors such as perchlorate and thiocyanate.

## 17.32

*Answer:* E    Urinary bladder

Cyclophosphamide is a nitrogen mustard alkylating agent, used to treat various types of cancer and some autoimmune disorders. It is a 'prodrug', being converted in the liver to active forms that have chemotherapeutic activity. The main use of cyclophosphamide is in combination with other chemotherapy agents in the treatment of lymphomas, some forms of leukaemia and some solid tumours. It is a chemotherapy drug that works by slowing or stopping cell growth. It also works by decreasing the immune system's response to various diseases.

pharmacology

The main effect of cyclophosphamide is due to its metabolite, phosphoramide mustard. This metabolite is only formed in cells which have low levels of aldehyde dehydrogenase (ALDH). Phosphoramide mustard forms DNA cross-links between (inter-strand) and within (intra-strand) DNA strands at guanine N-7 positions. This leads to cell death.

Cyclophosphamide is relatively non-toxic as ALDHs are present in relatively large concentrations in bone marrow stem cells, liver and intestinal epithelium. ALDHs protect these actively proliferating tissues against the toxic effects phosphoramide mustard and acrolein by converting aldophosphamide to carboxyphosphamide, which does not give rise to the toxic metabolites (phosphoramide mustard and acrolein). Many people taking cyclophosphamide therefore have no have serious side-effects. Side-effects that can occur, however, include nausea and vomiting, bone marrow suppression, stomach ache, diarrhoea, darkening of the skin/nails, alopecia and lethargy. Haemorrhagic cystitis is a common complication, but this can be prevented by ensuring an adequate fluid intake and with sodium 2-mercaptoethane sulphonate, which is a sulphhydryl donor and binds acrolein. Cyclophosphamide is itself carcinogenic, potentially causing transitional cell carcinoma of the bladder as a long-term complication.

## 17.33

*Answer: C*     Piperacillin

Piperacillin is an extended-spectrum beta-lactam antibiotic of the ureidopenicillin class. It is normally used with a beta-lactamase inhibitor such as tazobactam, a combination which is commercially available as Tazocin®. The combination has activity against many Gram-positive and Gram-negative pathogens and anaerobes, including *Pseudomonas aeruginosa*. Piperacillin/tazobactam is administered intravenously. Its main uses are in the intensive care setting (pneumonia, peritonitis), in the treatment of some diabetes-related foot infections and as empirical therapy in febrile neutropenia (eg after chemotherapy).

## 17.34

*Answer: A*    Azlocillin

Azlocillin is an acylampicillin antibiotic with an extended spectrum of activity and greater in vitro potency than the carboxypenicillins. Azlocillin is similar to mezlocillin and piperacillin. It demonstrates antibacterial activity against a broad spectrum of bacteria, including *Pseudomonas aeruginosa* and, in contrast to most cephalosporins, also exhibits activity against enterococci.

## 17.35

*Answer: E*    Oral vancomycin

Three antibiotics are effective against *Clostridium difficile*. Metronidazole 500 mg orally three times daily is the drug of choice, because of superior tolerability, lower price and comparable efficacy. Oral vancomycin 125 mg four times daily is second-line therapy, but is avoided due to theoretical concerns of converting intestinal flora into vancomycin-resistant organisms. However, it is used in the following cases: when there has been no response to oral metronidazole; when the organism is resistant to metronidazole; when the patient is allergic to metronidazole; when the patient is either pregnant or younger than 10 years of age; and when the patient is critically ill because of *C. difficile* diarrhoea (the duration of diarrhoea is reduced to 3 days, compared with 4.6 days with metronidazole). Vancomycin must be administered orally because intravenous administration does not achieve minimum therapeutic concentrations in the gut lumen. Thirdly, the use of linezolid might also be considered.

## 17.36

*Answer: B*    Methicillin-resistant *Staphylococcus aureus*

Linezolid is a synthetic antibiotic, the first of the oxazolidinone class, used for the treatment of infections caused by multiresistant bacteria, including streptococci and methicillin-resistant *Staphylococcus aureus* (MRSA). It was the first commercially available oxazolidinone antibiotic and is usually reserved for the treatment of serious bacterial infections where older antibiotics have failed due to antibiotic resistance. Conditions such as skin infections or nosocomial pneumonia where methicillin or penicillin resistance is found are indications for linezolid use. Compared with the older antibiotics it is quite expensive.

The drug works by inhibiting the initiation of bacterial protein synthesis. Linezolid is effective against Gram-positive pathogens, notably *Enterococcus faecium*, *S. aureus*, *Streptococcus agalactiae*, *Streptococcus pneumoniae* and *Streptococcus pyogenes*. It has almost no effect on Gram-negative bacteria and is only bacteriostatic against most enterococci. Linezolid has also been used to treat tuberculosis.

## 17.37

*Answer: D* Inhibits initiation of bacterial protein synthesis

Linezolid works on the initiation of protein synthesis. It does this by stopping the 30S and 50S subunits from binding together. Linezolid binds onto the 50S subunit, close to the peptidyl transferase and chloramphenicol binding sites. This then stops the interaction with the 30S subunit.

## 17.38

*Answer: D* Erythromycin

Erythromycin is a macrolide antibiotic which has an antimicrobial spectrum similar to or slightly wider than that of penicillin, and is often used for people who have an allergy to penicillins. For respiratory tract infections, it has better coverage of atypical organisms, including *Mycoplasma* and *Legionella* organisms It is also used to treat outbreaks of *Chlamydia* infections, syphilis, acne and gonorrhoea.

pharmacology

## 17.39

*Answer: E*    Inhibits translocation of peptides

Erythromycin prevents bacteria from growing by interfering with their protein synthesis. Erythromycin binds to the 23S rRNA molecule in the 50S subunit of the bacterial ribosome, blocking the exit of the growing peptide chain, thus inhibiting the translocation of peptides.

## 17.40

*Answer: C*    Inhibit DNA replication and transcription

Quinolones are bactericidal drugs, actively killing bacteria. Quinolones inhibit the bacterial DNA gyrase or the topoisomerase IV enzyme, thereby inhibiting DNA replication and transcription. Quinolones can enter cells easily and therefore are often used to treat intracellular pathogens such as *Legionella pneumophila* and *Mycoplasma pneumoniae*. DNA gyrase is the target for many Gram-negative bacteria; topoisomerase IV is the target for many Gram-positive bacteria.

## 17.41

*Answer: D*    Inhibits DNA-dependent RNA polymerase

Rifampicin is a bactericidal drug of the rifamycin group. It is a semisynthetic compound derived from *Amycolatopsis mediterranei* (formerly known as *Streptomyces mediterranei*). Rifampicin is typically used to treat mycobacterial infections, including tuberculosis and leprosy; and also has a role in the treatment of methicillin-resistant *Staphylococcus aureus* (MRSA) infections, in combination with fusidic acid. It is used in prophylactic therapy against *Neisseria meningitidis* (ie meningococcal) infection.

It is also used to treat infections by *Listeria* species, *Neisseria gonorrhoeae*, *Haemophilus influenzae* and *Legionella pneumophila*. For these non-standard indications, sensitivity testing should be performed, if possible, before starting rifampicin therapy. Rifampicin resistance develops quickly during treatment and rifampicin

pharmacology

monotherapy should not be used to treat these infections – it should always be used in combination with other antibiotics.

Rifampicin inhibits DNA-dependent RNA polymerase in bacterial cells by binding its beta subunit, thus preventing transcription of messenger RNA (mRNA) and subsequent translation to proteins. Its lipophilic nature makes it a good drug for treating the meningitis form of tuberculosis, which requires distribution to the central nervous system and penetration through the blood–brain barrier.

### 17.42

*Answer: E*   Prevents the translocation of elongation factor G from the ribosome

Fusidic acid is an antibiotic that is used particularly for eye and skin infections. It works by interfering with bacterial protein synthesis, specifically by preventing the translocation of elongation factor G (EF-G) from the ribosome, although it works only on Gram-positive bacteria such as *Staphylococcus aureus*, streptococci and *Corynebacterium minutissimum*. Because it primarily inhibits their reproduction (as opposed to killing them directly) it is bacteriostatic.

### 17.43

*Answer: E*   Obstructs the formation of the bacterial cell wall

Ethambutol is a bacteriostatic antimycobacterial drug prescribed to treat tuberculosis. It is usually given in combination with other antituberculosis drugs such as isoniazid, pyrazinamide and rifampicin. Bacteriostatic against actively growing tubercle bacilli, it works by obstructing the formation of the cell wall. Mycolic acids attach to the 5′-hydroxyl groups of D-arabinose residues of arabinogalactan and form mycolyl-arabinogalactan-peptidoglycan complexes in the cell wall. Disruption of arabinogalactan synthesis inhibits the formation of this complex and leads to increased permeability of the cell wall.

## 17.44

*Answer: E*    Inhibits mycolic acid synthesis in the bacterial cell wall

Isoniazid (isonicotinyl hydrazine or INH) is a first-line antituberculosis medication used in the prevention and treatment of tuberculosis. Isoniazid is never used on its own to treat active tuberculosis because resistance quickly develops. Isoniazid is a prodrug and must be activated by bacterial catalase. It is activated by catalase-peroxidase enzyme katG to form isonicotinic acyl anion or radical. These forms will then react with a NADH radical or anion to form isonicotinic acyl-NADH complex. This complex will bind tightly to a ketoenoylreductase known as 'InhA' and prevents access of the natural enoyl-AcpM substrate. This mechanism inhibits the synthesis of mycolic acid in the mycobacterial cell wall.

Isoniazid reaches therapeutic concentrations in serum, cerebrospinal fluid, and within caseous granulomas. Isoniazid is metabolised in the liver by acetylation. There are two forms of the enzyme responsible for acetylation, so that some patients metabolise the drug more quickly than others. The metabolites are excreted in the urine. Doses do not usually have to be adjusted in patients who are in renal failure. Isoniazid is bactericidal to rapidly-dividing mycobacteria, but is bacteriostatic if the mycobacterium is slow-growing.

## 17.45

*Answer: A*    Enhances the effect of 5-fluorouracil

Folinic acid or leucovorin, generally administered as calcium folinate (or leucovorin calcium), is an adjuvant drug used in cancer chemotherapy involving the drug methotrexate. It is also used in synergistic combination with the chemotherapeutic agent, 5-fluorouracil. (Note that folinic acid is not the same as folic acid.) Folinic acid is a 5-formyl derivative of tetrahydrofolic acid. It is readily converted to other reduced folic acid derivatives (eg tetrahydrofolate). Because it does not require the action of dihydrofolate reductase for its conversion, it will be unaffected by inhibition of this enzyme by drugs such as methotrexate. This therefore allows for purine/pyrimidine synthesis to occur; so normal DNA replication and RNA transcription processes can proceed.

pharmacology

Folinic acid is administered at the appropriate time following methotrexate as part of a total chemotherapeutic plan, where it can 'rescue' bone marrow and gastrointestinal mucosal cells from methotrexate. There is no apparent effect on pre-existing methotrexate-induced nephrotoxicity, however. While not specifically an antidote for methotrexate, folinic acid can also be useful in the treatment of acute methotrexate overdose.

Folinic acid is used in combination with 5-fluorouracil for the treatment of colon cancer. In this case, folinic acid is not used for 'rescue' purposes; rather, it enhances the effect of 5-fluorouracil on the inhibition of thymidylate synthase. Folinic acid is also sometimes used to prevent the toxic effects of high doses of antimicrobial dihydrofolate reductase inhibitors such as trimethoprim and pyrimethamine.

## 17.46

*Answer: E*    FOLFOX

FOLFOX is a chemotherapy regimen used for the treatment of colorectal cancer, made up of the following drugs:

- FOL: fluorouracil (5-fluorouracil or 5-FU)
- F: folinic acid (leucovorin)
- OX: oxaliplatin (Eloxatin®).

Adjuvant treatment in patients with stage III colon cancer is recommended for 12 cycles, every 2 weeks. The recommended dose schedule (given every 2 weeks) is as follows:

**Day 1:** oxaliplatin (Eloxatin®) 85 mg/m intravenous infusion in 250–500 ml 5% dextrose and leucovorin 200 mg/m intravenous infusion in 5% dextrose, both given over 120 minutes at the same time in separate bags using a Y-line, followed by 5-FU 400 mg/m intravenous bolus given over 2–4 minutes, followed by 5-FU 600 mg/m intravenous infusion in 500 ml 5% dextrose (recommended) as a 22-hour continuous infusion.

**Day 2:** Leucovorin 200 mg/m intravenous infusion over 120 minutes, followed by 5-FU 400 mg/m intravenous bolus given over 2–4 minutes, followed by 5-FU 600 mg/m intravenous infusion in 500 ml 5% dextrose (recommended) as a 22-hour continuous infusion.

Premedication with anti-emetics, including 5-HT$_3$ blockers with or without dexamethasone, is recommended.

## 17.47

*Answer: A*  ABVD

ABVD is a chemotherapy regimen used in the first-line treatment of Hodgkin's lymphoma. It consists of concurrent treatment with the chemotherapy drugs, adriamycin, bleomycin, vinblastine and dacarbazine. One cycle of ABVD chemotherapy is typically given over 4 weeks, with two doses in each cycle (on day 1 and day 15). All four of the chemotherapy drugs are given intravenously. ABVD chemotherapy is usually given in an outpatient setting.

Typical dosages for one 28-day cycle of ABVD are as follows:

- Adriamycin 25 mg/m$^2$ intravenously on day 1 and on day 15

- Bleomycin 10 mg/m$^2$ intravenously on day 1 and on day 15

- Vinblastine 6 mg/m$^2$ intravenously on day 1 and on day 15

- Dacarbazine 375 mg/m$^2$ intravenously on day 1 and on day 15.

The total number of cycles given depends upon the stage of the disease and on how well the patient tolerates chemotherapy. Doses might be delayed because of neutropenia, thrombocytopenia or other side-effects.

## 17.48

*Answer: C*  CHOP

CHOP is the acronym for a chemotherapy regimen used in the treatment of non-Hodgkin's lymphoma, comprising cyclophosphamide, hydroxyrubicin (adriamycin), Oncovin® (vincristine) and prednisone.

pharmacology

This regimen can also be combined with the monoclonal antibody rituximab if the lymphoma is of B-cell origin (R-CHOP or CHOP-R). Typically, courses are administered at an interval of 3 weeks. A staging computed tomographic scan is generally performed after three cycles to assess whether the disease is responding to treatment. In patients with a history of cardiovascular disease, the doxorubicin (which is cardiotoxic) is often considered to be too great a risk and is omitted from the regimen. The combination is then referred to as 'COP' or 'CVP'.

## 17.49

*Answer: D*   Inhibition of T-cell activation

Methotrexate competitively and reversibly inhibits dihydrofolate reductase (DHFR), an enzyme that is part of the folate synthesis metabolic pathway. The affinity of methotrexate for DHFR is about one thousand times that of folate for DHFR. Dihydrofolate reductase catalyses the conversion of dihydrofolate to the active tetrahydrofolate. Folic acid is needed for the de novo synthesis of the nucleoside thymidine, required for DNA synthesis. Methotrexate, therefore, inhibits the synthesis of DNA, RNA, thymidylate and proteins.

Methotrexate acts specifically during DNA and RNA synthesis, and it is therefore cytotoxic during the S-phase of the cell cycle. Logically, it therefore has a greater toxic effect on rapidly dividing cells (such as malignant and myeloid cells, but also gastrointestinal and oral mucosal cells), which replicate their DNA more frequently, and thus inhibits the growth and proliferation of both cancerous and non-cancerous cells, leading to the therapeutic and toxic effects respectively.

Lower doses of methotrexate have been shown to be very effective for the management of rheumatoid arthritis, Crohn's disease and psoriasis. In these cases inhibition of DHFR is not thought to be the main mechanism, which is thought to be the inhibition of enzymes involved in purine metabolism, leading to accumulation of adenosine, or the inhibition of T-cell activation and suppression of intercellular adhesion molecule expression by T cells.

## 17.50

*Answer: A*    Cross-linking of DNA

Cisplatin, cisplatinum or cis-diamminedichloroplatinum(II) (CDDP) is a platinum-based chemotherapy drug used to treat various types of cancers, including sarcomas, some carcinomas (eg small-cell lung cancer and ovarian cancer), lymphomas and germ cell tumours. It was the first member of its class, which now also includes carboplatin and oxaliplatin. Its mechanism of action is as follows: a chlorine ligand in cisplatin can undergo slow displacement with water molecules, in a process known as 'aquation'; the aqua ligand is highly reactive, allowing cisplatin to coordinate a base in DNA, and a subsequent cross-link is formed after loss of the second chlorine ligand. Cisplatin acts by crosslinking DNA in several different ways, making it impossible for rapidly dividing cells to duplicate their DNA for mitosis. The damaged DNA sets off DNA repair mechanisms, which activate apoptosis when repair proves impossible.

pharmacology

# INDEX

(The number in bold indicates section and the number in italics indicates question number)